Veteran Suicide

A PUBLIC HEALTH IMPERATIVE

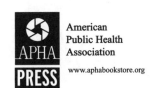

American
Public Health
Association
www.aphabookstore.org

Edited by
Robert M. Bossarte, PhD

WASHINGTON, D.C. ● 2013

American Public Health Association
800 I Street, NW
Washington, DC 20001-3710
www.apha.org

Georges C. Benjamin, MD, FACP, FACEP (Emeritus), Executive Director

Printed and bound in the United States of America
Production Editor: Teena Lucas
Typesetting: The Charlesworth Group
Cover Design: Alan Giarcanella
Printing and Binding: Victor Graphics, Baltimore, MD

Library of Congress Cataloging-in-Publication Data

Veteran suicide : a public health imperative / edited by Robert M. Bossarte, PhD.
p. cm.
Includes bibliographical references
ISBN 978-0-87553-211-0 (alk. paper)
1. Veterans--Suicidal behavior--United States. 2. Veterans--Mental health--United States. 3. Suicide--United States--Prevention. 4. War neuroses--United States. 5. Military psychiatry--United States. I. Bossarte, Robert M.
HV6545.7.V48 2013
362.28086'970973--dc23

2013011532

TABLE OF CONTENTS

PART VIII – WARNING SIGNS FOR SUICIDE

Foreword

Over the past several years, the Department of Veteran Affairs (VA) has increased mental health staffing and implemented a number of new elements to the VA suicide prevention program, including a national toll-free Veterans Crisis Line, enhanced care packages for high-risk patients, and mandatory safety planning to promote management of periods with increasing risk. We are starting to see positive results from these efforts, however, our work as a public health community is not complete, and recent data suggest that the urgency of our task has increased. Despite our efforts Veterans continue to die by suicide.

In 2012, the *American Journal of Public Health* published a Supplement dedicated to the topic of suicide among Veterans of military service. The publication of this issue emphasize awareness of the national importance of this problem and demonstrated response from public health, clinical, and scientific communities. Since the issue, the work has continued. In 2010, more than 38,000 Americans died from suicide, and the VA has estimated that approximately 21% of all suicides reported that year were Veterans. Despite a decrease in the percentage of suicides identified as Veterans, the VA has also estimated that the number of those with history of military service who die from suicide each day has increased along with the rate of suicide in the US general population. These increases identify similarities in rates of suicide among Veterans and members of surrounding communities and emphasize that the burden of suicide is not borne by Veterans alone.

Earlier this year, the VA released a Suicide Data Report summarizing information obtained through agreements with US states and territories, internal reports of suicide events among those receiving care from the Veterans Health Administration, and the national toll-free Veterans Crisis Line. Results from analyses of data included in this report provide early evidence of the impact of recently implemented suicide prevention initiatives and justifies efforts to improve existing programs and identify innovative solutions for effective risk identification and management.

The research represented by the collection of manuscripts included in this volume is an important step towards addressing the national problem of suicide and a reminder that even one death by suicide is too many. It is tragic when a citizen of the United States willingly puts themselves in harm's way and survives, only to later die by suicide. Our efforts to understand and intervene are important and life saving.

Janet Kemp, RN, PhD
VA National Mental Health Program Director
Suicide Prevention and Community Engagement

Introduction

In March 2012, the *American Journal of Public Health* published a Supplement dedicated to the topic of suicide among Veterans of military service. The manuscripts included in that Supplement, and now included in this volume, reported on results from some of the largest and most recent studies of suicide risk among those with history of US military service to date. The broad range of reports on research studies, clinical strategies, and policy initiatives included in the Supplement are representative of the complex and multifaceted characteristics of suicide and highlight the importance of this public health crisis.

Results from studies of the prevalence of suicide ideation, attempt, and mortality provide a foundation for understanding changes in suicide risk over time or differences among those with and without history of US military service that may be associated with a common exposure or shared characteristic. Population-based studies of suicide risk, such as those included in this volume, represent the cornerstone of a public health approach to suicide prevention by identifying groups with increased risk and evaluating the impact of universal strategies to promote help-seeking or increase access to care among those experiencing distress.

Clinically oriented studies, including reassessment of symptoms of psychiatric disorders or recognition of risk among patients being treated in primary care settings, provide evidence of the value of the integration of clinical strategies to identify and address risk across multiple settings.

The continued evaluation of variability in rates of suicide among Veterans provides an opportunity to confirm findings reported by previous studies and enhance our understanding of characteristics of risk among those who have served. Studies of suicidal behaviors among previously understudied populations, such as sexual minority and transgender Veterans, provide opportunities for the development of innovative and targeted programs across all Veteran groups.

The current volume of results from studies comes at a time of increased national awareness of suicide among Veterans and a desire to adequately support those who have served. Last year, the 2012 National Strategy for Suicide Prevention identified members of the armed forces and Veterans as groups with evidence of increased risk for suicide. Among the first priority areas listed by the National Strategy were objectives to transform health care systems to significantly reduce suicide and promote efforts to change public conversation about suicide and suicide prevention. The first steps toward achieving these goals are an increased understanding of the prevalence and characteristics of suicide and the identification of evidence-based strategies to reduce risk among those with history of military service. The collection of reports included in this volume provide an opportunity to achieve these goals by raising awareness of characteristics of suicide among Veterans and providing a foundation for the development of innovative and integrated strategies to prevent additional loss of life.

PART I
Letters

Suicide Prevention is a Winnable Battle

Eric D. Caine, MD

At the heart of the challenge posed by suicide, attempted suicide, and their antecedent risks (e.g., trauma, interpersonal violence, drinking and drug use, family turmoil, work-related difficulties, depression) is the question of whether suicide really is preventable. This is especially true now for veterans and active duty personnel, for whom the nation has been challenged as never before, to support service personnel returning from combat with new or more intense problems not routinely encountered in the past.

Here are 10 reasons why suicide prevention is possible:

1. SUICIDE IS UNAVOIDABLE AS A PUBLIC HEALTH CHALLENGE

Suicide continues to increase in the United States to the point that it has become unavoidable as a public health challenge—it is now the tenth leading cause of death. It is associated with greater mortality and morbidity than other recognized priorities for injury prevention. The need is great, and a necessary national urgency is emerging. In September 2010, Health and Human Services Secretary Kathleen Sebelius and Department of Defense Secretary Robert M. Gates commissioned the National Action Alliance for Suicide Prevention, a public–private partnership now co-chaired by the Secretary of the Army John McHugh and former Senator Gordon Smith. This points directly to the nation's building commitment and deepening resolve to frankly address the challenge.

2. SUICIDE PREVENTION EFFORTS CAN SUCCEED

Suicide prevention efforts can succeed: we know how to make a difference by providing the vision, the will, and the support.

The systematic implementation of national strategies for suicide prevention has been associated with robust reductions in suicide—e.g., World Health Organization (WHO) data showed decreases of more than 20% in the United Kingdom and more than 30% in Finland during the past two decades.[1] Suicide in Denmark declined from 1600 to 600 individuals per year (M. Nordentoft, personal communication, September 2011), which was associated with robust means control efforts (i.e., elimination of barbiturates from the country's pharmacopeia, substitution of less toxic second generation antidepressants for first generation compounds, use of catalytic converters in automobiles, and removal of carbon monoxide from domestic cooking gas) and enhanced clinical follow-up services of individuals who survived their "index" suicide attempt or were deemed clinically unstable and "at risk." Each national program involved multilayered initiatives that were inclusive of broader universal and selective efforts (e.g., changing laws about alcohol intoxication and clarifying and enforcing policies regarding the safe design of psychiatric inpatient services) and indicated interventions such as post–emergency room (ER) or inpatient aftercare.

The US Air Force suicide prevention program, a multilayered array of initiatives, demonstrated that a public health approach saved lives involving multiple forms of violent death—suicide, homicide, and accidental death—as it targeted antecedent morbidity (e.g., family violence, alcohol use, financially related tensions) using a "common risk" strategy.[2,3] Of note, this program did not focus on means restriction; by necessity, service personnel have access to many weapons and a culture of safety is deeply ingrained.

US health care systems that defined "boundaried" populations showed that it was possible to deploy multipronged approaches that altered outcomes, including suicide and attempted suicide—when the entire system is committed to implementing and sustaining the changes.[4,5]

The WHO Suicide Prevention of Suicidal Behaviors—Multisite Intervention Study (SUPRE-MISS) randomized controlled trial reported that post-ER interventions with attempters reduced subsequent suicides (although not all subsequent attempts reported were in its published data).[6]

The Taiwan National Suicide Surveillance System demonstrated that a public health surveillance program, including mandatory registration of attempts followed by widely applied aftercare, was associated with reduced attempts and deaths (Lee MB et al., unpublished data, 2011).

3. SOCIETY MEMBERS ARE OWED THE BEST INTERVENTIONS

A society owes its members the best interventions that current knowledge can support, especially when applied in a cost-effective fashion. Where there is sufficient political will power, action to save lives is feasible even when all causes are not known, especially when using public health approaches to prevention and early intervention. The nation has had significant success with HIV/AIDS; it can muster the same commitment to reducing suicide by focusing on socially important "presuicidal" conditions and behaviors that have public health significance.

4. SUICIDE IS ONE OF SEVERAL OVERLAPPING RISKS

Suicide and attempted suicide reflect one of several sets of adverse outcomes arising from overlapping or common risks, including, among others, interpersonal violence and homicide, and accidental death because of motor vehicle accidents or drug ingestion ("overdose"). There are many survivor groups, community organizations, and governmental agencies that separately deal with such risks, largely in isolation from each another.[7] Acting together, they would have the potential to profoundly influence social priorities that could prevent a broad swath of mortality and morbidity.

5. THERE ARE OPPORTUNITIES FOR FUTURE EFFECTIVE ACTION

A fair accounting of the burdens of suicide in the Unites States—and a candid appraisal of the shortcomings of past and recent efforts—reveals many opportunities for future effective action. From a public health perspective, these can be applied at broader, intermediate, and individual levels in a developmental framework—as part of a well-conceived mosaic of preventive and therapeutic interventions that share a public health philosophy. These interventions involve contextual social and community initiatives to comple-ment indicated clinical activities for individuals, the latter largely being built on mental health perspectives.

6. SUICIDE CAN BE PREVENTED

At the individual level, suicide can be prevented readily—*if* there is the ability to intervene in a timely fashion before someone reaches the "edge of the cliff." As a multidetermined outcome, there are frequent opportunities to change individuals' life trajectories before they become acutely or severely distressed and "suicidal." Distal interventions are relevant to individuals as well as broader communities and segments of society.

7. STIGMA SURROUNDING SUICIDE IS STILL A BARRIER

Although the stigma associated with frankly discussing suicide, self-harming behaviors, and interpersonal victimization has diminished greatly over the past two decades, allowing more open consideration of complex and potentially embarrassing problems, it continues as a powerful force. Suicide remains a frightening and devastating way to end life; at an individual and family level, it may be a forbidden topic. Yet discussions of suicide prevention now serve to mobilize broad concern and cooperative efforts to build essential "action coalitions." It is now possible to candidly consider centrally important issues— firearm safety, suicide among populations that have fewer advocates, and the weighing and balancing of population and individual perspectives—when such discussions were too sensitive or "off limits" only a few years ago. Such discussions will be essential for building a foundation for future prevention initiatives.

8. IMPROVED SURVEILLANCE CAN REDUCE SUICIDE MORTALITY

Taken together, research indicates that improved surveillance, when linked to action, can reduce the mortality and morbidity of suicide and attempted suicide. Put succinctly: suicides and suicide attempts can be counted—repeated measurement can drive accountability and quality improvement.

9. PREVENTION AND SUPPORT EFFORTS ARE GROWING STRONGER

Many individuals and agencies are committed to preventing suicide, attempted suicide, and their antecedent risk factors; they now are in a position to actively and creatively respond to galvanizing leadership, knowledge, guidance, and technical support.

10. THE TIME TO ACT IS NOW

The timing is right! The next generation of the National Strategy for Suicide Prevention (NSSP 2.0) is now being developed.

It is notable that the Department of Veterans Affairs and Department of Defense have embarked on a variety of initiatives to lessen suicide among those whom they serve. Each organization faces distinct challenges. The experiences of others—in bounded systems akin to the Veterans Health Administration and each of the military services, or more open systems such as countries—have much to teach us. However, one thing is certain: this is a winnable battle!

ABOUT THE AUTHOR

Eric D. Caine is with the Department of Psychiatry, Center for the Study and Prevention of Suicide, University of Rochester Medical Center, Rochester, NY, and the VA Center of Excellence for Suicide Prevention, Canandaigua, NY.

ACKNOWLEDGMENTS

Discussions with Yeates Conwell and Jerry Reed were centrally important to developing a draft of this editorial. Comments from many colleagues, particularly Kerry Knox, Catherine Cerulli, Kenneth Connor, Wendi Cross, Paul Duberstein, Robert Bossarte, and Peter Wyman, were important for shaping and sharpening key ideas.

REFERENCES

1. World Health Organization. Mental Health. Available at: http://www.who.int/mental_health/prevention/suicide/country_reports/en/index.html. Accessed September 25, 2011.

2. Knox KL, Litts DA, Talcott GW, Feig JC, Caine ED. Risk of suicide and related adverse outcomes after exposure to a suicide prevention programme in the US Air Force: cohort study (abstract). *BMJ*. 2003;327(7428):1376.

3. Knox KL, Pflanz S, Talcott GW, Campise RL, Lavigne JE, Bajorska A, et al. The US Air Force Suicide Prevention Program: implications for public health policy. *Am J Public Health*. 2010;100(12):2457–2463.

4. Coffey CE. Building a system of perfect depression care in behavioral health. *Jt Comm J Qual Patient Saf.* 2007;33(4):193–199.

5. Coffey DE. Pursuing perfect depression care. *Psychiatr Serv.* 2006;57(10):1524–1526.

6. Fleischmann A, Bertolote JM, Wasserman D, De Leo D, Botega NJ, De Silva J, et al. Effectiveness of brief intervention and contact for suicide attempters: a randomized controlled trial in five countries. *Bull World Health Organ.* 2008;86(9):703–709.

7. Caine ED, Knox KL, Conwell Y. Public health and population approaches for suicide prevention. In: Cohen NL, Galea S, eds. *Population Mental Health: Evidence, Policy, & Public Health Practice.* London, New York: Routledge; 2011:303–338.

PART II
Editor's Choice

2

Preventing Suicide Is a National Imperative

A. Kathryn Power, MEd, and Richard McKeon, PhD, MPH

Preventing suicide is a national imperative (Goldsmith S, Pellmar T, Kleinman A, Bunney W. *Reducing Suicide: A National Imperative.* Washington, DC: National Acadamies Press; 2002.). Over 36 000 Americans die by suicide annually, another 1.1 million adults make suicide attempts, and over 8 million adults seriously consider suicide each year (Substance Abuse and Mental Health Services Administration [SAMHSA]. *2010 National Survey on Drug Utilization and Health.* Rockville, MD: SAMHSA; 2010.). In the past dozen years, there have been increasing efforts to reduce suicide's tragic toll, and suicide prevention has emerged as a national priority.

There is a special obligation to prevent suicide among those who have served our nation in the military, as well as to support their families. It is particularly poignant when we lose to suicide those who have risked their lives for the rest of us. In the words of former Secretary of Defense Robert Gates, spoken when he and Secretary of Health and Human Services Kathleen Sebelius launched the National Action Alliance for Suicide Prevention, "It is always a horrible tragedy to see a service member safely off the battlefield, only to lose them to this scourge. We can, we must, we will do better."

This special issue of the *American Journal of Public Health* presents vibrant testimony to the many outstanding ways that we as a nation are working to do better. The articles represent different strands of a comprehensive public health approach to suicide prevention—our nation's best hope for saving lives. These studies cover a broad array of settings and interventions, including key components of a comprehensive approach, ranging from surveillance to clinical services to mental health enhancement, from emergency departments to primary care settings to suicide hotlines, from promotion of community integration to the reduction of sleep disturbance. They demonstrate the intensive efforts of the Department of Veterans Affairs (VA) and Department of Defense (DoD), as well as public and private partners around the country. As one example of these efforts, the VA has placed a suicide prevention coordinator in each of its medical centers in the country. The Substance Abuse and Mental Health Services Administration (SAMHSA) has been privileged to work with our Federal partners on these extraordinarily important efforts. SAMHSA's collaboration with VA to utilize the National Suicide Prevention Lifeline (1-800-273-TALK/8255) as the gateway to the Veteran's Crisis Line has led to this service being accessed by hundreds of thousands of veterans and their families and friends since its inception in 2007. SAMHSA also works closely with the VA and DoD to support our nation's military families, and through vehicles such as the Suicide Prevention Resource Center and the National Action Alliance for Suicide Prevention, helps ensure that the nation benefits from the knowledge gained through efforts such as those included in this special issue.

The DoD recently released a suicide prevention task force report called "The Challenge and the Promise." This title underscores the fact suicide is preventable, but that large-scale prevention requires sustained, focused effort. The authors of the studies in this special issue have met the challenge of providing important new information, and it is now up to the rest of us to meet the challenge, to put this knowledge into practice, and to fulfill the promise of preventing suicide among those who have risked everything to protect us.

ABOUT THE AUTHORS

A. Kathryn Power and Richard McKeon are with the Center for Mental Health Services, Suicide Prevention Branch, Substance Abuse and Mental Health Services Administration, Rockville, MD.

PART III
Editorials

3

Surveillance of Suicide and Suicide Attempts Among Veterans: Addressing a National Imperative

Janet Kemp, RN, PhD, and Robert M. Bossarte, PhD

In 2008, the Department of Veterans Affairs (VA) implemented a suicide event reporting system designed to collect standardized information on all suicide attempts reported to VA clinicians and suicide prevention coordinators in VA medical centers and outpatient facilities. Since that time, the VA has collected information on nearly 46 000 suicide attempts, and the suicide event reporting system has transitioned from an aggregate spreadsheet submitted monthly to an electronic reporting system capable of achieving near "real time" surveillance of suicide events among veterans. The VA's suicide event reporting system, known collectively as the Suicide Prevention Applications Network (SPAN), and complimentary programs such as the Department of Defense's (DoD's) Suicide Event Reporting system (DoDSER), represent vertical advances in the surveillance of suicide and provide a foundation for the development of similar efforts among broader segments of the US general population. However, these systems alone are not sufficient to fill existing gaps in the availability of timely and comprehensive data on suicide-related events among members of the broader US general population.

The need for improved and expanded surveillance of suicide and suicide attempts is well recognized. The 2001 National Strategy for Suicide Prevention

(NSSP)[1] called for improved systems for collecting data on suicide and suicide attempts and included objectives to implement a national violent death reporting system, increase the utility of hospital data, and increase the number of states that produce annual reports on suicide and suicide attempts using information from multiple linked data systems. The Institute of Medicine's (IOM's) 2002 report on reducing suicide similarly called for the "sustained and systematic collection, analysis, and dissemination of accurate information on the incidence, prevalence, and characteristics of suicide and suicide attempts" and noted "serious inadequacies in the availability and quality" of information on suicide and similar limitations associated with of data on suicide attempts.[2] The 2010 document "Charting the Future of Suicide Prevention" reviewed progress toward achieving the goals set forth in the 2001 National Strategy for Suicide Prevention. In a 2010 review of progress data and surveillance, the Charting the Future report supported the 2002 IOM report conclusion that there exists significant deficiencies in the availability of data on nonfatal suicidal behavior and concluded that the NSSP goal of achieving regular systematic reporting of suicide and suicide attempts is still occurring on a "very limited" basis.[3]

Models for comprehensive data systems that provide a foundation for surveillance of suicide exist internationally in the population registries of Denmark[4] and more locally in population-specific efforts such as mandatory reporting of suicide attempts among youth in Oregon.[5] However, US public health agencies have been slow to respond to calls for standardization of data elements and integrated systems for surveillance of suicide. Limitations associated with the availability of population registries or event reporting are compounded by differences in terminology that complicate comparisons across systems or populations.

The suicide event reporting systems established by the Department of Veterans Affairs (SPAN) and Department of Defense (DoDSER) provide templates for the continued expansion of suicide event reporting that is consistent with existing calls for action. As reported by Gahm et al.,[6] DoDSER is an event-based reporting system collecting systematic information on a standardized set of variables for all suicide events known to the Department of Defense. Similarly, SPAN collects information on a standardized set of variables for all suicide events (fatal and nonfatal) known by VA providers. Importantly, officials for both systems have agreed to collect information on suicide events using a single standardized suicide event nomenclature that was developed as a result of an integrated effort including partners from the VA, DoD, Centers for Disease Control and Prevention, and National Institutes of Health.[7] The adoption of a standardized nomenclature increases the utility of suicide event data by providing a mechanism for comparability across systems and time. Together these distinct but interrelated systems represent the most comprehensive information available for the surveillance of suicide among any single US population.

The efforts of the VA and DoD are necessary but not sufficient components of adequate suicide surveillance. In 2010, the Action Alliance for Suicide Prevention was formed as a public–private partnership with the primary mission of revisiting the goals of the 2001 National Strategy and advancing suicide prevention in the United States.[8] Once again, addressing gaps in the availability of data for the surveillance of suicide and suicide attempts has been identified as a priority for prevention programs. The surveillance systems implemented in the VA and DoD provide a foundation for the development of comparable systems among broader segments of the US general population. Together, these systems will provide the information necessary for the identification of emerging risk populations, changes in characteristics or context associated with increased risk, and the evaluation of suicide prevention needed for the development of effective and evidence-based programs.

Since October 1, 2008, the Department of Veterans Affairs has recorded information on nearly 46 000 suicide events among more than 38 000 individuals. Information from the SPAN system has been used to inform clinical management of high risk Veterans, identify periods of increased risk, measure the impact of prevention programs on suicide and suicide attempts, and identify changes in the distribution of risk across populations and time. Additional efforts include the assessment of risk for suicide and suicide attempt, including an emphasis on the impact of prevention programs on repeat suicide attempts. Over time, information obtained from SPAN, linked with data from DoDSER and comparable surveillance systems, is expected to provide the single-most comprehensive source of information on the identification and management of suicide risk available to clinicians and public health professionals. In 2008, suicide was once again a top ten leading cause of death in the US general population. The time for action is now. The development of comparable surveillance systems for veterans and others who do not receive care from the VA is needed for the adequate and timely assessment of suicide and improved clinical management for those with established risk. The systems implemented by the VA and DoD provide a foundation for integrated and active suicide surveillance, but should not stand alone. Addressing the challenge of suicide prevention will require interagency synergism to enhance and extend existing VA and DoD efforts.[9] Comparable systems, utilizing a common nomenclature, are needed to supplement these systems and support our national effort to reduce the burden of suicide.

ABOUT THE AUTHORS

Janet Kemp is with the Office of Mental Health Services Director, Suicide Prevention, Department of Veterans Affairs, Washington, DC. Robert M. Bossarte is with the VISN 2 Center of Excellence for Suicide Prevention, Canandaigua, NY.

CONTRIBUTORS

J. Kemp and R. M. Bossarte coauthored the manuscript.

REFERENCES

1. Department of Health and Human Services. *National Strategy for Suicide Prevention: Goals and Objectives.* Rockville, MD: US Department of Health and Human Services, Public Health Service; 2001.

2. Goldsmith S, Pellmar T, Kleinman A, Bunney W, editors. *Reducing Suicide: A National Imperative.* Washington, DC: National Academies Press; 2002.

3. Suicide Prevention Resource Center and SPAN USA. *Charting the Future of Suicide Prevention: A 2010 Progress Review of the National Strategy and Recommendations for the Decade Ahead.* Newton, MA: Education Development Center, Inc; 2010.

4. Jakobsen IS, Christiansen E. Young people's risk of suicide attempts in relation to parental death: a population-based register study. *J Child Psychol Psychiatry.* 2011;52(2):176–183.

5. Oregon Youth Suicide Prevention Program [website]. Available at: http://egov.oregon.gov/DHS/ph/ipe/ysp/index.shtml. Accessed December 14, 2011.

6. Gahm GA, Reger MA, Kinn JT, Luxton DD, Skopp NA, Bush NE. Addressing the surveillance goal in the National Strategy for Suicide Prevention: the Department of Defense Suicide Event Report. Am J Public Health. 2012;102(Suppl 1):S24–S28.

7. US Department of Veterans Affairs. Self-Directed Violence Classification System (Nomenclature). VISN 19 Mental Illness, Education, and Clinical Center. Available at: http://www.mirecc.va.gov/visn19/education/nomenclature.asp. Accessed December 15, 2011.

8. AASP. Action Alliance for Suicide Prevention. Available at: http://www.actionallianceforsuicideprevention.org. Accessed December 15, 2011.

9. Harrell M, Berglass N. Losing the Battle: The Challenge of Military Suicide. Washington, DC: Center for a New American Security; 2011.

4

Preventing Suicide by Preventing Lethal Injury: The Need to Act on What We Already Know

Matthew Miller, MD, ScD, MPH

As I write this, all US troops are returning from Iraq, and many from Afghanistan. With rates of suicide having doubled among active duty soldiers since 2005,[1] preventing suicide has become a high-visibility, high-priority issue for the military and the Veterans Health Administration (VHA). Since most of our troops, once separated from the military, will be cared for by practitioners beyond the VHA, these statistics are of also of immediate concern to the broader public health community. Unfortunately, for all the physical, emotional, and psychological benefits that leaving a war zone may confer, returning home has its own problems and, in and of itself, is no guarantee that suicide risk will decline. Indeed, even at the height of recent conflicts, three of four suicides occurred here in the United States (and one out of three occurred among soldiers who had never deployed).

In light of where (in their homes), when (during acute financial, interpersonal, and legal crises), and how (with privately owned firearms) most suicides among current and former military personnel occur, it is incumbent upon us to give high priority to prevention strategies that greatly decrease the likelihood of death for those suicidal acts that could not be averted. In the United States, this means reducing access to household firearms—the method used in more suicides among Americans than all other methods combined.

One reason that it is vitally important to focus attention on improving the odds of surviving a suicide attempt is that although it is easy to identify high risk groups, such as persons with depression or substance use disorders, it is extremely difficult to prospectively identify either who among a high-risk group will die by suicide or when bearable suffering will deteriorate into a suicidal crisis. As a result, many suicidal acts will offer, at best, a narrow window for prevention. In one study of near-lethal suicide attempts, for example, 24% of attempters took less than 5 minutes between the decision to kill themselves and the actual attempt (70% took less than one hour).[2]

It stands to reason that even with dedicated resources, such as the Veterans Affairs' (VA's) 24-hour hotline, preventing any given suicide attempt will be difficult, even as mental health and drug treatment services may reduce the likelihood of suicide attempts in high-risk groups overall. Moreover, surviving an attempt matters, not simply because 90 out of 100 people who would have been dead of a gunshot are instead alive but also because at least 80 of the 90 who survived their attempt will not go on to die by suicide thereafter. Indeed, a review of more than 70 studies that followed suicide attempters over time found that, on average, only 7% eventually died by suicide.[3]

Unfortunately, despite an unequivocal statement by an international panel of suicide experts that reducing access to highly lethal means is one of only two suicide prevention approaches with a sound empirical basis,[4] few practitioners, including psychiatrists, appear to discuss firearm safety with suicidal patients,[5] let alone with patients who are at heightened risk but not actively suicidal. Reasons for this reticence may include not being familiar with the scientific evidence, uncertainty about what to say and how to say it, and discomfort with the prospect of such a discussion. An additional impediment may be that there are no formal procedures in place to help physicians and patients act quickly on a patient's decision to temporarily remove firearms from the home. When informal arrangements fail or are difficult to make, there is no reliable alternative to fall back on. For example, few police departments have mechanisms in place to accept and temporarily store firearms for citizens.

In the following sections, I briefly note additional findings from the literature that physicians and others who engage patients in conversations about lethal means might want to know. I conclude with three actionable suggestions that would help reduce the toll of suicide among the men and women who have served our country in recent years.

THE SCIENTIFIC EVIDENCE

The scientific literature convincingly demonstrates that the ready availability of highly lethal means—not just the intent of the victim—determines whether many suicidal acts prove fatal.[6] There are over a dozen case–control studies in the peer-reviewed literature in the United States, all of which have found that a gun in the home is associated with an increased risk of suicide, not only for the gun owner but also for other members of the household, such as his spouse and children. The increase in risk is large, typically two to ten times that in homes without guns, depending on the sample population (e.g., higher for adolescents than for older adults) and how the firearms are stored. The association between guns in the home and the risk of suicide is attributable to a large increase in the risk of suicide by firearms, which is not counterbalanced by a reduced risk of nonfirearm suicide. Of vital importance for targeting prevention efforts is the fact that the increased risk of suicide is not explained by increased psychopathology, suicidal ideation, or suicide attempts among members of gun-owning households. Indeed, the greatest relative risk appears to be among persons without known psychopathology.

Ecologic studies in the United States have also shown a strong association between rates of household gun ownership and rates of completed suicide—attributable, as found in the case–control studies, to the strong association between firearm prevalence and firearm suicide without a counterbalancing association between firearm ownership levels and rates of nonfirearm suicide.[6] Studies from other countries also illustrate the dominant role that readily available, highly lethal means can play in determining suicide mortality rates. For example, during the 1950s, nearly half of all suicides in the United Kingdom were because of carbon monoxide gas from coal burning ovens. As homes replaced coal with detoxified gas over the next 2 decades, rates of suicide by gas fell in effect to zero without offsetting increases in rates of nongas suicide. Consequently (and critically), overall rates of completed suicide dropped substantially for both men and women (by approximately 30%).[7] In Sri Lanka, where pesticide poisoning was the dominant method used in suicide deaths, a ban on the most toxic pesticides resulted in a dramatic decline in pesticide suicides and overall suicides, without significant changes in rates of suicide from other mechanisms.[8] Most recently, suicide among the Israeli Defense Forces fell by 40% after an injury prevention policy reduced soldiers' access to firearms on weekends.[9] The decline in suicides was because of a decrease in weekend firearm suicides, with no significant change in weekday suicide rates or any compensatory increase in nonfirearm suicides.

THREE ACTIONABLE SUGGESTIONS

The recent, unprecedented increase in suicide rates among our troops has effectively undone the historically protective effect of serving in the military, the so called "health warrior effect," at least with respect to suicide. With suicide rates among soldiers now on par with rates among comparable members of the general population who never served, it is incumbent upon the public health community to identify actions that empirical research suggests can save lives today. To this end, I have three high priority recommendations. First, discussions about household firearms and other lethal means should be undertaken with all patients who are in a high-risk group (e.g., those with depression, drug and alcohol problems, histories of interpersonal violence), not only with patients who are actively suicidal. Ideally these conversations should take place at a time when a patient is better able to act in his own enlightened self-interest. Tversky and Kahneman called this strategy of precommittment a Ulysses contact,[10] referring to Ulysses' prescient decision to have himself bound to his ship's mast prior to venturing within earshot of the Siren's irresistible call.

Second, the military, the VHA, and the broader medical community should do what it takes to create a trusted mechanism for the safe removal and temporary storage of firearms that a patient wishes out of his home. For the military, the infrastructure is already in place to do so. For the VHA, creating a mechanism to effect the timely transfer of firearms for safekeeping is a logical next step for their ambitious firearm safety program, which already includes efforts to distribute gun safety locks and educational material to veterans and their families (and firearm safety interventions for patients with dementia).

Third, the federal government and others should promote serious interdisciplinary research that aims to determine how to optimally communicate firearm safety messages and otherwise operationalize what we *already* know can save lives.

CONCLUSION

Preventing suicidal behavior and the suffering that leads to desperate action has proven extremely difficult. But lives can still be saved, in the short run and the long run, if vested parties resist political arguments about the impossibility of reducing access to firearms and instead commit to the achievable goal of enabling the kind of enlightened self interest that Ulysses' choice epitomized. After all, Ulysses survived where myriad others perished, not because he found the Siren's calls less compelling, but because he anticipated his inability to resist voices urging him toward death—and took steps to avert disaster.

ABOUT THE AUTHOR

Matthew Miller is with the Harvard Injury Control Research Center, Department of Health Policy and Management, Harvard School of Public Health, Boston, MA.

REFERENCES

1. Department of Defense. The Challenge and the Promise: Strengthening the Force, Preventing Suicide and Saving Lives: Final Report of the Department of Defense Task Force on the Prevention of Suicide by Members of the Armed Forces. Available at: http://www.health.mil/dhb/downloads/Suicide%20Prevention%20Task%20Force%20final%20report%208-23-10.pdf. Accessed April 19, 2011.

2. Simon OR, Swann AC, Powell KE, Potter LB, Kresnow MJ, O'Carroll PW. Characteristics of impulsive suicide attempts and attempters. *Suicide Life Threat Behav.* 2001;32(Suppl):49–59.

3. Owens D, Horrocks J, House A. Fatal and non-fatal repetition of self-harm. Systematic review. *Br J Psychiatry.* 2002;181:193–199.

4. Mann JJ, Apter A, Bertolote J, et al. Suicide prevention strategies: a systematic review. *JAMA.* 2005;294:2064–2074.

5. Price JH, Kinnison A, Dake JA, Thompson AJ, Price JA. Psychiatrists' practices and perceptions regarding anticipatory guidance on firearms. *Am J Prev Med.* 2007;33(5):370–373.

6. Miller M, Azrael D, Barber C. Suicide mortality in the United States: the importance of attending to method in understanding population-level disparities in the burden of suicide. *Annu Rev Public Health.* Published online ahead of print on April 4, 2011.

7. Kreitman N. The coal gas story. United Kingdom suicide rates, 1960–71. *Br J Prev Soc Med.* 1976;30:86–93.

8. Gunnell D, Fernando R, Hewagama M, Priyangika WD, Konradsen F, Eddleston M. The impact of pesticide regulations on suicide in Sri Lanka. *Int J Epidemiol.* 2007;36:1235–1242.

9. Lubin G, Werbeloff N, Halperin D, Shmushkevitch M, Weiser M, Knobler HY. Decrease in suicide rates after a change of policy reducing access to firearms in adolescents: a naturalistic epidemiological study. *Suicide Life Threat Behav.* 2010;40:421–424.

10. Tversky A, Kahneman D. The framing of decisions and the psychology of choice. *Science.* 1981;211(4481):453–458.

5

Suicide Prevention for Veterans and Active Duty Personnel

Kerry L. Knox, PhD, and Robert M. Bossarte, PhD

A considerable body of research has identified correlates of suicide at the genetic, neurologic, psychological, social, and cultural levels. Among risk characteristics identified in existing studies, current or former military service has emerged as a topic of considerable scientific and public interest. Of those who die from suicide, veterans and active duty military personnel represent a select group with considerable heterogeneity in individual characteristics and life histories. Such heterogeneity in individuallevel characteristics and precipitating events carries with it the potential to obfuscate relationships between individual risk factors, experiences uniquely associated with military service, and social and cultural factors. Despite these challenges, results from existing studies suggest that history of military service is an element worthy of consideration in efforts to address the complex and multifaceted nature of intentional self-harm. Given the intricate etiology of suicide and limitations of current data systems, it is not surprising that uncertainty surrounds the exact nature of the relationships between history of military service and suicide.[1] Moreover, the unique experiences of different military cohorts may play a key role as major contextual factors given the diverse range of exposures experienced by different cohorts.

It is our position that an appropriate response to any evidence of increased risk for suicide among veterans and active duty service members include a multifaceted prevention strategy that considers both traditional markers of individual risk for suicide and those that are universally represented, without consideration of individual history.[2,3] Universal strategies, such as public education campaigns and toll-free crisis lines, provide opportunities to increase awareness, facilitate access, and promote use of crisis services among those experiencing distress. At the same time, targeted approaches in those who have served and especially subpopulations who may bear a disproportionate burden of risk are critically needed. We also are keenly aware of the need to identify and provide immediate intervention to those who are in imminent danger of taking their own lives. Taken together, these prevention strategies embody a public health approach to prevention. A public health approach has been shown to be promising because, in part, of the overlapping influence of strategies at each level. At the same time, it avoids piecemeal approaches that may not, by their very nature, be sustainable.[2] By way of example, a public health approach should include universal programs designed to promote seeking help and access to services among those in distress (ideally before they are at imminent risk for suicide), the implementation of systems to inform clinical decisions and understand outcomes among those with demonstrated risk, and the development and evaluation of clinical approaches to reduce risk for self-directed violence among unique clinical groups that have already experienced signs and symptoms (such as suicide attempts and reattempts).

The articles in this issue provide the most current and comprehensive picture of what we know about the epidemiology, assessment, and prevention of suicide from clinical and population-based perspectives. They include a reanalysis of data from the National Health Interview Survey by Miller et al.,[4] accompanying commentaries by Miller et al.[5] and Kaplan et al.,[6] and an editorial by Gibbons et al.,[7] which reflect the ongoing debate regarding both the nature of the data available on suicide in veterans and methodological approaches for calculating estimates of risk associated with veteran status. This debate underscores the need for improved data sources to estimate the burden of suicide and suicidal behaviors in veterans and military populations and the challenges posed by a lack of integration among existing data systems. It is worth noting the difficulty in identifying the incidence or characteristics of suicide among veterans who have not received services from the Veterans Health Administration (VHA), and in ascertaining whether these veterans bear a significantly different risk for suicide than veterans seen within the VHA health care system.

Based on evidence largely from postmortem research using psychological autopsy methods, many who die by suicide bear a tremendous burden of risk associated with psychopathology. However, a study of suicide among veterans who received VHA services also suggested that many of those who died from suicide did not carry a diagnosis at the time of their death,[8] suggesting the need for continued efforts to promote help seeking and treatment among those experiencing distress. There are a number of articles in this supplement that focus on specific risk factors that appear to increase the risk of suicidality among veterans and military personnel, including sleep disorders (Pigeon et al.[9]), substance abuse (Ilgen et al.[10]), and depression (Britton et al.[11]). In an editorial in this supplement, Conner and Bossarte[11] argue that clinical services, rather than being in opposition to public health approaches to suicide prevention, are a fundamental component of public health approaches to reducing deaths and associated morbidity from suicide. Finally, assessment of suicidal behaviors is a constant challenge to the field of suicide prevention in general. McCarthy et al.[12] describe the first use of a clinical assessment tool that resulted in a public health impact through providing early identification and support to airmen that potentially could reduce suicidal behaviors.

In summary, much as the Framingham study found in its early decades, collaborative efforts between clinicians and epidemiologists provide a foundation for changing the cultural norms associated with a major public health problem. Treating groups at high risk for suicide is a necessary, but insufficient response to suicide. Strategies designed to engage entire populations, with and without consideration of individual risk characteristics, may ultimately have the biggest impact.[13] The promise of a population strategy is eloquently discussed by Katz,[14] who provides one hypothesis for how a public health approach may result in reduced mortality because of suicide in veterans. This supplement represents an effort on the part of many to bring together divergent perspectives from those who are working daily to acquire a better understanding of what works for preventing suicide in those who have served our country. The considerable interest shown in this supplement is a tribute to all who have served in the military and we, as do all Americans, thank them for their service. We deeply hope that this supplement will serve as a catalyst for continued research that will improve the lives of our veterans, and reduce the morbidity and mortality because of suicide in those who have served in the military.

ABOUT THE AUTHORS

Kerry L. Knox and Robert M. Bossarte are with the Department of Veterans Affairs, Canandaigua, NY, and the Department of Psychiatry, Center for the Study and Prevention of Suicide, the University of Rochester Medical Center, Rochester, NY.

CONTRIBUTORS

K. L. Knox took the lead in writing the article. R. M. Bossarte contributed to revisions of the initial article. Both authors contributed to the intellectual content of this editorial and approved the editorial.

ACKNOWLEDGMENTS

The Department of Veterans Affairs Veterans Integrated Services Network 2 (VISN) Center of Excellence for Suicide Prevention supported the preparation of this special supplement.

The guest editors would like to sincerely thank the authors of the individual articles, editorials, and commentaries, the reviewers, and the *AJPH* editors and staff.

We owe special thanks for the tremendous support that the VISN 2 Center of Excellence for Suicide Prevention received from the Department of Veterans Affairs Offices of Mental Health Services and Mental Health Operations. Specifically, we thank Antonette Zeiss, PhD; Sonja Batten, PhD; Janet Kemp, PhD; and Mary Schohn, PhD, for their ongoing and tireless support of the Center's activities.

We gratefully acknowledge our academic affiliate, the University of Rochester Medical Center, Department of Psychiatry, and especially the Department's Center for the Study and Prevention of Suicide.

We also thank the staff and investigators at the VISN 2 Center of Excellence for Suicide Prevention, especially Lisa Lochner, Kathy Main, and Annie Nolan for facilitating the administrative aspects of this project.

REFERENCES

1. Bossarte R, Claassen CA, Knox K. Veteran suicide prevention: emerging priorities and opportunities for intervention. *Mil Med.* 2010;175(7):461–462.

2. Knox KL, Litts DA, Talcott GW, Feig JC, Caine ED. Risk of suicide and related adverse outcomes after exposure to a suicide prevention programme in the United States Air Force. Cohort study. *BMJ*. 2003;327:1376.

3. Knox KL, Pflanz S, Talcott GW, Campise RL, Lavigne JE, Bajorska A, et al. The Air Force Suicide Prevention Program: implications for public health policy. *Am J Public Health*. 2010;100(12):2457–2463.

4. Miller M, Barber C, Young M, Azrael D, Mukamal K, Lawler E. Veterans and suicide: a reexamination of the National Death Index–linked National Health Interview Survey. *Am J Public Health*. 2012;102(Suppl 1):S154–S159.

5. Miller M, Azrael D, Barber C, Mukamal K, Lawler E. A call to link data to answer pressing questions about suicide among veterans. *Am J Public Health*. 2012;102(Suppl 1):S20, S22.

6. Kaplan MS, McFarland BH, Huguet N, Newsom JT. Estimating the risk of suicide among US veterans: how should we proceed from here? *Am J Public Health*. 2012;102(Suppl 1):S21, S23.

7. Gibbons RD, Brown CH, Hur K. Is the rate of suicide among veterans elevated? *Am J Public Health*. 2012;102(Suppl 1):S17–S19.

8. Ilgen MA. Bohnert AS, Ignacio RV, McCarthy JF, Valenstein MM, Kim HM, et al. Psychiatric diagnoses and risk of suicide in veterans. *Arch Gen Psychiatry*. 2010;67(11):1152–1158.

9. Pigeon WR, Britton PC, Ilgen MA, Chapman B, Conner KR. Sleep disturbance preceding suicide among veterans. *Am J Public Health*. 2012;102(Suppl 1):S93–S97.

10. Ilgen MA, Conner KR, Roeder KM, Blow FC, Austin K, Valenstein M. Patterns of treatment utilization before suicide among male veterans with substance use disorders. *Am J Public Health*. 2012;102(Suppl 1):S88–S92.

11. Britton PC, Ilgen MA, Valenstein M, Knox K, Claassen CA, Conner KR. Differences between veteran suicides with and without psychiatric symptoms. *Am J Public Health*. 2012;102(Suppl 1):S125–S130.

12. McCarthy MD, Thompson SJ, Knox KL. Use of the Air Force Post-Deployment Health Reassessment for the identification of depression and posttraumatic stress disorder: public health implications for suicide prevention. *Am J Public Health*. 2012;102(Suppl 1):S60–S65.

13. Knox KL, Conwell Y, Caine ED. If suicide is a public health problem, what are we doing to prevent it? *Am J Public Health.* 2004;94:37–45.

14. Katz I. Lessons learned from mental health enhancement and suicide prevention activities in the Veterans Health Administration. *Am J Public Health.* 2012;102(Suppl 1):S14–S16.

6

Precedence for Integration of Clinical Services in Public Health Initiatives

Kenneth R. Conner, PsyD, and Robert M. Bossarte, PhD

Reduction of suicide is widely recognized as a public health priority, and reports of elevated rates among veteran and military populations have received considerable attention. Clinical services, including effective management of behavioral disorders, psychotherapy, and the use of pharmaceutical agents, have been identified as important elements in a comprehensive approach to the prevention of suicide.[1] Nonetheless, the proper role of clinical services in suicide prevention programs remains unclear, with a perceived tension between diagnosis- or symptom-driven clinical management and more universal approaches. However, such tension is more likely a function of the many challenges to implementing effective clinical services to address suicide risk, including the relative lack of evidence-based clinical therapies to prevent suicide deaths, stigma associated with behavioral disorders (e.g., mood disorders, substance use disorders), and low service utilization and adherence to treatment, than inconsistencies between the missions of clinical science and population health. We view such challenges as a call to create systems of care that are more inclusive and effective in meeting the needs of individuals vulnerable to suicide than a justification for divorcing clinical services from a comprehensive public health approach to suicide. Many of the major public health achievements of the 20th century, such as the eradication of smallpox and global reductions in the incidence and consequence of paralytic poliomyelitis (polio), relied on clinical services to identify and protect vulnerable populations. For example, the eradication of smallpox would not have been possible without safe and effective strategies for vaccine delivery, and reductions in polio (while similarly related to safe and effective vaccine administration) resulted from enhanced clinical and laboratory surveillance to identify vulnerable populations and pockets of vaccine resistance.[2]

DEPARTMENT OF VETERANS AFFAIRS' INTEGRATION OF CLINICAL SERVICES IN SUICIDE PREVENTION

The Department of Veterans Affairs (VA) provides an illustration of integrating clinical services in a multifaceted approach to reduce suicide. The approach includes an "enhanced care package" for veterans identified as high risk or potential risk, with use of evidence-based and promising interventions, including Safety Planning, the "caring letter program," increased follow-up, and care monitoring and tracking by the Suicide Prevention Coordinators located at each site. The approach also features universal strategies to enhance access to services and availability of treatment of vulnerable veterans, such as the National Veterans Crisis Line and Chat Service. These and other clinically based initiatives demand rigorous study to document their effectiveness and to inform continuous improvement. Consistent with a public health framework, each of these initiatives addresses veterans' suicidal thoughts and behaviors regardless of underlying behavioral disorders that may be contributing to risk. A public health perspective also demands attention to the primary methods leading to suicide fatalities, with firearms used in the majority of cases.[3] In response, VA clinical training materials stress the importance of addressing means safety when working with suicidal patients, including in treatment planning.[4] A public health perspective also requires that the settings where high-risk individuals are concentrated be targeted in preventive efforts.[5] Along these lines, veterans discharged from inpatient psychiatric care after an attempt and those who receive treatment of a suicide attempt are routinely placed on the "high-risk list," with their records flagged and the enhanced care package initiated.

RATIONALE FOR ADDRESSING BEHAVIORAL DISORDERS IN SUICIDE PREVENTION IN CLINICAL SETTINGS

A focus on addressing suicidal thoughts and behavior regardless of underlying disorders does not rule out parallel efforts to study and prevent suicide in diagnostic populations. Because of exposure to combat, stress of deployment, and other factors, military service members and veterans experience sleep disturbances, traumatic brain injury, posttraumatic stress disorder, substance use disorders, mood disorders, and other behavioral health difficulties at high rates during deployment to warzones and after return to home.[6–8] Accordingly, clinically informed research on these and other correlates of suicide is needed to inform treatment development efforts. The need to integrate clinical services to treat behavioral disorders and to prevent suicide is underscored by the strong etiological link between behavioral disorders and suicide.[9] A recent national cohort study of veterans who received Veterans Health Administration services reported that approximately half (46%) of veteran suicide decedents had a history of one or more behavioral health disorders.[10] Although the study was excellent, it likely underestimated the prevalence of behavioral disorders because the diagnoses were made months or years before the eventual suicides. Psychological autopsy studies that focused on the last weeks of life indicate that about 90% of suicide decedents in the United States and other western nations had one or more behavioral health disorders.[11]

Because of the role of behavioral disorders in suicide, each major US report on suicide has recognized the critical role that clinical care providers play in suicide prevention.[8,12,13] Although major behavioral disorders, including mood disorders and schizophrenia, confer increased risk for many causes of premature death, they confer massive risk for suicide in particular.[14] Moreover, suicide is unlike many other public health challenges, such as drinking, where the bulk of injury, death, and societal cost occur in individuals who engage in hazardous or harmful drinking (e.g., binge drinking pattern) but do not meet criteria for alcohol dependence.[15] In contrast, suicide decedents overwhelmingly meet full criteria for alcohol dependence, major depression, or other behavioral health conditions.[9,11] Accordingly, sound delivery of evidence-based care for behavioral health conditions that confer risk for suicide in and of itself is an important element of a comprehensive suicide prevention strategy. In this regard, treatment of depression stands out as having an evidence base in suicide prevention,[1] with a need to study the potential role of prevention in treatments for other conditions (e.g., substance use disorders[16]).

ABOUT THE AUTHORS

Kenneth R. Conner and Robert M. Bossarte are with the Veterans Integrated Services Network (VISN) 2 Center of Excellence for Suicide Prevention, Canandaigua, NY, and the Department of Psychiatry, University of Rochester, Rochester, NY.

CONTRIBUTORS

K. R. Conner conceived and led development of the editorial. R.M. Bossarte contributed to the editorial.

ACKNOWLEDGMENTS

We thank Janet Kemp, PhD, Peter Britton, PhD, and Wil Pigeon, PhD, for their comments and edits.

REFERENCES

1. Mann JJ, Apter A, Bertolote J, et al. Suicide prevention strategies: a systematic review. *JAMA*. 2005;294:2064–2074.

2. Dowdle WR, Mayer LW, Steinberg KK, Ghiya ND, Popovic T, Global Polio Eradication, Task Force for Global Health, Decatur, Georgia. Laboratory contributions to public health. *MMWR Surveill Summ*. 2011;60:27–34.

3. McCarthy JF, Blow FC, Ignacio RV, Ilgen MA, Austin KL, Valenstein M. Suicide among patients in the veterans affairs health system: rural–urban differences in rates, risks, and methods. *Am J Public Health*. 2012;102(suppl 1): S111–S117.

4. Stanley B, Brown GK. *The Safety Plan Treatment Manual to Reduce Suicide Risk: Veteran Version*. Washington, DC: Department of Veterans Affairs; 2008.

5. Valenstein M, Kim HM, Ganoczy D, et al. Higher-risk periods for suicide among VA patients receiving depression treatment: prioritizing suicide prevention efforts. *J Affect Disord*. 2009;112:50–58.

6. Hoge CW, Castro CA, Messer SC, McGurk D, Cotting DI, Koffman RL. Combat duty in Iraq and Afghanistan, mental health problems, and barriers to care. *N Engl J Med*. 2004;351:13–22.

7. Milliken CS, Auchterlonie JL, Hoge CW. Longitudinal assessment of mental health problems among active and reserve component solidiers returning from the Iraq war. *JAMA*. 2007;298:2141–2148.

8. US. Department of Defense. *Department of Defense Task Force on the Prevention of Suicide by Members of the Armed Forces*. Washington, DC: Department of Defense; 2010.

9. Nock MK, Borges G, Bromet EJ, Cha CB, Kessler RC, Lee S. Suicide and suicidal behavior. *Epidemiol Rev*. 2008;30:133–154.

10. Ilgen MA, Bois C, Ignacio RV, et al. Psychiatric diagnoses and risk of suicide in veterans. *Arch Gen Psychiatry*. 2010;67:1152–1158.

11. Cavanagh JTO, Carson AJ, Sharpe M, Lawrie SM. Psychological autopsy studies of suicide: a systematic review. *Psychol Med*. 2003;33:395–405.

12. Institute of Medicine. *Reducing Suicide: A National Imperative*. Washington, DC: The National Academies Press; 2002.

13. US. Public Health Service. *The Surgeon General's Call to Action to Prevent Suicide*. Washington, DC: Department of Health and Human Services; 1999.

14. Laursen TM, Munk-Olsen T, Nordentoft M, Mortensen PB. Increased mortality among patients admitted with major psychiatric disorders: a register-based study comparing mortality in unipolar depressive disorder, bipolar affective disorder, schizoaffective disorder, and schizophrenia. *J Clin Psychiatry*. 2007;68:899–907.

15. Monteiro MG. *Alcohol and Public Health in the Americas: A Case for Action*. Washington, DC: PAHO; 2007.

16. Ilgen MA, Jain A, Lucas E, Moos RH. Substance use-disorder treatment and a decline in attempted suicide during and after treatment. *J Stud Alcohol Drugs*. 2007;68:503–509.

7

Facilitating Treatment Engagement During High-Risk Transition Periods: A Potential Suicide Prevention Strategy

Lisa A. Brenner, PhD, and Sean M. Barnes, PhD

The Departments of Defense (DoD) and Veterans Affairs (VA) have made it a priority to combat suicide. Each of the military services and the VA have developed educational campaigns to reduce the stigma associated with reporting emotional distress, raise awareness of the risk of suicide, and teach military personnel, veterans, and their families suicide prevention strategies. Within the DoD and VA, significant resources have been leveraged toward studying and implementing both public health and clinical intervention strategies. These resources have also fostered significant collaborative efforts between individuals in the DoD and VA.

Within the Veterans Health Administration (VHA) vital components of the suicide prevention program are the Veterans Crisis Line and online chat service. Strategies for assessing, identifying, and tracking those at increased risk for suicide have been implemented. Moreover, at VA Medical Centers and large Community Based Outpatient Clinics, Suicide Prevention Coordinators are in place to ensure that veterans at high risk receive needed counseling and services.

Despite these advances, rates of suicide within the military and among veterans support enhancing current efforts. In 2001, for every 100 000 individuals serving in the military, 9.9 died by suicide.[1] By 2009, military suicide rates rose to 18.3 per 100 000 with 1.3 per 100 000 deaths still under investigation.[1] Suicide continues to be a concern for military personnel, even after returning to civilian life. In fiscal year 2010, veterans made nearly 15 000 suicide attempts, with 18 veterans dying by suicide every day.[2]

Facilitating treatment engagement, particularly during high-risk periods of transition, might be an important means of reducing suicide. Valenstein et al.[3] conducted a retrospective cohort study of 887 859 VA patients receiving care for depression, and calculated suicide rates for five sequential 12-week periods after treatment events (e.g., psychiatric hospitalization, new antidepressant starts). Findings suggested that the highest risk period for suicide among VA patients was in the 12-week period after psychiatric hospitalization. Although the suicide rate for all time periods was 114 per 100 000 person-years, the rate after psychiatric hospitalization was 568 deaths per 100 000 person-years. In support of these results, Hunt et al.[4] found that among members of the general population, 43% of suicides after inpatient psychiatric treatment occurred within the first month after discharge. The first week after discharge was noted as being a particularly high-risk period. Knox et al.[5] highlighted the risk for suicide after acute psychiatric services (e.g., care in Emergency Department [ED]), the reality that a visit to the ED might be the "sole point of contact" for an individual, and the importance of using the contact to engage individuals in care; thereby facilitating a transition from crisis to outpatient services.

Research also suggested that transitions associated with life events increased risk for suicidal behavior. For example, Binswanger et al.[6] conducted a retrospective cohort study of all inmates from the Washington State Department of Corrections. Results supported an increased rate of suicide in the two weeks after being released from prison (136 deaths by suicide per 100 000 person-years). After the first 2 weeks, the rate dropped to 69 deaths by suicide per 100 000 person-years. Other life transitions associated with increased risk for death by suicide included job loss,[7] divorce or romantic breakup,[8,9] and physical injuries or illnesses.[7,10]

Of particular import to DoD and VHA providers are data that suggested periods of increased risk during deployment and postdischarge. Warner et al.[11] explored suicidal thoughts and behaviors among US soldiers over a 15-month deployment cycle and found three distinct time periods of increased suicidality. The first occurred around month two and was hypothesized as being in response to separation from families and friends. A second peak was noted after six months in theater. The authors indicated this was a common time for using leave (e.g., two weeks back in the United States with family and friends), and suggested that upon return to the combat zone, soldiers might experience increased stress and feelings of isolation. The final peak was noted around month 12, in close proximity to the end of deployment when individuals might be increasingly focused on stressors at home. In the United Kingdom, Kapur et al.[12] examined the rate for suicide among individuals who left the Armed Forces (1996–2005) and found that among men under the age of 25 years, the risk of suicide was two to three times higher than the risk for the general and serving populations (same age groups).

Moreover, Brenner et al.[13] conducted a qualitative study of potential suicide risk factors (burdensomeness, belongingness, and acquired ability) among returned combat veterans, which explicated some potential causes of postdischarge suicide risk. Many of these were related to the need to re-establish or redefine occupational, social, and recreational roles. The veterans interviewed described a loss of sense of self and purpose postdischarge. Many veterans found it difficult to leave their well-defined and meaningful military roles to re-establish their place in the civilian world. Veterans also reported a heightened sense of burdensomeness and described struggling to provide their families with financial and emotional support. Many also reported feeling disconnected from civilians. This was in contrast to the sense of belongingness they felt when among those in the military or other veterans. During the course of the interviews veterans linked perceived burdensomeness and a failed sense of belongingness with a desire for death.[14]

With the growing recognition of the risk associated with stressful life transitions, researchers have begun developing engagement strategies to decrease negative outcomes. Early work in this area expanded the notion of treatment by focusing on supporting patients in their transition from an inpatient psychiatric setting to their home environment.[15] Motto and Bostrom[15] explored the impact of sending caring letters on suicide prevention among 843 patients who refused ongoing outpatient care. The focus of the letters, each of which was worded differently, was an "expression of concern that the person was getting along all right and invited a response if the patient wished to send one."[15(p829)] The authors hypothesized that the letters would decrease patients' sense of isolation and enhance their sense of connectedness. Findings suggested that those who received letters had lower suicide rates than a control group in all five years of the study. The authors did not report rates of treatment re-engagement. However, they noted that an incidental benefit of the contact program, which might have contributed to the outcome, was that patients who received the caring letters occasionally turned to project personnel for help re-entering the health care system.

Several other more recent engagement strategies also added to the evidence base for assisting patients during times of transition. Work by Davis et al.[16] suggested that outreach (i.e., letters, face-to-face contact, telephone calls) might result in individuals with severe mental illness returning to care. Preliminary findings from a VA hospital ED project, SAFE VET, suggested that targeted follow-up might increase treatment engagement in terms of outpatient services.[5] An integral component of SAFE VET is the Acute Services Coordinator, who is a resource to the veteran during the transition period and facilitates engagement in outpatient care. Moreover, work by Verwey et al.[17] highlighted the potential positive impact of home-based assessment postdischarge from hospital psychiatric emergency services. Lastly, in addition to tracking suicidal thoughts and behaviors, Warner et al.[11] implemented a deployment cycle-specific suicide prevention plan that included targeted interventions during periods of increased risk. As noted previously, these high-risk periods seemed to coincide with deployment-related transitions.

Because heightened stress could be anticipated during times of transition, such events might mark opportune times for prevention and intervention. Findings presented in this editorial support identifying individuals during periods of transition and implementing treatment engagement protocols as a means of enhancing current suicide prevention efforts. Actual interventions indicated might vary in terms modality and intensity (e.g., psychoeducation, caring letter, outpatient mental health treatment). Based on the needs of the population, a focus on increasing psychosocial functioning might also be warranted (e.g., employment services). An example of such a program is the VHA's Health Care for Re-entry, which was "designed to address the community re-entry needs of incarcerated veterans."[18] Although initial evidence exists regarding treatment engagement during periods of transition as a suicide prevention strategy, further work in this area is required to establish efficacy and effectiveness. It is hoped that continued efforts to maximize treatment engagement during high-risk transitional periods will enhance clinicians' ability to care for those who have served our country.

ABOUT THE AUTHORS

Lisa A. Brenner and Sean M. Barnes are with the Veterans Integrated Service Network 19, Mental Illness Research, Education and Clinical Center, Denver Veteran Affairs Medical Center, Denver, CO, and the University of Colorado Denver, School of Medicine, Denver.

Note. The views expressed in this article are those of the authors and do not necessarily represent the views of the Department of Veterans Affairs.

CONTRIBUTORS

Both authors contributed equally to the conception, research, and development of this editorial.

REFERENCES

1. Department of Defense Personnel & Procurement Statistics. Military casualty information. Available at: http://siadapp.dmdc.osd.mil/personnel/CASUALTY/castop.htm. Updated December 12, 2011. Accessed November 10, 2011.

2. Department of Veterans Affairs. *Fact Sheet: VA Suicide Prevention Program Facts about Veteran Suicide.* Washington, DC: Dept of Veterans Affairs Office of Patient Care Services Office of Mental Health Services; 2011.

3. Valenstein M, Kim HM, Ganoczy D, et al. Higher-risk periods for suicide among VA patients receiving depression treatment: prioritizing suicide prevention efforts. *J Affect Disord.* 2009;112(1-3):50–58.

4. Hunt IM, Kapur N, Webb R, et al. Suicide in recently discharged psychiatric patients: a case-control study. *Psychol Med.* 2009;39(3):443–449.

5. Knox KL, Stanley B, Currier GW, Brenner LA, Ghahramanlou-Holloway M, Brown GK. An emergency based brief intervention for veterans at risk for suicide (SAFE VET). *Am J Public Health.* 2012;10(s1).

6. Binswanger IA, Stern MF, Deyo RA, et al. Release from prison–a high risk of death for former inmates. *N Engl J Med.* 2007;356(2):157–165.

7. Duberstein PR, Conwell Y, Conner KR, Eberly S, Caine ED. Suicide at 50 years of age and older: perceived physical illness, family discord and financial strain. *Psychol Med.* 2004;34(1):137–146.

8. Kposowa AJ. Marital status and suicide in the National Longitudinal Mortality Study. *J Epidemiol Community Health.* 2000;54(4):254–261.

9. Thoresen S, Mehlum L. Suicide in peacekeepers: risk factors for suicide versus accidental death. *Suicide Life Threat Behav.* 2006;36(4):432–442.

10. Brown SL, Vinokur AD. The interplay among risk factors for suicidal ideation and suicide: the role of depression, poor health, and loved ones' messages of support and criticism. *Am J Community Psychol.* 2003;32(1-2):131–141.

11. Warner CH, Appenzeller GN, Parker JR, Warner C, Diebold CJ, Grieger T. Suicide prevention in a deployed military unit. *Psychiatry.* 2011;74(2):127–141.

12. Kapur N, While D, Blatchley N, Bray I, Harrison K. Suicide after leaving the UK armed forces–a cohort study. *PLoS Med.* 2009;6(3):e26.

13. Brenner LA, Gutierrez PM, Cornette MM, Betthauser LM, Bahraini N, Staves PJ. A qualitative study of potential suicide risk factors in returning combat veterans. *J Ment Health Couns.* 2008;30(3):211–225.

14. Joiner TE. *Why People Die by Suicide.* Cambridge, England: Harvard University Press; 2005.

15. Motto JA, Bostrom AG. A randomized controlled trial of postcrisis suicide prevention. *Psychiatr Serv.* 2001;52(6):828–833.

16. Davis CL, Kilbourne AM, Pierce JR, et al. Reduced mortality among VA patients with schizophrenia or bipolar disorder lost to follow-up and engaged in active outreach to return to care. *J Public Health.* 2012;10(s1).

17. Verwey B, van Waarde JA, Bozdag MA, van Rooij I, de Beurs E, Zitman FG. Reassessment of suicide attempters at home, shortly after discharge from hospital. *Crisis.* 2010;31(6):303–310.

18. United States Department of Veterans Affairs. Health care re-entry Veterans services and resources. Available at: http://www.va.gov/HOMELESS/Reentry.asp. Updated August 29, 2011. Accessed November 10, 2011.

8

Lessons Learned From Mental Health Enhancement and Suicide Prevention Activities in the Veterans Health Administration

Ira Katz, MD, PhD

This publication of a special issue of the *American Journal of Public Health,* which focuses on suicide in veterans and service members, is occurring when America has been at war for over a decade. Over this time, suicide in veterans and service members has become a national concern. This can be documented in a number of ways. For one, a search of the Medline database for articles indexed under the expanded subject heading "suicide" and the text words "veteran" or "veterans" identified one article in the year 2000 and three in 2001, but 23 in 2009 and 33 in 2010. For another, a search of the *New York Times* archives for "veteran" and "suicide" followed by review of the citations identified three articles referring to suicide among American veterans in 2000 and one in 2001, but 11 in 2009 and 15 in 2010. Perhaps most significantly, the 2001 US National Strategy for Suicide Prevention[1] did not address suicide in military and veteran populations. However, the National Action Alliance for Suicide Prevention, the public–private partnership charged with revising the strategy, was structured to ensure relevant input. The partnership's public sector cochair is the Secretary of the Army; it includes representatives of the Department of Defense (DoD), the Department of Veterans Affairs (VA), and relevant support groups on its Executive Committee; and it has formed a work group on military and veterans issues.

There are a series of possible reasons for the recognition of suicide in military and veteran populations as a national priority. As Operation Enduring Freedom and Operation Iraqi Freedom (OEF/OIF), the wars in Afghanistan and Iraq, have gone on, suicide rates have increased in active duty service members, including those who have recently returned from deployment. The American public has responded, in part, to support the troops, and, in part, to ensure that America recognizes the full measure of the costs of war. A number of stories of individual suicides have been widely reported; each one speaks for itself, demonstrating the tragedy and suffering associated with each death. Specifically for VA, there have been a substantial number of reports of problems with mental health services and calls for improvement. There have also been reports recognizing the innovative nature of the VA's programs for suicide prevention. One summary of recent activities[2] stated, "In the past few years the Department of Veterans Affairs has become one of the most vibrant forces in the US suicide prevention movement, implementing multiple levels of innovative and state of the art interventions, backed up by a robust evaluation and research capacity." Anticipating the formation of the National Action Alliance for Suicide Prevention and the revision of the National Strategy for Suicide Prevention, the same document included the recommendation to: "Evaluate and assess practices being implemented in the VA for dissemination to the broader healthcare delivery system.[1,2]

The VA's current suicide prevention program began with the approval of its Mental Health Strategic Plan by the Under Secretary for Health in 2004. The plan was motivated by the recommendations of the 2003 release of the report of the President's New Freedom Commission on Mental Health,[3] and by early recognition of the mental health problems facing veterans returning from Afghanistan and Iraq. It included 242 actions that could be factored into 6 domains, including increasing access and capacity, integrating mental health with primary care, transforming mental health specialty care into recovery-oriented services, and implementing evidence-based practices, as well as prioritizing services for returning veterans and suicide prevention. To promote the implementation of the strategy, VA established the Mental Health Initiative as a way to complement its usual mechanisms for funding clinical services with targeted funding for mental health enhancements. This led to an increase in core mental health staff on a national level by 50%, from about 14 000 in 2005 to 21 000 by the end of 2010; approximately half of the increase occurred between 2005 and the end of 2008, and half since then. Moreover, as a means for translating a time-limited strategic plan into the sustained operation of enhanced programs, the strategy led to approval of the *Handbook on Uniform Mental Health Services in VA Medical Centers and Clinics*,[4] a policy document that specifies requirements for those services that must be available to all veterans with mental health conditions, and those that must be provided at each medical center and at very large, large, mid-sized, and small community-based outpatient clinics.

Implementation of VA's suicide prevention program was based on the principle that prevention requires ready access to high quality mental health services within the health care system, supplemented by two additional components; first, public education and awareness promoting engagement for those who need help, and second, availability of specific services addressing the needs of those at high risk. Implementation began approximately one year after the Mental Health Initiative was established, after enhancements in access and capacity for the mental health system were already moving ahead. Establishing the program included creating a national office for suicide prevention, partnering with the Substance Abuse and Mental Health Services Administration and its Lifeline to add a centrally located veterans' call center to the national 800–273-TALK crisis line and funding suicide prevention coordinators with support staff in each VA medical center and in the largest of the outpatient clinics. The crisis line has been the focus for public information campaigns that promoted use of the crisis line for veterans. Thus, it serves as a tangible symbol for the availability of VA as a source for care as well as a component of VA services. Responders in the VA crisis center can access medical records of those seeking help, and they can refer them to the suicide prevention coordinator at the closest VA medical center. The suicide prevention coordinators at each facility receive referrals from the crisis line, facilitate coordination and care of suicidal patients within the facility, and conduct outreach to providers and stakeholders in the community. Thus, VA's program includes two types of hub and spoke networks to help veterans engage in care. The national system includes the crisis center as a hub and the suicide prevention coordinators as spokes. The local systems include the suicide prevention coordinators as hubs and both VA and community providers as spokes.

Other actions included policy requirements for screening all VA patients for mental health conditions at least annually, with follow-up evaluations of the risk for suicide in those who screen positive; for identifying veterans at high risk for suicide and for ensuring that they receive enhanced care; and for using safety planning[5] as an intervention for those at high risk. Additional components of the system included two centers for research, education, and clinical innovation, and extensive evaluation activities within the office of suicide prevention and in the mental health program. Parts of the system that are still evolving include collaborations with the DoD; extensions of the crisis line to include Internet chat and texting services, a self-assessment component on the Internet, and systems for surveillance for suicide attempts.

It is important to evaluate the impact on veterans of all that has happened since the start of OEF/OIF. At this time, there are no definitive national listings of veterans across eras of service, and it is not possible to determine the annual count or rate for deaths from suicide among the entire veteran population. However, data are available for veterans who have utilized clinical services in the Veterans Health Administration (VHA), the VA's health care system (see McCarthy et al.[6] for methods). For veterans utilizing VHA services, rates and standardized mortality ratios (rates relative to age- and gender-matched people from the US population) decreased from fiscal year 2001, before the start of the war in Afghanistan, to 2008, the most recent year for which data were available as of the end of fiscal year 2011 (Figures 1 and 2). During this time, the number of veterans served per year increased from approximately 4.0 million to 5.3 million, and the number of suicides increased from 1609 to 1909. The suicide rate decreased by 9%, and the standard mortality ratio by 14%. The decrease appeared to begin in 2002 or 2003, before the VA Mental Health Strategic Plan, the Mental Health Initiative, and the implementation of VA's current program for suicide prevention. Rates and standard mortality ratios remained more or less constant since 2003, during a period of intense improvements in mental health and suicide prevention activities.

What events in 2002 or 2003 could explain the decrease in suicide rates in VHA? It is possible to develop two hypotheses, one related to specific legislation and the other to a "yellow ribbon" effect related to increases in community support. The Veterans Millennium Health Care Act (Public Law 106–117), enacted in 1999 and implemented over subsequent years, provided for increases in VHA services, including mental health services and other

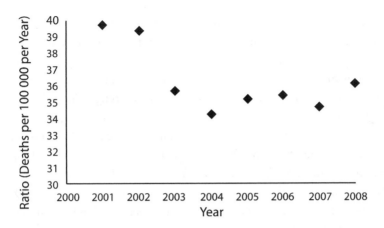

Figure 1. Suicide rates for veterans using Veterans Affairs (VA) health care relative to other age- and gender-matched Americans: 2001-2008.

benefits. However, the increases were modest relative to subsequent enhancements. Moreover, the need for the Mental Health Strategic Plan and subsequent enhancements were apparent to VA leadership through evaluations of the system after the act was implemented. Therefore, the yellow ribbon hypothesis appears to be more likely. According to this hypothesis, the

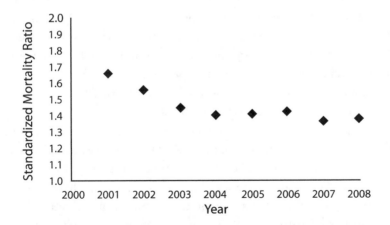

Figure 2. Standardized mortality ratios for veterans using VA health care relative to other age- and gender-matched Americans: 2001-2008.

decrease in suicide rates that began in 2002 or 2003 could be attributed to the start of the war, the way that it changed the public's view of military service and of veterans, and, probably, the way it led to changes in veterans' perceptions of the way America valued their history of service. Conceptually, this hypothesis is supported by models in which strengthening the sense of belonging to a valued community or group can protect against suicide.[7] Empirically, it is supported by observations that perceived social support (including community support) is associated with decreased suicidal ideation in National Guard Members returning from OEF/OIF.[8]

The yellow ribbon hypothesis suggests a number of secondary questions: do the increased rates of suicide in active duty personnel reflect the sum of opposing effects, a direct effect that is increasing rates, and an indirect effect mediated through increased support that is decreasing rates? Have the hypothesized yellow ribbon effects been persistent, or were they responsible for the initiation of a decline in suicide that has been sustained through other factors, such as clinical programs? What will happen at the end of the wars in Afghanistan and Iraq if there are decreases in public support for service members and veterans?

Regardless of the reasons for the decline in suicide rates, the substantial changes that occurred before the implementation of VA's mental health enhancements and its suicide prevention program complicate VA's evaluations of these programs. VA is continuing to follow rates as data from additional years become available. It is also pursuing other strategies, including evaluations of specific subpopulations and studies of the associations between regional variability in program implementation and outcomes. At the same time, it continues to enhance its suicide prevention activities.

Assuming for moment that the yellow ribbon hypothesis is valid, there may be important lessons to be drawn from the observed decrease in suicide rates. First, it may be important to reframe the discussion of the war-related increases in national concerns about the health and well-being of service members and veterans as previously summarized. In a sense, the increase in national concerns about service members and veterans may have constituted an intervention. In this context, supporting our troops and our veterans is not only a matter of patriotism; it is a matter of public health. Second, the magnitude of the yellow ribbon effects observed in veterans appears to be at least as great as the effects of large-scale and broad-based interventions in an integrated health care system. Therefore, observation from the VA during a unique era in our nation's history may provide support for the importance of public health models for suicide prevention. Key questions that remain are about how the yellow ribbon hypothesis can be tested, and, if validated, how the findings can be translated into generalizable public health interventions.

ABOUT THE AUTHOR

Ira Katz is with the University of Pennsylvania, Philadelphia, PA, and the Veterans Health Administration, Washington, DC.

ACKNOWLEDGMENTS

Analyses of suicide rates and standard mortality ratios were conducted by the VA Serious Mental Illness Treatment Resource and Evaluation Center, Ann Arbor, MI.

Note. I. Katz is an employee of the Department of Veterans Affairs The opinions expressed in this editorial are those of the author. They do not necessarily reflect policies or positions of the Department of Veterans Affairs.

REFERENCES

1. Department of Health and Human Services. National Strategy for Suicide Prevention: Goals and objectives for action. Public Health Service. Publication ID SMA01-3517, 2001. Available at: http://www.SAMHSA.gov/prevention/suicide.aspx. Accessed January 3, 2012.

2. Suicide Prevention Resource Center and Suicide Prevention Action Network USA. Charting the Future of Suicide Prevention: A 2010 Progress Review of the National Strategy and Recommendations for the Decade Ahead. Available at: http://library.sprc.org. Accessed January 3, 2012.

3. President's New Freedom Commission on Mental Health. Final Report to the President. 2003. Publication ID SMA03–3832. Available at: http://govinfo.library.unt.edu/mentalhealthcommission/reports/reports.htm. Accessed January 3, 2012.

4. Department of Veterans Affairs. Veterans Health Administration. Uniform Mental Health Services in VA Medical Centers and Clinics. Handbook 1160.01. 2008. Available at: http://www.va.gov/vhapublications/index.cfm. Accessed January 3, 2012.

5. Department of Veterans Affairs. SPRC Best Practices Registry: Section III. Adherence to Standards. Safety Plan Treatment Manual to Reduce Suicide Risk. Veterans: Veteran Version. 2011. Available at: http://www2.sprc.org/sites/sprc.org/files/SafetyPlan.pdf. Accessed January 3, 2012.

6. McCarthy JF, Valenstein M, Kim HM, Ilgen M, Zivin K, Blow FC. Suicide mortality among patients receiving care in the Veterans Health Administration health system. *Am J Epidemiol.* 2009;169:1033–1038.

7. Van Orden KA, Witte TK, Cukrowicz KC, Braithwaite SR, Selby EA, Joiner TE. The interpersonal theory of suicide. *Psychol Rev.* 2010;117:575–600.

8. Pietrzak RH, Goldstein MB, Malley JC, Rivers AJ, Johnson DC, Southwick SM. Risk and protective factors associated with suicideal ideation in veterans of Operations Enduring Freedom and Iraqi Freedom. *J Affect Disord.* 2010;123:102–107.

9

Is the Rate of Suicide Among Veterans Elevated?

Robert D. Gibbons, PhD, C. Hendricks Brown, PhD, and Kwan Hur, PhD

The article by Miller et al.[1] in this issue of the *Journal* raises new questions about Kaplan et al.'s[2] findings regarding the elevated rate of suicide among America's veterans. The original findings, which were based on data from the National Health Interview Survey (NHIS) for 1986 to 1994 and linked to the National Death Index (NDI) for 1986 to 1997 (using 12 weighted criteria: social security number, first and last names, middle initial, race, gender, marital status, birth date [day, month, and year], and state of birth and residence), found a two-fold increased risk of suicide among veterans relative to nonveterans (hazards ratio [HR] = 2.13; 95% confidence interval [CI] = 1.14, 3.99), adjusted for age, marital status, living arrangement, race, education, family income, employment status, region, time since last doctor visit, self-rated health, and body mass index. No effects were seen for other causes of death. The new study, which expanded the data acquisition period through 2000 with mortality data from the date of interview through 2006, found no increased risk of suicide among veterans when the data were adjusted for differences in age, race, and survey year (HR = 1.1; 95% CI = 0.96, 1.29). The article by Miller et al. also attempted to replicate the earlier analysis using an updated dataset and confirmed the earlier finding of a significant effect of veteran status on suicide, but of a smaller magnitude (HR = 1.33; 95% CI = 1.03, 1.71). The fully adjusted model using the expanded data yielded a somewhat marginal effect (HR = 1.18; 95% CI = 1.02, 1.36).

So what is the difference? As noted by Miller et al.,[1] Kaplan et al.[2] used a restricted-use mortality data file, whereas they used a public-use file. They were not able to reproduce the same marginals that Kaplan et al.[2] used, and the findings were not numerically identical. We attempted the same analysis as Miller et al. and found that the earlier marginal frequencies and findings were not reproducible using the current dataset. Something has clearly changed with the dataset since the time of the original study. We know of no definitive way to validate one version of this dataset over another, so we are unable to comment on the accuracy of either of these datasets. Instead, this editorial focuses on what we believe to be more extensive data that are publically available to address this question of suicide risk among veterans. It should be noted that because of the rarity of suicide, the first study that relied on NHIS interviews later linked to NDI death records from the time of interview through 1997 was based on analysis of only 508 suicides. The newer study with NDI data through 2006 had 1317 suicides, still a relatively small number. To add perspective, there were 34 598 suicides in the United States in 2007 (the most current year reported by the Centers for Disease Control and Prevention), with 26 615 among male adults aged 18 years and older. Thus, both the previous and new analyses were based on a nationally representative but still small proportion of the population.

The question of whether veterans are at increased risk of suicide remains a critical one, and as noted by the 2008 Blue Ribbon Working Group on Suicide Prevention[3] and the two studies reviewed here, the results are equivocal. In an attempt to obtain a more definitive answer, we took another route than the two previous studies and relied on the most complete enumeration available on suicides. The National Violent Death Reporting System (NVDRS),[4] provides standardized and detailed data (including veteran status—current or former military) on all violent deaths—including confirmed and uncertain suicides— for 16 states (Alaska, Colorado, Georgia, Kentucky, Maryland, Massachusetts, New Jersey, New Mexico, North Carolina, Oklahoma, Oregon, Rhode Island, South Carolina, Utah, Virginia, and Wisconsin) from 2005 to 2008. We examined cases for men aged 17 years and older, which included a total of 27 391 deaths classified as confirmed suicides. In 2005, these 16 states represented 27% of the total adult male population in the United States.[5] Among suicide victims, 24.6% were identified as current or former military ("Has the person served in the US Armed Forces?"). Note that this estimate included active military, during which time there were 854 suicides.[6] Assuming that active duty suicides are equally distributed to the NVDRS and non-NVDRS states, the estimated number of suicides in the 16 NVDRS states for current military was 0.27 854 = 231. As such, the number of suicide deaths among veterans not in active service in the NVDRS states was 6750 − 231 = 6519 or 6519 / (27 391 − 231) = 24.0% of all adult male suicide deaths, where 6750 was the total number of active and former military suicides in the 16 NVDRS states (see Table A, available as a supplement to the online version of this article at http://www.ajph.org). This estimate was slightly biased (downward) because it was adjusted for suicides among both males and females among the active military (although we would expect few suicides among females). To obtain the proportion of veterans in the population, we used data from the 2009 American Community Survey,[7] which indicated that 18.6% of the adult male US population (17 years and older) were veterans. This represented an overall risk ratio of 24.0 / 18.6 = 1.29, which was similar to the crude risk ratio of 26.2 / 18.8 = 1.39 reported by Miller et al.[1]

However, a quite different picture was seen when the data were stratified by age. Subtracting out the 231 suicides in amounts proportional to the age distribution of men in the active military[8] revealed that for the youngest group (age 17–24 years), the relative risk was 3.84, indicating that risk of suicide was almost four times higher among the youngest veterans compared with same age group among men without military service (Table 1 and Figure 1). Between the ages of 25 to 75 years, the relative risk was fairly constant at approximately 1.5 and then decreased to 1.36 for veterans aged 75 years or older; all relative risks were highly significant by conventional statistical tests. The absolute magnitude of the risk per 100 000 is presented in Table 1 and Figure 2. Unlike nonveterans, in whom the highest risk of suicide was for those older than 75 years (24 per 100 000), the youngest veterans, aged 17–24 years, had the highest risk (61 per 100 000). These data revealed that there was a strong age-by-veteran status interaction in terms of suicide, with veterans of recent military actions being at much higher relative and absolute risk of suicide than veterans of less recent wars or conflicts. These results, which were based on 16 states' data in the NVDRS, are likely representative of the entire US population because the overall percentage of veterans (men and women) in the 16 NVDRS states (10.6%) was quite similar to the entire United States (9.3%).[9]

Table 1. Number of Suicides, Populations at Risk, Rates, and Relative Risk Among Males: 16 States, National Violent Death Reporting System, 2005–2008

Age, y	No. of Suicides Among Veterans	No. of Veterans In 16 States	Veterans, Rate per 100 000 per Year	No. of Suicides Among Nonveterans	No. of Nonveterans In 16 States	Nonveterans, Rate per 100 000 per Year	Relative Risk (95% CI)
17–24	161	65 974	61.01	2827	4 442 150	15.91	3.84 (3.26, 4.51)
25–34	329	302 379	27.20	3490	4 997 418	17.46	1.56 (1.39, 1.75)
35–44	748	544 281	34.36	4068	4 804 281	21.17	1.62 (1.50, 1.76)
45–54	1186	808 175	36.69	4249	4 852 566	21.89	1.68 (1.57, 1.79)
55–64	1413	141 2933	25.00	2041	2 969 481	17.18	1.46 (1.36, 1.56)
65–74	1046	1 094 061	23.90	865	1 424 385	15.18	1.57 (1.44, 1.72)
≥ 75	1636	1 269 990	32.20	595	627 695	23.70	1.36 (1.24, 1.49)
Total	6519	5 497 793	29.64	18 135	24 117 976	18.80	1.58 (1.53, 1.62)

Note. CI = confidence interval.

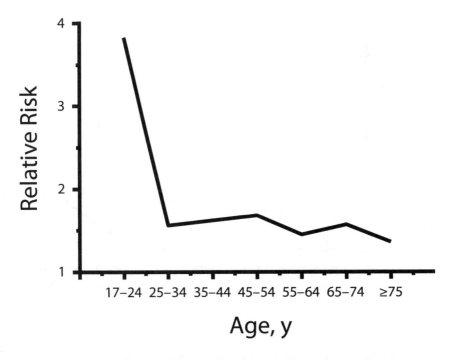

Figure 1. Relative Risk of Suicide as a Function of Veteran Status and Age.

The articles by Miller et al. and Kaplan et al.,[1,2] which yielded contradictory results, both treated age as a main effect in their statistical models (i.e., they compared the difference in suicide rates between veterans and nonveterans adjusting for the effect of age on suicide rate). The analyses that we performed revealed that age moderated the relationship between veteran status and suicide, and as a consequence, the two articles might be biased by differences between the age distributions of the two veteran cohorts. There were several plausible explanations for the clear age differences seen with veterans' risk for suicide. First, each age cohort in the military experienced unique military, medical, mental health, sociopolitical, and personal contexts that had profound effects on their lives and potentially on the rate of suicide across the life course. Second, it was also possible that the increased absolute and relative suicide risk observed in the youngest veterans had less to do with the specific conflicts in which they were engaged and more to do with factors experienced by returning military from all conflicts. It might simply be that suicide risk was highest

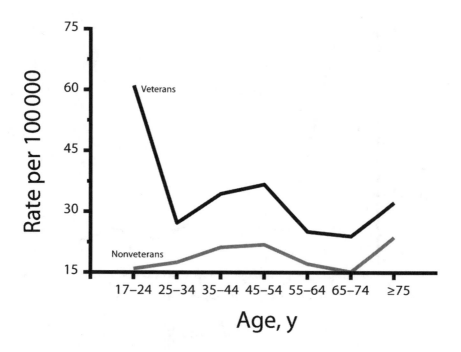

Figure 2. Suicide Rate per 100 000 in Male Veteran and Nonveterans.

directly after (or during) military service. Older veteran cohorts might have already experienced large losses because of suicide, and what we observed was a more modest residual suicide rate that was closer to that observed for nonveterans. This is a serious limitation of survey-based studies, such as the two reviewed here, in that those veterans at highest risk might have been selectively censored because they had died by suicide before the survey. Also, age was measured at the time of the survey and might have provided little information regarding the actual timing of a person's military service and the nature of that service.

Because the data we reported here did not capture lifetime history of suicide, our finding of higher suicide rates among younger veterans in recent years could not by itself distinguish between the two possibilities found in the studies we reviewed.[10] If we do take the two reported findings of the NCIS–NDI studies at face value and append our results, there was a suggestion that the elevated rate of suicides in years immediately after military service began to lessen.

ABOUT THE AUTHORS

Robert D. Gibbons is with the Departments of Medicine, Health Studies and Psychiatry, Center for Health Statistics, University of Chicago, Chicago, IL. C. Hendricks Brown is with the Prevention Science and Methodology Group, Center for Family Studies, Department of Epidemiology and Public Health, University of Miami, Miami, FL. Kwan Hur is with the Center for Medication Safety, Pharmacy Benefit Management Services, Hines VA Hospital, Hines, IL, and the Center for Health Statistics, University of Chicago, Chicago.

CONTRIBUTORS

All three authors worked on the conceptualization, analysis, writing, and revision of the editorial.

ACKNOWLEDGMENTS

This work was supported by the National Institute of Mental Health (grant MH8012201).

REFERENCES

1. Miller M, Barber C, Young M, Azrael D, Mukamal K, Lawler E. Veterans and suicide: a reexamination of the National Death Index–linked National Health Interview Survey. *Am J Public Health.* 2012;102(Suppl 1):S154–S159.

2. Kaplan MS, Huguet N, McFarland BH, Newsom JT. Suicide among male veterans: a prospective population-based study. *J Epidemiol Community Health.* 2007;61(7):619–624.

3. Department of Veterans Affairs. *Report of the Blue Ribbon Work Group on Suicide Prevention in the Veteran Population.* Washington, DC: US Department of Veterans Affairs; 2008.

4. Centers for Disease Control and Prevention. National Violent Death Reporting System (NVDRS). Available at: http://www.cdc.gov/violenceprevention/nvdrs. Accessed August 8, 2011.

5. US Census Bureau. Projections of the population by age and sex of states: 1995–2025. Available at: http://www.census.gov/population/projections/state/stpjage.txt. Accessed August 8, 2011.

6. US Department of Defense Personnel and Procurement Statistics. Military casualty information. Department of Defense. December 2011. Available at: http://siadapp.dmdc.osd.mil/personnel/CASUALTY/castop.htm. Accessed August 8, 2011.

7. US Department of Veteran Affairs, National Center for Veterans Analysis and Statistics. Profile of veterans: 2009. Data from the American Community Survey. January 2011. Available at: http://www.va.gov/vetdata/docs/SpecialReports/Profile_of_Veterans_2009_FINAL.pdf. Accessed August 8, 2011.

8. Defense Manpower Data Center. US Military active duty demographic profile. September 2008. Available at: http://www.slideshare.net/pastinson/us-military-active-duty-demographic-profile-presentation. Accessed August 8, 2011.

9. US Census Bureau. The 2011 Statistical Abstract. Veterans by sex, period of service, and state, 2008. Available at: http://www.census.gov/compendia/statab/2010/tables/10s0508.xls. Accessed August 8, 2011.

10. Nesselroad JR, Baltes PB, eds. *Longitudinal Research in the Study of Behavior and Development*. New York: Academic Press; 1979.

PART IV

On the Other Hand

10

A Call to Link Data to Answer Pressing Questions About Suicide Risk Among Veterans

Matthew Miller, MD, MPH, ScD, Deborah Azrael, PhD, Catherine Barber, MPA, Kenneth Mukamal, MD, MPH, and Elizabeth Lawler, DSc

OUR PAPER IN THE CURRENT issue of *Journal*[1] makes the case that male veterans of conflicts prior to Operation Iraqi Freedom and Operation Enduring Freedom (OIF/OEF) have an age- and race-adjusted suicide risk that is modestly, but not significantly, higher than risk among male nonveterans. Our estimate is consistent with findings from prior military cohort studies[2-6] but not with findings from Kaplan et al. 2007,[7] who, using the same underlying data set, found a statistically significant and greater than 2-fold increase in suicide risk among male veterans.

Because both our study and Kaplan's use the National Health Interview Survey-National Death Index (NHIS-NDI) linked database (and we attempted, unsuccessfully, to replicate Kaplan's findings), our study unavoidably challenges the validity of Kaplan's. Unfortunately, Robert Gibbons, PhD, declined the opportunity to adjudicate between our findings[8] and concludes that "there is no way to comment on the accuracy" of the 2 sets of results, despite his and our inability to replicate the higher risk observed by Kaplan et al. Clearly, had Gibbons requested the datasets and analytic code from both published studies, it would have been possible to ascertain whether differences in the analytic datasets, analytic strategy, or simple human error explained these differences. Because Gibbons chose not to undertake this effort, the most transparent way to resolve the issue is for the NHIS to conduct a reanalysis and report the findings. We have done so and urge Kaplan to do the same.

Instead of offering the specific findings of his own reanalysis of the current NHIS-NDI data set, Gibbons uses his editorial to explore rates of suicide among men identified by the National Violent Death Reporting System (NVDRS)[9] as current or former members of the US military. We feel obliged to respond to this new analysis, both because our long involvement with the development of NVDRS (C. B. and D. A. codirected its pilot and are familiar with its strengths and limitations) leads us to question whether the NVDRS can currently identify veterans with accuracy and because Gibbons conflates 3 important but distinct issues in his analysis: suicide risk among veterans of OIF/OEF, risk among younger veterans (irrespective of conflict), and risk among those recently separated from active military duty (irrespective of conflict and age).

NVDRS is a rich dataset, but without linking NVDRS records to Department of Defense (DOD) data to determine which decedents were truly veterans (according to the same definition used in the US veteran population estimates), findings from NVDRS are problematic when used to answer questions about suicide risk among veterans.

In short, suicide decedents categorized by NVDRS as having served in the military will correctly include current active duty personnel (which Gibbons attempts to adjust for, as we demonstrate next) but may also incorrectly include persons who never served as active duty personnel, such as decedents who, at the time of death, were current or former National Guard or Reserves but were never activated, civilians serving in the military, or people in training for the military. Because this overestimation occurs only among decedents, it leads to overestimates of risk among veterans, particularly among the youngest cohort, for whom it is also problematic to separate out recency of service from age–group related effects.

To his credit, Gibbons tries to subtract out known active duty suicides from suicides identified as ever having served. However, as exemplified by the ways in which he distributes active duty suicides across NVDRS versus non-NVDRS states (and across age strata), Gibbons makes assumptions that further bias his estimates. For example, Gibbons distributes active duty suicides evenly across NVDRS and non-NVDRS states, despite the fact that several of the states with the largest active duty populations are non-NVRDS states. The estimate of the risk of veteran suicide among the youngest age group may be further exaggerated because Gibbons distributes the military suicides according to the age distribution of military enrollment rather than according to the observed distribution of military suicides by age group (which would attribute a greater proportion of suicides, approximately half, to the youngest age stratum).[10] Mitigating this bias, to some extent, is the fact that Gibbons subtracts out all active duty suicides, including those that occured abroad, when, in fact, deaths abroad are not counted in NVDRS statistics.

Understanding the risk of suicide among recently separated veterans, especially veterans of the Iraq and Afghanistan conflicts, is of pressing concern given the unprecedented increase in rates of suicide in the active US armed forces since 2005. This issue, however, is not relevant to the discrepancies between our study and Kaplan's, both of which used (NHIS) data based on interviews that not only do not specify period of service but also took place before these wars began. Moreover, the issue cannot be resolved using unlinked NVDRS data. It can be answered, however, if data routinely collected by the DOD are linked to NVDRS data or to the NDI. Indeed, Kang and Bullman[2,4–6] have published first-rate analyses along these lines on select populations of veterans. Following their lead, data from the DOD, the NDI, and the NVDRS could readily be linked not only retrospectively (DOD, NDI), allowing resolution of the historical issue of suicide risk among veterans remote from military service but also prospectively (DOD, NDI, NVDRS, and possibly VHA), thus providing an ongoing surveillance system that would enable policymakers and health care providers to make decisions aimed at saving lives based on unbiased risk assessment.

ABOUT THE AUTHORS

Matthew Miller, Deborah Azrael, and Catherine Barber are with the Harvard Injury Control Research Center, Harvard School of Public Health, Boston, MA. Kenneth Mukamal is with the Department of Medicine, Beth Israel Deaconess Medical Center, Boston. Elizabeth Lawler is with the Massachusetts Veterans Epidemiology Research and Information Center, VA Cooperative Studies Program, VA Boston Healthcare System, Boston, and the Division of Aging, Brigham and Women's Hospital, Harvard Medical School, Boston.

CONTRIBUTORS

M. Miller wrote the initial draft of this study. All coauthors provided critical editorial and substantive feedback as well as original and ongoing interpretation of the data presented.

ACKNOWLEDGMENTS

This material and the effort by E. Lawlor is based upon work supported by the Department of Veterans Affairs, Veterans Health Administration, Office of Research and Development, VA Clinical Science Research and Development Service. This material is also the result of work supported with resources and the use of facilities at the VA Boston Healthcare System, Boston MA and the resources of the VA Cooperative Studies Program. Funding for M. Miller, D. Azrael, and C. Barber was provided, in part, by the Joyce and Bohnett foundations.

REFERENCES

1. Miller M, Barber C, Young M, Mukamal K, Lawler L. Veterans and suicide: a reexamination of the National Death Index–linked National Health Interview Survey. *Am J Public Health.* 2012;102(Suppl 1):S154–S159.

2. Kang HK, Bullman TA. Mortality among US veterans of the Persian Gulf War. *N Engl J Med.* 996;335(20):1498–1504.

3. Watanabe KK, Kang HK. Military service in Vietnam and the risk of death from trauma and selected cancers. *Ann Epidemiol.* 1995;5(5):407–412.

4. Kang HK, Bullman TA. Risk of suicide among US veterans after returning from the Iraq or Afghanistan war zones. *JAMA.* 2008;300(6):652–653.

5. Kang HK, Bullman TA. Mortality among US veterans of the Persian Gulf War: 7-year follow-up. *Am J Epidemiol.* 2001;154(5):399–405.

6. Kang HK, Bullman TA. Is there an epidemic of suicides among current and former US military personnel? *Ann Epidemiol.* 2009;19(10):757–760.

7. Kaplan MS, Huguet N, McFarland BH, Newsom JT. Suicide among male veterans: a prospective population-based study. *J Epidemiol Community Health.* 2007;61(7):619–624.

8. Gibbons RD, Brown CH, Hur K. Is the rate of suicide among veterans elevated? *Am J Public Health.* 2012;102(Suppl 1):S17–S19.

9. Centers for Disease Control and Prevention. National Violent Death Reporting System. Last updated July 13, 2011. Available at: http://www.cdc.gov/violenceprevention/nvdrs. Accessed January 5, 2012.

10. Kinn JT, Luxton DD, Reger MA, Gahm GA, Skopp NA, Bush NE. *DoDSER: Department of Defense Suicide Event Reporting: Calendar Year 2010 Annual Report.* Washington, DC: National Center for Telehealth and Technology; 2011. Available at: http://t2health.org/sites/default/files/dodser/DoDSER_2010_Annual_Report.pdf. Accessed January 5, 2012.

11

Estimating the Risk of Suicide Among US Veterans: How Should We Proceed From Here?

Mark S. Kaplan, DrPH, Bentson H. McFarland, MD, PhD, Nathalie Huguet, PhD, and Jason T. Newsom, PhD

SUICIDE IS A MAJOR PUBLIC health problem. In 2008, suicide ranked as the 10th leading cause of death and claimed more than 33 000 American lives, according to the Centers for Disease Control and Prevention. There are important differences in suicide rates across population subgroups. For example, military veterans account for only 10% of US adults,[1] but completed about 20% of suicides in 2008.[2] According to the Department of Veterans Affairs (VA) Office of the Inspector General,[3] 1000 veterans who receive care from the VA and as many as 5000 of all veterans die by suicide every year.

In a groundbreaking prospective study involving data from the 1986 to 1994 National Health Interview Surveys (NHIS) linked to the 1986 to 1997 National Death Index (NDI), Kaplan et al.[4] showed that men who served in the military were twice as likely as were nonveterans to complete suicide even after adjustment for numerous established suicide risk factors. A key feature of the Kaplan et al.[4] analysis was its treatment of competing risks of death from causes other than suicide. There was no evidence that veterans had elevated death rates that were because of natural causes or accidents. In a follow-up analysis of data from the National Violent Death Reporting System (NVDRS), McFarland et al.[5] showed that suicide risk was 3 times greater among former military women aged 18 to 34 years than among women who had never served.

In addition, McCarthy et al.[6] found that male (43 of 100 000) and female (10 of 100 000) VA patients had higher crude suicide rates than did nonveteran men (23 of 100 000) and women (5 of 100 000).

However, some studies have found no connection between military service and suicide.[7,8] Findings may vary because analyses of the risk of suicide among veterans have differed in statistical methods (e.g., standardized mortality ratio versus relative risk), inclusion of confounders, representativeness of the samples, and military branch or exposure to combat.[9] Moreover, nearly all survival analyses used the date of a particular survey as the time of origin, a far less precise measure than discharge date. Using expanded linked NHIS–NDI data to include a longer follow-up period, Miller et al.[10] found that veterans were not at a significantly higher risk of suicide than were nonveterans in the general population after adjusting for a limited number of covariates (race, age, and survey years). The longer follow-up appears to weaken the relative risk of suicide because a reanalysis using a shorter period shows that veterans have a significantly higher suicide hazard than do nonveterans.[10] Gibbons et al.[11] confirmed this finding and suggested that the discrepancy may be partially explained by age differences possibly associated with variation in service era and exposure to combat. Thus, more needs to be learned about aspects of service that may put veterans at a higher risk of suicide.

Indeed, numerous issues have complicated studies of suicides among veterans, and, thus, existing estimates of suicide risk among veterans are likely to be only rough approximations of actual risk. As noted in the 2008 report of the Blue Ribbon Work Group on Suicide Prevention in the Veteran Population, there may be misclassification in ascertainment of veteran status on death records, deceased veterans as compared with nonveteran decedents may be more likely to be correctly classified as suicides, and analyses may improperly adjust for demographics. Furthermore, it is important to appreciate that military service has been highly selective since the end of conscription in 1973, which may lead to a "healthy warrior" effect.[9,10] This type of selection implies that veterans' suicide rates (with all else being equal) would be expected to be lower than those of the general population. In other words, it may be difficult to find groups within the general population who would be appropriate comparisons to veterans.

One speculation has been that misclassification may account for elevated suicide risk among veterans, but recent work suggests this possibility is unlikely.[12]

Gibbons et al.[11] and Kaplan et al.[12] used the NVDRS to assess the risk of suicide among veterans of different age groups. The studies found similar, but not identical, risk estimates using 2 different analytic approaches to adjust for the problematic ascertainment of veteran status on death certificates. Gibbons et al.[11] adjusted the suicide count down by the proportion of men who were on active duty. Kaplan et al.[13] used a more conservative approach, adjusting the veteran suicide rate with a broader estimate of the military population, including those who were veterans, on active duty, in the reserves, or in the National Guard. Regardless of the adjustment approach, both studies showed that veterans, especially younger men, were at a significantly higher risk of suicide than were nonveterans. And, in a supplementary analysis, Kaplan et al.,[13] with data from the National Mortality Followback Survey, showed that relatively few decedents (10% or less) who were identified as veterans on death certificates were on active duty at the time of their deaths. Nonetheless, as the Blue Ribbon Work Group noted, there remains a need for a "consistent approach to describing the rates of suicide and suicide attempts in veterans."

How should we proceed from here? First, it is crucial to recognize the importance of suicide among veterans. In the *Army Health Promotion, Risk Reduction and Suicide Prevention Report 2010*, General Peter Chiarelli (the Vice Chief of Staff of the US Army) explained: "These are not just statistics; they are our Soldiers." Second, we need to understand that this concern is not restricted to persons within the VA because most veterans do not use VA health or mental health care facilities. Consequently, studies that focus on people in the general population rather than rely on VA clinical samples are key. Third, improved study design and data collection can facilitate the development and evaluation of public health programs that are designed to improve the lives of those who have served. Finally, although the data are imperfect, the evidence concerning higher-than-expected suicide rates in the veteran population is undeniable. We urge policymakers and clinicians to remain ever vigilant for suicide among men and women with military service. To quote Martha Bruce, "any suicide is an unnecessary tragedy."[9]

ABOUT THE AUTHORS

Mark S. Kaplan is with the School of Community Health, Portland State University, Portland, OR. Bentson H. McFarland is with the Department of

Psychiatry, Oregon Health and Science University, Portland. Nathalie Huguet is with the Center for Public Health Studies, Portland State University, Portland. Jason T. Newsom is with the Institute on Aging, Portland State University, Portland.

CONTRIBUTORS

All the authors participated in the conceptualization and writing of the column and approved the final version.

REFERENCES

1. US Census Bureau. American Community Survey, 2008. Available at: http://factfinder.census.gov. Accessed December 05, 2011.

2. Sundararaman R, Panangala SV, Lister SA. Suicide prevention among veterans. CRS Report for Congress, 2008. Available at: http://www.fas.org/sgp/crs/misc/RL34471.pdf. Accessed December 05, 2011.

3. Department of Veterans Affairs Office of Inspector General. *Healthcare Inspection: Implementing VHA's Mental Health Strategic Plan Initiatives for Suicide Prevention.* Washington, DC: VA Office of Inspector General; 2007.

4. Kaplan MS, Huguet N, McFarland BH, Newsom JT. Suicide among male veterans: a prospective population-based study. *J Epidemiol Community Health.* 2007;61:619–624.

5. McFarland BH, Kaplan MS, Huguet N. Self-inflicted deaths among women with US military service: a hidden epidemic? *Psychiatr Serv.* 2010;61:1177.

6. McCarthy JF, Valenstein M, Kim HM, et al. Suicide mortality among patients receiving care in the Veterans Health Administration Health System. *Am J Epidemiol.* 2009;169:1033–1038.

7. Kang HK, Bullman TA. Is there an epidemic of suicides among current and former US military personnel? *Ann Epidemiol.* 2009;19:757–760.

8. Miller M, Barber C, Azrael D, et al. Suicide among US veterans: a prospective study of 500,000 middle-aged and elderly men. *Am J Epidemiol.* 2009;170:494–500.

9. Bruce ML. Suicide risk and prevention in veteran populations. *Ann N Y Acad Sci.* 2010;1208:98–103.

10. Miller M, Barber C, Young M, Azrael D, Mukamal K, Lawler E. Veterans and suicide: a reexamination of the National Death Index–linked National Health Interview Survey. *Am J Public Health.* 2012;102(Suppl 1):S154–S159.

11. Gibbons RD, Brown CH, Hur K. Is the rate of suicide among veterans elevated? *Am J Public Health.* 2012;102(Suppl 1):S17–S19.

12. Kaplan MS, Huguet N, McFarland BH. The effects of misclassification biases on veteran suicide rate estimate. Paper presented at: American Public Health Association 139th Annual Meeting and Exposition; October 29–November 2, 2011; Washington, DC.

13. Kaplan MS, McFarland BH, Huguet N, Valenstein M. Suicide risk and precipitating circumstances among young, middle-aged, and older male veterans. *Am J Public Health.* 2011;102(Suppl 1):S131–S137.

PART V
Commentaries

12

Addressing the Surveillance Goal in the National Strategy for Suicide Prevention: The Department of Defense Suicide Event Report

Gregory A. Gahm, PhD, Mark A. Reger, PhD, Julie T. Kinn, PhD, David D. Luxton, PhD, Nancy A. Skopp, PhD, and Nigel E. Bush, PhD

The US National Strategy for Suicide Prevention (National Strategy) described 11 goals across multiple areas, including suicide surveillance. Consistent with these goals, the Department of Defense (DoD) has engaged aggressively in the area of suicide surveillance.

The DoD's population-based surveillance system, the DoD Suicide Event Report (DoDSER) collects information on suicides and suicide attempts for all branches of the military. Data collected includes suicide event details, treatment history, military and psychosocial history, and psychosocial stressors at the time of the event.

Lessons learned from the DoDSER program are shared to assist other public health professionals working to address the National Strategy objectives.

THE US NATIONAL STRATEGY for Suicide Prevention[1] (National Strategy) provided a framework for action in the United States. This "roadmap" directed a coordinated approach to suicide prevention for both public and private sectors that has guided efforts to modify attitudes, policies, and services. The National Strategy was published in 2001 and included 11 goals in areas that range from developing broad-based support for suicide prevention to improving entertainment and news media portrayals of suicidal behavior.

Goal 11 was "Improve and Expand Surveillance Systems" and was the focus of this article.

Since the release of the National Strategy, the military has experienced a rising suicide rate,[2] and Department of Defense (DoD) leaders have dedicated significant effort toward improving all areas of the suicide prevention mission, including surveillance approaches.[3] The DoD surveillance program provides an example of one approach to addressing surveillance challenges related to suicide. The purpose of this article was to review the DoD's suicide surveillance program, the DoD Suicide Event Report (DoDSER), and suggest how this effort can inform broader public health initiatives seeking to address some of the surveillance concerns detailed in the National Strategy.

DOD SUICIDE EVENT REPORT

Historically, the military services (Air Force, Army, Navy, Marine Corps) collected suicide surveillance data through separate systems. Each system had its own strengths and limitations. Aggregated DoD-level analyses were not possible because the same data points were not collected with standardized items. In addition, it was not possible to compare the services' data.

The DoD identified a standardized suicide surveillance system as a key goal. In the first phase of development, a collaborative plan was developed to synchronize surveillance efforts across services while also seeking to maintain flexibility to address service-specific needs. The general requirements included a web-based data management application, analytic reporting features, and standardized data collection items. The data collection process was developed to build on processes the services had used previously. The Army's surveillance software was optimized to meet the needs for the DoDSER application. Barriers and facilitators of success are described in the section on "Lessons for Other Public Health Initiatives."

Data Collection

The ultimate objective of the DoDSER program is to provide data that can help refine suicide prevention approaches and ultimately prevent suicides. To accomplish this, the military services ask designated professionals to collect standardized records after suicides and other suicide behaviors, review the records for information related to the DoDSER items, and submit the information via the secure online web application (Figure 1). DoDSERs are submitted for suicides as determined by the Armed Forces Medical Examiner System, and for suicide attempts that result in a hospitalization or evacuation from a combat theater; suicide attempts are defined by the Centers for Disease Control and Prevention (CDC) Self Directed Violence Classification System. Data collected includes detailed demographics, suicide event details, treatment history, military and psychosocial history, and information about other potential risk factors, such as psychosocial stressors at the time of the event. The comprehensive nature of the DoDSER can be seen in the summary of the DoDSER items in Table 1. The items are reviewed annually in collaboration with the services and updated on January 1 of each year. Additional details about the development and implementation of the DoDSER system and data collection process have been reported elsewhere.[4]

The following section reviews the National Strategy's assessment of the status of suicide surveillance in the United States. We then describe some of the National Strategy surveillance objectives and how the DoDSER program attempts to address some of the concerns for the DoD.

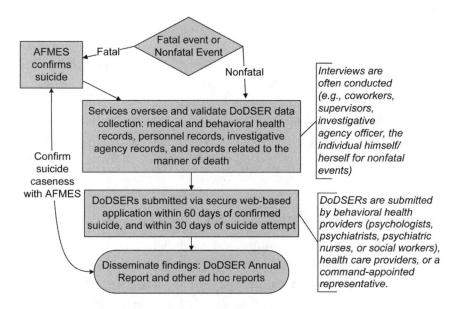

Figure 1. Department of Defense Suicide Event Report (DoDSER) process flowchart.

Note. AFMES = Armed Forces Medical Examiner System.

SUICIDE SURVEILLANCE CHALLENGES AND OBJECTIVES IN THE NATIONAL STRATEGY

The National Strategy defined surveillance as "the ongoing, systematic collection, analysis and interpretation of health data with timely dissemination of findings."[1(p204)] Quality surveillance data can be used to "track trends in rates, to identify new problems, to provide evidence to support activities and initiatives, to identify risk and protective factors, to target high risk populations for interventions, and to assess the impact of prevention efforts."[1(p117)]

The National Strategy provided a brief review of the status of suicide surveillance at the time of its writing and noted numerous concerns. For instance, there were significant limitations noted for the use of death certificates for surveillance purposes. Death certificates had misclassifications of deaths and suicides, a limited amount of information included, and missing information. Suicide prevention efforts would be improved by the availability of more comprehensive and systematically collected information.

Problems associated with existing sources of information on suicide attempts (e.g., trauma registries and uniform hospital discharge datasets) were also documented. Most of the problems with these data sources resulted from the fact that they were designed for other purposes. Therefore, the resulting data had problems, such as incomplete case capture or incomplete information about the circumstances surrounding the suicide attempt. In addition, systems utilized different definitions for a "suicide attempt" and other self-harm behaviors, therefore creating problems with standardization, comparison, and synthesis of data.

Based on these problems, several objectives were set related to suicide surveillance. The following section provides an overview of the objectives and how DoDSER addressed some of the concerns for the DoD.

National Strategy Objectives and the DoDSER

Enhance the quality and quantity of data available.
Overall, the surveillance goals were "designed to enhance the quality and quantity of data available at the national, state, and local levels on suicide and attempted suicide and ensure that the data are useful for prevention purposes."[1(p120)] To that end, the National Strategy aimed to increase the routine collection of information for follow-back studies on suicides. Follow-

back studies include data such as information about the decedent, event details, and antecedents of the suicide, which are collected from several sources, such as a review of records and personal interviews. To address the need for more comprehensive suicide data, the National Strategy promoted the development of a national reporting system that would supplement death certificate data with other sources of information, such as medical examiner and law enforcement records.

The DoDSER system was developed to improve the quality and quantity of data available for the DoD. As described previously, the DoDSER collects comprehensive information, including event details and antecedents from a variety of records and personal interviews. In response to the challenge to provide useful data for both national and local needs, the DoDSER software was developed to provide user-defined reports. Individuals with local or "national" (service or DoD-wide) responsibilities can select DoDSER variables of interest and generate numeric and graphical outputs to support suicide prevention needs related to their region of responsibility.

Increase the number of hospitals that collect information about self-harm behaviors.

The National Strategy noted that hospital data on suicide behaviors could provide an extremely valuable tool for suicide research and surveillance. The National Strategy focused on the use of external cause of injury codes from the *International Classification of Diseases, Tenth Revision*[5] *(ICD-10)*, as a mechanism to obtain additional hospital data on suicides and self-inflicted injuries.

The DoDSER system was launched in 2008 and initially required data collection for only suicides. In 2010, however, the requirement expanded to include suicide attempts that "require hospitalization or evacuation from the wartime theater."[6] Some services exceeded this standard and collected DoDSER data on other self-harm behaviors. Typically, the individual collecting the data coordinates closely with (or works on) an inpatient psychiatric ward. All of the applicable items described in the box on this page are collected for suicide attempts consistent with the National Strategy's intent of expanding surveillance capabilities for suicide attempts requiring hospitalization.

List of variables included in the 2010 DoDSER

Event Information
Event type
Suicide (suicide, suicide attempt,
   self harm, suicidal ideation)
Event date
Event time

Patient Information
Name
Social security number
Date of birth
Sex
Racial category
Specific ethnic group
Current marital status
Education
Religious preference
Residence
Resided alone
Have minor children
Involved in community support

Military Information
Component/Military status
Primary job code
Working in primary job code
Duty status
Pay grade
Permanent duty station
Permanent duty assignment
Unit identification code
Date of entry into the military
Date of rank
Assigned to warrior transition unit
Length of time in unit
Geographic location of event
Setting

Event Information
Hospitalization (inpatient outpatient
mental health evaluation/treatment
evacuation)
Primary method used
Alcohol used during the event
Drugs used during the event
Intended to die

Self-inflicted injuries
Death-risk gambling
Planned/premeditated
Observed and intervened
Suicide note
Communicated self harm
Primary motivation for suicidal
   behavior for suicide behavior
Duty environment /status
Sequence of events

Medical History
Seen in medical treatment facility
Utilized substance abuse services
Utilized family advocacy program
Utilized chaplain services
Utilized outpatient behavioral
   health Utilized inpatient
   behavioral health
History of traumatic brain injury
List psychiatric diagnoses
List psychotropic medications
Prior self injurious events
Received suicide prevention trainings
Elaborate on treatment history

Military History
Court martial proceedings
Article 15
Administrative separation proceed-
ings
AWOL/Unexcused absence
Medical evaluation board
Civil legal problems
Non-selection for advanced schooling,
   promotion, or Command
Elaborate on life stressors

Deployment History
How many deployments
Deployment location (most recent
   last 3)
Start dates
End dates
Rest & Recuperation Dates
Obtained a waiver to deploy

Experienced direct combat
Had orders to deploy
Suicide event related to deployment
Describe additional relevant info

Personal History
Victim of
Physical abuse or assault
Sexual abuse or assault
Emotional abuse or assault
Sexual harassment
Perpetrator of
Physical abuse or assault
Sexual abuse or assault
Emotional abuse or assault
Sexual harassment
Life Stressors
Childhood/developmental History
History of
Failed intimate relationship
Failed relationship other
Spousal suicide
Family suicide
Suicide by friend
Death of spouse or family member
Death of friend
Physical health problem
Chronic spousal or family severe
   illness
Excessive debt or bankruptcy
Job problems
Supervisor or coworker issues
Poor work performance review or
   evaluation
Unit or workplace hazing
Family history of mental illness
Gun in home or immediate
   environment
Elaborate on additional details

Provider Information
Respondent's qualifications and
contact information

Increase the use of annual reports on suicide and suicide attempts.

The National Strategy aimed to increase the number of states that produced an annual report that described the magnitude of the problem. It argued that annual reports would help track trends, identify new problems, and prioritize prevention refinements.

The DoD's National Center for Telehealth and Technology (T2) led the effort to develop the DoDSER program and is required to produce a comprehensive annual report.[6] At the time of this writing, three annual reports have been completed and released publically as a resource for the public health community (available at http://www.t2health.org).

Increase knowledge about suicide behaviors in the population.

Obtaining population-based estimates of even the basic frequency of suicide attempts is extremely challenging. The National Strategy sought to increase the number of nationally representative surveys that include items about suicide behaviors to help fill this gap.

The DoDSER program has not attempted to conduct a national survey, but a small proof-of-concept study to collect DoDSER control data, including history of previous self-harm behaviors, was conducted. In the initial phase, soldiers were randomly selected from a large Army installation to conduct a DoDSER interview and provide permission to review their records. The business process was refined, and a second iteration was initiated at the time of this writing. Successful collection of DoDSER control data would provide an extremely valuable resource for analyzing suicide risk factors.

Conduct pilot projects that link data from separate systems.

Linking datasets from separate surveillance systems can increase valuable analytic options exponentially. The National Strategy acknowledged the administrative and privacy barriers posed by this objective and also recommended potential solutions, such as probabilistic matching procedures.

The DoDSER is similar to the CDC National Violent Death Reporting System (NVDRS). Both systems use some similar data sources and seek to provide more comprehensive information about suicides than is typically contained in death certificates. The NVDRS eventually hopes to provide national representation, and it is now operational in 18 states. T2 is currently collaborating with the CDC to conduct probabilistic matching studies of the

DoDSER and NVDRS data to examine how the systems may inform one another. Early results support the value of such approaches.

LESSONS FOR OTHER PUBLIC HEALTH INITIATIVES

Internal and external reviews of the DoDSER program identified a number of strengths and growth opportunities. In its short history since 2008, the program has undergone systematic reviews by the Congressionally mandated DoD Suicide Prevention Task Force,[3] the RAND Corporation review of the DoD's suicide prevention program,[7] and others. In general, these reports praised the DoDSER program as an important advancement in the DoD, and all offered helpful recommendations. The DoDSER system has undergone continuous quality improvement based on these reviews and other DoD experiences with the system. The following section describes some of the primary lessons learned. This information is intended to assist other public health professionals seeking to implement surveillance programs that are consistent with the National Strategy.

Collaborative Partnerships Are Key to the Implementation Phase

Implementation of a new population-based surveillance program is daunting. Challenges range from resourcing, to privacy requirements, to policy needs. Numerous stakeholders and complex business processes must be addressed appropriately. The success of the implementation phase of the DoDSER program was due in large part to a unique collaborative team that shared a vision for what was needed. Each of the services' suicide prevention program managers played a key role in consensus decisions that focused on the primary needs of the services while demonstrating flexibility on secondary issues. Assistance was provided by the corresponding privacy office and by DoD policymakers and leadership. Significant concerns by any one of a number of groups could have hindered or halted the development of the DoDSER program. Building consensus among key stakeholders early in the implementation phase is critical to success.

Prioritize Resources for Information Management/Information Technology Requirements

An active population-based surveillance system (e.g., one that does not simply rely on existing administrative data) requires a data collection methodology involving numerous individuals over a huge geographic area. Before the development of the DoDSER, several of the military services attempted surveillance procedures without a software tool. All of these efforts proved very challenging, and some failed. For the DoDSER program, a web application provides a key data collection solution for the worldwide surveillance mission; DoDSERs are submitted from Europe, Iraq, Afghanistan, and other locations around the world. The software also serves as a platform to provide users other resources. The skills required for software development, frequent software refinements, and database management suggests that information management and information technology expertise should not be underestimated.

Standardization of an Active Surveillance System Is Challenging

The most common DoDSER recommendation from the systematic reviews of the DoD's suicide prevention program was to improve standardization. Formal research can often create carefully controlled, standardized data collection procedures, but operational surveillance programs face additional challenges and must make multiple tradeoffs. To help improve standardization, the DoDSER program recently added a multimedia training module to the web application, refined the coding manual, and piloted a standardized nomenclature shared by the DoD, Department of Veterans Affairs, and CDC. Identifying feasible approaches to ensure high quality data must be a top priority for any surveillance program.

Weigh the Advantages and Disadvantages of Using Existing Systems and Personnel

The DoDSER system leverages existing DoD personnel to perform data collection responsibilities. This approach has major advantages. The program is extremely cost effective since the use of dedicated personnel to conduct interviews and analyze records would require a major investment. In addition, the current solution permitted the DoD to launch the program several years ahead of other models that would have required staffing solutions. The disadvantages are primarily associated with the fact that DoDSER data collection is an "extra duty." Behavioral health providers, for example, sometimes manage heavy case loads and manage multiple priorities. The services' DoDSER program managers must frequently contact providers to emphasize the importance of timely, accurate data submission. These limitations can be mitigated by requesting feedback from personnel, ensuring the data have local value, and working to obtain and maintain "buy in." Cooperation can be increased when data collectors know how the data are used, or better yet, can access and use the data themselves.

Plan to Educate Consumers of the Data

As described previously, one of the primary surveillance goals of the National Strategy was to address the need for more comprehensive data. When reporting surveillance data, it is always important to educate those using the data about the limitations and interpretive considerations inherent in the data. In a comprehensive system where some data are highly objective and reliable and other data are more subjective, the challenge is amplified. The DoDSER system represents a reasonable approach to collecting information about a topic that is extremely difficult to study, with a strong emphasis on carefully educating consumers of the data.

Intense Administrative Challenges Are Worth the Effort

The experience with the DoDSER data supports the National Strategy priorities; surveillance data are extremely valuable and the challenges are "worth it." DoDSER data has been used extensively to try to improve suicide prevention in the DoD. For example, the DoD Suicide Prevention Task Force Report cited DoDSER data to support numerous recommendations that will reshape the suicide prevention programs in the DoD. In addition, the National Institute of Mental Health and the Army are partnering to conduct the Army Study to Assess Risk and Resilience in Service Members (Army STARRS), the largest suicide study ever conducted in the military. The DoDSER data are serving as one of their most important datasets for their retrospective study. Furthermore, the DoDSER data are used routinely to support senior leaders' decisions, as well as the efforts of the services' Suicide Prevention Programs.

CONCLUSION

The National Strategy's surveillance goal aimed to increase the quality and quantity of suicide surveillance data. The DoD worked rapidly in recent years to launch a surveillance program that was consistent with many of the

National Strategy's objectives. The lessons learned from this initiative might be useful to other public health initiatives, as well as to leaders who are reviewing and revising the National Strategy for the future.

ABOUT THE AUTHORS

The authors are with the National Center for Telehealth and Technology (T2), Tacoma, WA.

CONTRIBUTORS

All of the authors contributed to the development and refinement of the DoDSER program. All authors contributed to the conceptualization of the paper. G. A. Gahm and M. A. Reger led the writing of the article. All authors provided critical reviews.

ACKNOWLEDGMENTS

Many individuals and organizations facilitated the development and implementation of the DoDSER program. We are grateful to the services' behavioral health providers and Command appointed representatives who collect and verify suicide event data and later complete DoDSERs. We also thank the services' Suicide Prevention Program Managers (SPPMs) and DoDSER Program Managers who oversee the DoDSER data collection process to ensure data integrity and program compliance. In particular, Major Michael McCarthy (Air Force SPPM), Amy Millikan (Manager, Behavioral and Social Health Outcomes Program), Walter Morales (Army SPPM), John Wills (Army DoDSER Program Manager), Lieutenant Commander Andrew Martin (Marine Corps SPPM), and Lieutenant Commander Bonnie Chavez (Navy SPPM) are integral to DoDSER program success. We are also indebted to Lynne Oetjen-Gerdes and Captain Joyce Cantrell, MD, MPH, of the Mortality Surveillance Division of the Armed Forces Medical Examiner System for their support of the DoDSER program.

REFERENCES

1. National Strategy for Suicide Prevention. *Goals and Objectives for Action. Center for Mental Health Services (US); Office of the Surgeon General (US).* Rockville, MD: US Public Health Service; 2001.

2. Kuehn BM. Soldier suicide rates continue to rise: military, scientists work to stem the tide. *JAMA.* 2009;301(11):1111–1113. doi:10.1001/jama.2009.342

3. The Challenge and the Promise: Strengthening the Force, Preventing Suicide and Saving Lives: Final Report of the Department of Defense Task Force on the Prevention of Suicide by Members of the Armed Forces. Available at: http://www.health.mil/dhb/downloads/Suicide%20Prevention%20Task%20Force%20final%20report%208-23-10.pdf. Accessed April 19, 2011.

4. Luxton DD, Skopp NA, Kinn JT, et al. DoD Suicide Event Report: Calendar Year 2009 Annual Report. National Center for Telehealth & Technology, 1–198. 2010. Available at: http://t2health.org/programs/dodser. Accessed November 27, 2011.

5. *International Classification of Diseases, 10th Revision.* Geneva, Switzerland: World Health Organization; 1980.

6. Deputy Under Secretary of Defense (Plans), Performing the Duties of the Under Secretary of Defense (Personnel and Readiness) Memorandum, "Standardized Reporting of Department of Defense Suicides and Department of Defense Suicide Event Report," October 14, 2009.

7. Ramchand R, Acosta J, Burns RM, Jaycox LH, Pernin CG. *The War Within: Preventing Suicide in the U.S. Military.* Monograph. Santa Monica, CA: Rand Corporation, 2011.

13

Using Science to Improve Communications About Suicide Among Military and Veteran Populations: Looking for a Few Good Messages

Linda Langford, ScD, David Litts, OD, and Jane L. Pearson, PhD

Concern about suicide in US military and veteran populations has prompted efforts to identify more effective prevention measures.

Recent expert panel reports have recommended public communications as one component of a comprehensive effort. Messaging about military and veteran suicide originates from many sources and often does not support suicide prevention goals or adhere to principles for developing effective communications.

There is an urgent need for strategic, science-based, consistent messaging guidance in this area. Although literature on the effectiveness of suicide prevention communications for these populations is lacking, this article summarizes key findings from several bodies of research that offer lessons for creating safe and effective messages that support and enhance military and veteran suicide prevention efforts.

FROM 2006 TO 2010, THERE were more than 1300 suicide deaths among members of the United States military, with increasing rates in the Marines and Army.[1,2] Some studies also suggest that suicide rates are higher among veterans than among the general population, although findings are mixed.[3,4] In response, various expert panels have conducted reviews and released reports with recommendations for strengthening suicide prevention efforts among military and veteran populations.[1,5,6] Citing the multifactorial causality of suicidal behavior and the evidence that comprehensive interventions can successfully reduce suicide,[7,8] these reports advocate for multiple, coordinated interventions to reduce risk, promote protective factors, and enhance overall wellness, skills, and resiliency.

Each of these reports emphasizes the importance of public communications (i.e., messaging). For example, two of the 18 recommendations issued in the 2010 report of the Department of Defense (DoD) Task Force on the Prevention of Suicide by Members of the Armed Forces include messaging components: "develop strategic communications that promote life, normalize help-seeking behaviors, and support DoD suicide prevention strategies" and "reduce stigma and overcome military and cultural leadership barriers to seeking help."[1] Similarly, one of the eight findings outlined in the 2008 report of the US Department of Veterans Affairs (VA) Blue Ribbon Work Group on Suicide Prevention in the Veteran Population is as follows: "The VA should continue to pursue opportunities for outreach to enrolled and eligible veterans, and to disseminate messages to reduce risk behavior associated with suicidality."[6]

These reports also describe deficiencies in communications efforts. The DoD report revealed that messaging often fails to promote effective solutions and may contribute to the problem:

> Messages from senior leaders regarding suicide, suicide prevention, resilience, health, and readiness frequently do not sufficiently support— and sometimes significantly detract from—suicide prevention efforts. The news media commonly report on suicide in ways that contribute to suicide risk.[1]

Specific problems include using talking points that suggest military suicides are more common than they actually are, that reflect a sense of hopelessness about solutions, and that miss opportunities to promote positive prevention messages.

According to the VA report, "Efforts to improve accurate media coverage and disseminate universal messages to shift normative behaviors to reduce population suicide risk behavior are not being fully pursued."[6] Specifically, the authors noted that media coverage may unintentionally discourage veterans from seeking services. Although little research has analyzed this message content systematically, one study in which newspaper reports on military and civilian suicide deaths were compared showed that articles about military or veteran suicides were more likely to mention failed psychological treatment.[9]

Importantly, the DoD and VA create only a small proportion of messages disseminated about military and veteran suicide. The news media are important message sources. Communications are created by each service, suicide prevention coordinators, and other veteran- and military-related organizations. Still other materials and messages are conveyed by civilian entities operating at multiple levels.

Given this landscape, there is a need for dissemination of research-based messaging guidance that all stakeholders can use to improve military and veteran suicide communications. Although research on message effectiveness for these audiences is lacking, a robust science base exists that can inform these efforts. We provide an overview of findings from four areas of research that can guide messaging efforts: suicide-related and mental health–related campaigns, effective health communications, mental illness stigma, and safe messaging for suicide prevention.

SUICIDE- AND MENTAL HEALTH–RELATED CAMPAIGNS

Evaluations of mental health–related and suicide-related awareness and information campaigns are relatively rare and generally methodologically weak. Reviews indicate that some campaigns achieve short-term improvements in knowledge and attitudes but show limited behavioral changes when used alone.[10–12] Better results occur when media are combined with other programs.[10,13,14] For example, implementation of a four-level intervention that combined media with training and service components was associated with reductions in suicide in two German cities.[15]

Greater success also is associated with repeated exposure to messages through multiple types of media and with locally organized efforts that tailor messages to homogeneous populations.[10] Dumesnil and Verger noted that some campaigns are too ambitious, targeting entire populations, addressing many types of disorders, and pursuing numerous objectives.[10] They recommended focusing campaign goals, using diagnostic surveys and theoretical models to guide planning, increasing the specificity and clarity of messages, and using appropriate indicators to assess impact.

Some evidence suggests that informational messages promoting relatively straightforward actions can change behavior in broad populations.[16] Two local US campaigns publicizing crisis lines saw concomitant increases in call volume, although they were unable to verify whether the additional calls resulted from the campaign or represented high-risk individuals.[17,18] More complex messages may be effective under certain circumstances. In one study, emergency department personnel exposed to a poster and two-page triage guide increased self-reported knowledge and skills with respect to detecting and managing suicide risk. Importantly, the content was carefully designed and tested with the audience to be highly relevant and actionable in that context, rather than providing general information.[19]

Several reviews recommend that suicide-related messaging efforts be guided by the broader literature on health communications and social marketing.[10,12,14,20,21] The next section provides an overview of lessons from that research.

PRINCIPLES OF EFFECTIVE HEALTH COMMUNICATIONS

An extensive literature describes key lessons for effectively using communications to influence health. A 2006 review concluded that well-designed campaigns can yield small to moderate effects across large populations "*on the condition* that principles of campaign design are attended to."[22(p24)] These principles provide guidance about the process required to create effective messages as well as important considerations at each stage.

Strategic Planning

Communications are not a strategy, but rather a set of tools that can be used to support suicide prevention goals in numerous ways. Systematic planning is essential to ensure that messaging is used strategically and effectively.[20,23–25] In addition to diverse messengers, there is considerable heterogeneity between and within military and veteran populations.[26–29] Planning enables messages to be tailored to specific goals, audiences, and contexts.

Numerous communications planning models exist, each outlining a similar set of sequential steps.[23,30–33] Key tasks involve analyzing the situation, deciding how communications can support overall goals, defining specific audiences and behaviors, creating tailored messages, disseminating messages effectively, and conducting assessments. Using research to inform planning decisions at each stage (known as formative research) is essential.[22,23,34,35] Although planning may be more extensive for large-scale campaigns, these steps represent a set of strategic questions for any messaging effort. The answers will vary according to message developer, scope of the effort, goals, and other factors.

Analysis and Goal Setting

The initial strategy development stage often is overlooked. More effective communications are grounded in broad-based analyses that define the problem to be addressed, outline its causes and effective solutions, and identify existing efforts and gaps.[20,23,24] Research has shown that messages are more successful when they are developed as part of an overall prevention plan and work in sync with broader change goals.[24,36] Military and veteran suicide prevention encompasses many goals, for example increasing life skills and resiliency, promoting social connectedness, increasing help seeking, identifying and assisting individuals at risk, providing crisis services, increasing access to care, providing evidence-based care, and restricting access to lethal means.[1,5–7] Such analyses help to clarify priority goals and identify the changes needed to accomplish them.

Communication objectives should support these same goals and changes. Because more successful messages often work in sync with other programmatic efforts, a key question for message planners is, Which goals and activities can be enhanced by messaging?[23,24,36] Objectives should be specific and measurable.[23,35] Many campaigns seek to "raise awareness" of suicide; however, as noted, such a vaguely defined objective is ambiguous and unlikely to result in behavior change. Objectives should be closely tied to a specific behavior and its determinants (e.g., to promote help seeking, "increase the belief that counseling will help rather than hurt one's career").

One consideration is how best to leverage change. Many media campaigns target individuals' knowledge, attitudes, and behaviors. However, communications can also promote health by altering environmental factors such as public policies or organizational structures.[23,24,37] For example, messages could be used to build support for a policy designed to increase prevention funding[14] or to promote an organization's capacity to serve veterans. In addition, communications can enhance specific programs. For example, gatekeeper training could be augmented by messaging that reiterates the training content, provides supplemental resources, or cues participants to act. For example, the Army distributes ACE wallet cards that summarize the actions (Ask, Care,

Escort) taught in the training. The VA and other services use similar approaches; for example, Navy cards reinforce their ACT (Ask, Care, Treat) mnemonic. Ideally, communications should support evidence-based programs and services.

Messaging decisions will be shaped by the scope of the organization's work. For example, the VA funded a campaign to promote the availability of the Veterans Crisis Line, a national hotline and chat service that provides crisis intervention and serves as a conduit to care. A local behavioral health clinic conducting a similar analysis might decide to change its communications objective from increasing knowledge about suicide to publicizing the availability and efficacy of its evidence-based treatments. Before promoting a program or service, planners should ensure that it has the capacity to meet the resulting demand.[38]

Target Audiences and Behaviors

The next step is to define who needs to act and what they need to do.[25] The choice of audience is defined by who is well positioned to take action to achieve the established goals and objectives. Some messages take a direct approach (e.g., targeting veterans to call the VA). The best route of influence, though, may be indirect, for example targeting service members' or veterans' behavior through intermediaries such as friends, family members, coworkers, supervisors, or providers, or using messaging to prompt constituents to call policymakers.[37,39,40] In this case, the target audience is the intermediary (e.g., supervisors), and the desired behavior change must be appropriate to that audience (e.g., recognize and address early signs of stress in subordinates).

Messages are more effective when they are directed to well-defined audience "segments" rather than the general public.[22,23,30,41] Segments should be relatively homogeneous in their knowledge, attitudes, values, motivations, and other factors related to the desired behavior, and they should be reachable through similar media or other channels. The analysis often will suggest potential audience segments that can be refined and prioritized after additional audience research (as described in the next step). For military or veteran populations, possible segmentation factors include service branch, service era, deployment or postdeployment stage, rank, or location. Again, the deciding question is whether subgroup differences suggest the need for unique messages or channels.

It is also important to articulate the desired behavior change. If audiences are unwilling to engage in a behavior or the determinants are difficult to change, it may be advisable to choose a different behavior rather than seeking more persuasive ways to sell an unrealistic action.[30] Not all problems can be fixed by messaging.

Audience Research

Before developing messages, it is critical to conduct research to understand the problem and desired behavior from the audience's perspective. Methods include literature reviews, surveys, focus groups, and interviews.[23] The social marketing literature stresses the importance of highlighting benefits valued by the "customer" (the intended audience) that offset the tangible or intangible costs of taking action.[30,42] Other factors to explore include the audience's current beliefs and attitudes about the problem and the behavior, their general values and interests, and their perceptions of how others view the behavior.[23,34] It is the audience's current beliefs and perceptions—whether accurate or inaccurate—that shape their behavior. More effective messaging uses formal behavior change theories as an analytic framework to identify a full range of behavioral influences.[43-47] For example, the DoD-funded Real Warriors Campaign used the Health Belief Model, a theory that describes factors influencing health behavior, to guide its research about barriers to and motivators of help seeking in military populations.[48]

Message developers should also identify the audience's usual and trusted information sources and media usage. When multiple audiences are targeted, each audience and behavior should be analyzed separately.[23] Even if funds are lacking, planners should pursue creative ways to learn about and obtain feedback from audiences. Examples might include conducting intercept interviews at public places, speaking to existing groups, adding questions to surveys, or soliciting feedback through personal contacts.

Creative Brief and Evaluation Plan

The previous steps lay the groundwork for designing and implementing effective concepts, messages, and materials.[23,31-33,49] Experts recommend summarizing the background work into a communication strategy statement or creative brief that identifies the intended audience and behavior, the audience's perceived benefits and barriers, and supportive statements that make the benefits credible. It also lists possible settings, channels, and activities and describes the most appealing tone, look, and feel for that audience.[23,24,31] Program evaluation is a particular gap in the suicide messaging field.[10,14,20] Thus, the plan should also describe how the messaging will be assessed, including measurement of process, outcomes, and possible negative effects.[20,23,31,35]

Design and Delivery of Messages and Materials

Messages and materials should carry out the strategy and promote action.[50] Message content should be relevant, credible, and culturally appropriate for the target audience.[22,23,31] More effective materials include a "call to action" highlighting the desired behavior, why it is being advocated,[51] and the information needed to act.

More persuasive messages use the formative research to motivate action by conveying personally meaningful incentives to the audience. A common motivational approach emphasizes the dire negative consequences of inaction. However, experts caution that fear appeals can backfire.[52] Similarly, there is no evidence that statistics about the problem motivate behavior change. Recommended approaches include persuading the audience that they can perform the recommended action and that the action will be effective (efficacy messages), reducing perceived barriers to the behavior, promoting personally valued benefits of acting, and modeling needed skills.[23,29,31] Images, sounds, and spokespersons should appeal to the audience and match message objectives.[53]

Channels, or the means used to convey the message, should correspond to the nature of the message and behavior, available resources, channel strengths and weaknesses, and audience preferences.[22-24,31] For example, although 99% of younger veterans use the Internet, this percentage drops to 34% to 46% among those serving in 1955 or earlier.[54] Thus, reaching older veterans would require additional channels, such as mass media or organizations. Some channels may be unsuitable for certain efforts. For example, texting or e-mail might pose confidentiality concerns, whereas message boards require resources to monitor for crisis communications.[55] More effective campaigns achieve sufficient and repeated exposure to messages through a mix of channels.[22,24,56] Core messages should be consistent and reinforced across channels.[23,31]

Pretesting at Each Stage

It is essential to test concepts, messages, and materials with the audience before finalizing them to assess whether they accurately convey the intended meaning.[22,23,42] Although audience input is invaluable, experts caution against taking all feedback uncritically, noting that focus groups may favor approaches that are not supported by research.[24,53] Similarly, professional designers unfamiliar with behavior change research may create materials that undermine the message.[24,53] Pretesting assesses whether messages and materials are understood by the audience and accomplish the communications objectives.

In addition to these general principles, there are unique considerations associated with suicide messaging. Two such considerations are stigma and safety issues.

STIGMA

Because mental illness stigma is a barrier to treatment use, some communications efforts aim to reduce stigma.[8] These messages should be informed by the literature on stigma and related interventions. This research shows that stigma is multifaceted. For example, Corrigan et al. described cognitive, emotional, and behavioral components of stigma as follows.[57-59]

Stereotypes are collectively shared beliefs about a group (e.g., individuals with mental illness are unemployable). Prejudice occurs when people endorse a stereotype and generate negative reactions (yes, they are weak and unreliable). Discrimination is the associated behavioral response (I won't hire them). There are three main forms of stigma. Public stigma refers to beliefs, attitudes, and behaviors in the broader population, whereas self-stigma is the internalization of negative beliefs by group members, resulting in a diminished self-concept and failure to pursue goals. Label avoidance occurs when individuals do not acknowledge symptoms or seek services to avoid the negative consequences of being labeled with a diagnosis.[59]

Studies involving military and veteran populations underscore the multifaceted nature of stigma. For example, Hoge et al. found that service members who met criteria for a mental disorder were more likely than service members who did not meet these criteria to endorse barriers to service seeking, including several stigma-related factors.[60] Some barriers reflected attitudes (e.g., "I would be seen as weak"), whereas others signaled fear of discrimination (e.g., "It would harm my career"). Notably, many barriers reflected not stigma but logistical or structural issues (e.g., difficulty getting time off from work or scheduling an appointment). Subsequent studies have differentiated between stigma and barriers to care, which is a critical distinction in implementing appropriate interventions.[61–63] Other research describes help-seeking behavior as a multistage process: recognizing the need for help, believing symptoms are treatable, weighing costs and benefits of help-seeking, seeking care, and persisting with treatment. At each stage, behavior is influenced by both stigma-related and other factors, including beliefs about treatment effectiveness, availability and logistics of treatment, and others.[64–66]

Stigma interventions have taken 3 main forms: protest, education, and contact.[57] Protest, or criticizing problematic representations of mental illness, can alter corporate or media behavior but may lead to "rebound" and worsening of prejudicial attitudes. Education challenges inaccurate stereotypes with factual information. Outcomes from education alone typically are limited to short-term attitudinal changes.[58,67] Contact approaches involve face-to-face interaction with individuals in the stigmatized group (e.g., those using psychological services). Of the three approaches, contact appears to involve the greatest likelihood of sustained attitude and behavior change, although more testing of media-based interventions is needed.[57,68,69]

As with communications generally, experts recommend that anti-stigma messages address defined audiences with tailored messages.[67] While working through the strategic planning process described earlier, planners can use the stigma literature as a framework for deconstructing this concept and identifying specific stigma reduction goals. Again, these decisions are shaped by organizational context and mission and current efforts. One organization might address workplace discrimination against veterans with real or perceived mental health issues, whereas another might target families of service members in the "label avoidance" category with information about symptoms and skills to encourage seeking help.

Once planners have established a goal, audience, and behavior, the stigma literature can help pinpoint specific barriers to action and guide effective interventions. For example, if research showed that supervisors were concerned about the combat readiness of personnel receiving counseling, messaging might convey stories of individuals whose work performance improved after receiving help. Messaging to address label avoidance should deemphasize psychiatric diagnoses and jargon, for example by creating messages in which individuals describe in their own words their symptoms and the benefits of treatment. The VA's recently launched Make the Connection campaign uses this approach, featuring veterans telling their stories about acknowledging and receiving help with mental health and other issues.

SAFE MESSAGING FOR SUICIDE PREVENTION

Careful planning of suicide messaging is particularly critical because of the potential for harm. Research has shown that certain types of media coverage of individual suicides may spur imitative effects or "contagion" among vulnerable individuals by modeling or glamorizing suicidal behavior.[70-72] Increased risk is associated with the amount, duration, and prominence of coverage; details about suicide methods or locations; stories about well-known individuals; simplistic explanations; and information that encourages identification with the decedent.[72-75] One Austrian study revealed that newspaper articles emphasizing suicide research and statistics, which included characterizing suicide as an epidemic and reporting myths, were positively associated with suicide rates.[76] To address this problem, countries including the United States have created recommendations for media reporting on suicide, and evidence suggests that these recommendations can improve reporting practices.[70,77-79] Recommendations should be shared with news outlets and used when crafting talking points about military and veteran suicide.

Experts have translated these media recommendations into a list of dos and don'ts for information and educational materials about suicide.[80] Practices that may be harmful in suicide materials ("don'ts") include the following: "normalizing" suicide by presenting it as a common event, glorifying or romanticizing people who have died by suicide, focusing on personal details of people who have died by suicide, presenting overly detailed descriptions of suicide methods, and presenting suicide as inexplicable or resulting from stress only. (The full document, including a list of "dos," is available at the Suicide Prevention Resource Center's Web site.[80])

The recommendation to avoid normalizing suicide bears some elaboration. Social norms are unspoken rules about what is "normal" in a given social context.[44] The literature differentiates between descriptive norms, or perceptions of what most people do (behaviors), and injunctive norms, which describe perceptions about what the majority finds acceptable (attitudes). People often misperceive norms, overestimating unhealthy behaviors and attitudes and underestimating healthy norms.[81] Messages may contribute to problems by reinforcing misperceptions; conversely, they can convey existing healthy norms to correct misperceptions and support positive behavior.

Messaging about military and veteran suicides often conveys problematic norms. News is a story-driven medium, and many of the current narratives portray intractable problems, failed interventions, and individual suicides.[82] Educational messages frequently emphasize the extent of the problem. Although suicide is unquestioningly devastating, disproportionate attention to negative stories may normalize suicidal behavior and create hopelessness about solutions, thereby reinforcing the perception among distressed individuals that suicide is the only answer and leaving potential helpers discouraged or uncertain about what to do.[72,83]

Notably, these guidelines address public messaging, or content that will be seen by audiences that include individuals at risk for suicide. Some messages are aimed more narrowly at decision makers, for example policymakers or providers. In these contexts, it may make sense to convey the tragedy of suicide or provide statistics about suicidal behavior among constituents or patients. However, it is advisable to weigh the potential benefit against the possibility that the messages will be viewed by individuals at risk or disseminated more broadly.

As mentioned, the don'ts of safe messaging are matched by a corresponding list of dos, that is, content that may be helpful in designing prevention materials.[80] This list reflects general types of content supportive of prevention goals, such as providing information about available help and emphasizing the effectiveness of treatment. As noted, this content should be tailored to specific audiences and goals.

To our knowledge, only one study has assessed whether certain media content is associated with a reduced risk of suicide. In the earlier-mentioned Austrian study of newspaper stories, the "mastery of crisis" category—describing individuals with suicidal ideation who adopted coping strategies other than suicidal behavior—was negatively associated with suicide rates, although these articles also involved the least harmful reporting practices.[76] Surprisingly, the "expert opinion" category, which included stories providing contact information for services, was positively associated with suicide. However, these articles also tended to include harmful content, such as stating that suicide-related societal problems are increasing.[76] More research is needed to clarify these relationships; it is plausible that resources would be protective when coupled with mastery of crisis stories that model coping. One implication is that experts should avoid diluting helpful information with harmful messaging.

TOWARD MORE STRATEGIC AND EFFECTIVE MESSAGING

Fortunately, the problem of military and veteran suicide is mobilizing broad-based responses across governments, organizations, and communities. All stakeholders must see themselves as messengers and engage in careful communications planning based on the best available science. Existing research suggests guidance for developing messages that are more likely to contribute positively to military and veteran suicide prevention efforts and less likely to be counterproductive or harmful.

Systematic planning is essential. Message developers who are unfamiliar with the principles of effective communications can use the excellent step-by-step planning guides that exist.[23,31,32] The principles can help guide decision making regardless of the scope, budget, or level of the communications effort. Any messaging can benefit from establishing specific and realistic communications goals and articulating how these efforts complement or reinforce other program components; selecting a target audience and identifying a call to action; designing messages based on the audience's current behaviors, beliefs, values, and barriers to action; pretesting messages and materials; ensuring adequate exposure to messages; and assessing results.

During this process, message developers should attend to unique suicide messaging issues. The stigma literature can help planners select specific stigma reduction goals, audiences, and behaviors and identify stigma-related and non-stigma-related barriers to action. Avoiding clinical diagnoses in favor of lay language may be important when addressing label avoidance. Anti-stigma efforts can employ contact approaches—real stories of help and coping. This approach also avoids linking military or veteran populations with suicide. These associations may inadvertently increase stigma, which can feed discrimination and discourage help seeking. Similarly, rather than reiterating the extent to which stigma is a problem, we recommend focusing on solutions to stigma, such as countering barriers and promoting audience-identified benefits of acting. Accordingly, anti-stigma messages may never mention the word "stigma."

All suicide prevention communications should avoid potentially harmful content, including explicitly or implicitly characterizing suicide as a typical response to depression, stress, or other challenges service members and veterans may face. In fact, coping in ways other than attempting suicide is far more common. Other problematic content includes stories of individual suicides, details about suicide means or locations, romanticized or simplistic explanations, and presenting suicide as inexplicable or unpreventable. Messages can be accurate and honest about the prevalence of military and veteran suicide while avoiding descriptions suggesting the problem is uncontrollable or hopeless.

When appropriate, messages should provide concrete resources coupled with stories of individuals who struggled, reached out, and are now thriving, as well as accounts of individuals, groups, and leaders who are working proactively to increase their mental, physical, spiritual, and relational wellness. These messages acknowledge the thousands of service members and veterans who are finding ways to adaptively cope with the stresses of military service, including multiple combat deployments, to convey how truly common those behaviors are.

A comprehensive approach will include working with the news media. It is possible to educate journalists about media guidelines for safely reporting suicide, especially when they are approached as partners.[84,85] Providing the media with contacts and source materials they need to tell personal stories about early intervention, recovery, and resiliency may help create a more balanced picture of the mental health of military and veteran populations. Recognizing that stories about system failures and unsuccessful help seeking may be easier to find, we recommend that stakeholders proactively identify positive stories of effective actions by individuals and systems so that responses to media requests can include these examples along with available resources.

Communications are an important set of tools that, when used effectively, can advance and support research-based suicide prevention goals. Research will continue to build our knowledge about the effectiveness of specific messages for particular audiences and goals, but the information needed to plan safer and more effective communications efforts is already available. We owe it to service members and veterans to apply it.

ABOUT THE AUTHORS

Linda Langford and David Litts are with the Suicide Prevention Resource Center, Education Development Center Inc., Waltham, MA. Jane L. Pearson is with the National Institute of Mental Health, Bethesda, MD.

CONTRIBUTORS

L. Langford reviewed the communications, safe messaging, and stigma research and wrote the initial draft. D. Litts provided military- and veteran-specific research and message considerations and made extensive revisions. J. L. Pearson helped conceptualize the article, contributed insights from research on military and veteran suicide, and suggested revisions.

ACKNOWLEDGMENTS

The work of the Suicide Prevention Resource Center is supported by the Substance Abuse and Mental Health Services Administration. Jane L. Pearson's time was supported by the National Institute of Mental Health.

We thank the anonymous reviewers for their thoughtful feedback. Linda Langford and David Litts thank Reingold Inc. and Pat Corrigan for the opportunity to collaborate on and learn from the development of the Make the Connection campaign, funded by the US Department of Veterans Affairs.

Note. The views expressed in this article do not necessarily represent the views of the Substance Abuse and Mental Health Services Administration, the National Institute of Mental Health, the National Institutes of Health, the Department of Health and Human Services, or the United States government.

HUMAN PARTICIPANT PROTECTION

No protocol approval was needed because no human subjects were involved.

REFERENCES

1. Department of Defense Task Force on the Prevention of Suicide by Members of the Armed Forces. The challenge and the promise: strengthening the force, preventing suicide and saving lives. Available at: http://www.health.mil/dhb/downloads/ Suicide%20Prevention%20Task%20Force%20final%20report%208-23-10.pdf. Accessed September 10, 2012.

2. Kinn JT, Luxton DD, Reger MA, et al. Department of Defense suicide event report (DoDSER): calendar year 2010 annual report. Available at: http://t2health.org/sites/ default/files/dodser/DoDSER_2010_Annual_Report.pdf. Accessed September 10, 2012.

3. Bossarte RM, Claassen CA, Knox KL. Evaluating evidence of risk for suicide among veterans. *Mil Med.* 2010;175(10):703–704.

4. Miller M, Barber C, Azrael D, et al. Suicide among US veterans: a prospective study of 500,000 middle-aged and elderly men. *Am J Epidemiol.* 2009;170(4):494–500.

5. Ramchand R, Acosta J, Burns RM, Jaycox LH, Pernin CG. The war within: preventing suicide in the U.S. military. Available at: http://www.dtic.mil/cgi-bin/GetTRDoc?AD= ADA537090&Location=U2&doc=GetTRDoc.pdf. Accessed September 10, 2012.

6. US Dept of Veterans Affairs. Report of the Blue Ribbon Work Group on Suicide Prevention in the Veteran Population. Available at: http://www.mentalhealth.va.gov/ suicide_prevention/Blue_Ribbon_Report-FINAL_June-30-08.pdf. Accessed September 10, 2012.

7. Knox KL, Litts DA, Talcott WG, Feig JC, Caine ED. Risk of suicide and related adverse outcomes after exposure to a suicide prevention programme in the US Air Force: cohort study. *BMJ.* 2003;327(7428):1376–1378.

8. US Dept of Health and Human Services. National strategy for suicide prevention: goals and objectives for action. Available at: http://www.sprc.org/sites/sprc.org/files/ library/nsspsummary.pdf. Accessed September 10, 2012.

9. Edwards-Stewart A, Kinn JT, June JD, Fullerton NR. Military and civilian media coverage of suicide. *Arch Suicide Res.* 2011;15(4):304–312.

10. Dumesnil H, Verger P. Public awareness campaigns about depression and suicide: a review. *Psychiatr Serv.* 2009;60(9):1203–1213.

11. Francis C, Pirkis J, Dunt D, Blood RW, Davis C. Improving mental health literacy: a review of the literature. Available at: http://www.health.gov.au/internet/main/publishing.nsf/content/6A5554955150A9B9CA2571FF0005184D/$File/literacy.pdf. Accessed September 10, 2012.

12. Kelly CM, Jorm AF, Wright A. Improving mental health literacy as a strategy to facilitate early intervention for mental disorders. *Med J Aust.* 2007;187(7):S26–S30.

13. Hegerl U, Dietrich S, Pfeiffer-Gerschel T, Wittenburg L, Althaus D. Education and awareness programmes for adults: selected and multilevel approaches in suicide prevention. In: Wasserman D, Wasserman C, eds. *The Oxford Textbook of Suicidology and Suicide Prevention: A Global Perspective.* Oxford, England: Oxford University Press; 2009:495–500.

14. Pearson JL. Challenges in US suicide prevention public awareness programmes. In: O'Connor RC, Platt S, Gordon J, eds. *International Handbook of Suicide Prevention: Research, Policy and Practice.* New York, NY: John Wiley & Sons Inc; 2011:577–590.

15. Hegerl U, Mergl R, Havers I, et al. Sustainable effects on suicidality were found for the Nuremberg Alliance Against Depression. *Eur Arch Psychiatry Clin Neurosci.* 2010;260(5):401–406.

16. Hornik R. Introduction: public health communication: making sense of contradictory evidence. In: Hornik R, ed. *Public Health Communication: Evidence for Behavior Change.* Mahwah, NJ: Lawrence Erlbaum Associates; 2002:1–19.

17. Jenner E, Jenner LW, Matthews-Sterling M, Butts JK, Williams TE. Awareness effects of a youth suicide prevention media campaign in Louisiana. *Suicide Life Threat Behav.* 2010;40(4):394–406.

18. Oliver RJ, Spilsbury JC, Osiecki SS, et al. Brief report: preliminary results of a suicide awareness mass media campaign in Cuyahoga County, Ohio. *Suicide Life Threat Behav.* 2008;38(2):245–249.

19. Currier GW, Litts D, Walsh P, et al. Evaluation of an emergency department educational campaign for recognition of suicidal patients. *West J Emerg Med.* 2012;13(1):41–50.

20. Chambers DA, Pearson JL, Lubell K, et al. The science of public messages for suicide prevention: a workshop summary. *Suicide Life Threat Behav.* 2005;35(2):134–145.

21. Suicide Prevention Resource Center. Charting the future of suicide prevention: a 2010 progress review of the national strategy and recommendations for the decade ahead. Available at: http://www.sprc.org/sites/sprc.org/files/library/ ChartingTheFuture_Fullbook.pdf. Accessed September 10, 2012.

22. Noar SM. A 10-year retrospective of research in health mass media campaigns: where do we go from here? *J Health Commun.* 2006;11(1):21–42.

23. National Cancer Institute. Making health communication programs work. Available at: http://www.cancer.gov/pinkbook. Accessed September 10, 2012.

24. DeJong W. The role of mass media campaigns in reducing high-risk drinking among college students. *J Stud Alcohol Suppl.* 2002;14:182–192.

25. Salmon CT, Atkin C. Using media campaigns for health promotion. In: Thompson TL, Dorsey AM, Miller KI, Parrott R, eds. *Handbook of Health Communication.* Mahwah, NJ: Lawrence Erlbaum Associates; 2003:449–472.

26. Kaplan MS, McFarland BH, Huguet N, Valenstein M. Suicide risk and precipitating circumstances among young, middle-aged, and older male veterans. *Am J Public Health.* 2012;102(suppl 1):S131–S137.

27. McCarthy JF, Blow FC, Ignacio RV, et al. Suicide among patients in the Veterans Affairs health system: rural-urban differences in rates, risks, and methods. *Am J Public Health.* 2012;102(suppl 1):S111–S117.

28. Lindley S, Cacciapaglia H, Noronha D, Carlson E, Schatzberg A. Monitoring mental health treatment acceptance and initial treatment adherence in veterans. *Ann N Y Acad Sci.* 2010;1208(1):104–113.

29. Milliken CS, Auchterlonie JL, Hoge CW. Longitudinal assessment of mental health problems among active and reserve component soldiers returning from the Iraq war. *JAMA.* 2007;298(18):2141–2148.

30. Grier S, Bryant CA. Social marketing in public health. *Annu Rev Public Health.* 2005;26:319–339.

31. O'Sullivan GA, Yonkler JA, Morgan W, Merritt AP. A field guide to designing a health communication strategy. Available at: http://www.jhuccp.org/sites/all/files/ A%20Field%20Guide%20to%20Designing%20Health%20Comm%20Strategy.pdf. Accessed September 10, 2012.

32. US Centers for Disease Control and Prevention. CDCynergy planning tool. Available at: http://www.cdc.gov/healthcommunication/CDCynergy/. Accessed September 10, 2012.

33. Communications Resource Center, Substance Abuse and Mental Health Services Administration. Strategic communication planning: a workbook for Garrett Lee Smith Memorial Act state, tribal, and campus grantees. Available at: http://www.sprc.org/sites/sprc.org/files/library/GLSWorkbook.pdf. Accessed September 10, 2012.

34. Atkin C, Freimuth V. Formative evaluation research in campaign design. In: Rice RE, Atkin CK, eds. *Public Communication Campaigns*. 3rd ed. Thousand Oaks, CA: Sage Publications; 2001:125–145.

35. Flay BR. Evaluation of the development, dissemination and effectiveness of mass media health programming. *Health Educ Res*. 1987;2(2):123–129.

36. Wallack L, DeJong W. Mass media and public health: moving the focus from the individual to the environment. In: Martin SE, Mail P, eds. *Effects of the Mass Media on the Use and Abuse of Alcohol*. Bethesda, MD: National Institute on Alcohol Abuse and Alcoholism; 1995:253–268. NIH publication 95-3743.

37. Abroms LC, Maibach EW. The effectiveness of mass communication to change public behavior. *Annu Rev Public Health*. 2008;29:219–234.

38. Boeke M, Griffin T, Reidenberg DJ. The physician's role in suicide prevention: lessons learned from a public awareness campaign. *Minn Med*. 2011;94(1):44–46.

39. Atkin C. Theory and principles of media health campaigns. In: Rice RE, Atkin CK, eds. *Public Communication Campaigns*. 3rd ed. Thousand Oaks, CA: Sage Publications; 2001:49–68.

40. Hornik R, Yanovitzky I. Using theory to design evaluations of communications campaigns: the case of the National Youth Anti-Drug Media Campaign. *Commun Theory*. 2003;13(2):204–224.

41. Backer TE, Rogers EM, Sopory P. *Designing Health Communication Campaigns: What Works?* Thousand Oaks, CA: Sage Publications; 1992.

42. Gordon R, McDermott L, Stead M, Angus K. The effectiveness of social marketing interventions for health improvement: what's the evidence? *Public Health*. 2006;120(12):1133–1139.

43. Fishbein M, Cappella JN. The role of theory in developing effective health communications. *J Commun.* 2006;56(suppl 1):S1–S17.

44. Glanz K, Rimer BK, Viswanath K. *Health Behavior and Health Education: Theory, Research, and Practice.* 4th ed. San Francisco, CA: Jossey-Bass; 2008.

45. Wright K, Sparks L, O'Hair D. *Health Communication in the 21st Century.* Oxford, England: Blackwell Publishing; 2008.

46. Shemanski Aldrich R, Cerel J. The development of effective message content for suicide intervention: theory of planned behavior. *Crisis.* 2009;30(4):174–179.

47. Stecker T, Fortney J, Hamilton F, Sherbourne CD, Ajzen I. Engagement in mental health treatment among veterans returning from Iraq. *Patient Prefer Adherence.* 2010;4:45–49.

48. Defense Centers of Excellence for Psychological Health & Traumatic Brain Injury. Real Warriors Campaign presentation. Available at: http://www.dcoe.health.mil/Content/navigation/documents/SPC2010/Jan11/Real%20Warriors%20Campaign/DCoE_Comms_SuicidePrevention_%20Presentation_20100111_v9_Final.pdf. Accessed September 10, 2012.

49. Cho H, Salmon CT. Unintended effects of health communication campaigns. *J Commun.* 2007;57(2):293–317.

50. Goodman A. Why bad ads happen to good causes. Available at: http://www.agoodmanonline.com/bad_ads_good_causes/. Accessed September 10, 2012.

51. Murray-Johnson L, Witte K. Looking toward the future: health message design strategies. In: Thompson TL, Dorsey AM, Miller KI, Parrott R, eds. *Handbook of Health Communication.* Mahwah, NJ: Lawrence Erlbaum Associates; 2003:473–496.

52. Soames Job RF. Effective and ineffective use of fear in health promotion campaigns. *Am J Public Health.* 1988;78(2):163–167.

53. Russell CA, Clapp JD, DeJong W. Done 4: analysis of a failed social norms marketing campaign. *Health Commun.* 2005;17(1):57–65.

54. Westat. National survey of veterans, active duty service members, demobilized National Guard and Reserve members, family members, and surviving spouses. Available at: http://www.va.gov/vetdata/docs/SurveysAndStudies/NVSSurveyFinalWeightedReport.pdf. Accessed September 10, 2012.

55. Luxton DD, June JD, Kinn JT. Technology-based suicide prevention: current applications and future directions. *Telemed J E Health.* 2011;17(1):50–54.

56. Snyder LB, Hamilton MA. A meta-analysis of U.S. health campaign effects on behavior: emphasize enforcement, exposure, and new information, and beware the secular trend. In: Hornik R, ed. *Public Health Communication: Evidence for Behavior Change.* Mahwah, NJ: Lawrence Erlbaum Associates; 2002:357–383.

57. Corrigan PW, Shapiro JR. Measuring the impact of programs that challenge the public stigma of mental illness. *Clin Psychol Rev.* 2010;30(8):907–922.

58. Corrigan P. How stigma interferes with mental health care. *Am Psychol.* 2004;59(7):614–625.

59. Ben-Zeev D, Corrigan PW, Britt TW, Langford L. Stigma of mental illness and service use in the military. *J Ment Health.* 2012;21(3):264–273.

60. Hoge CW, Castro CA, Messer SC, et al. Combat duty in Iraq and Afghanistan, mental health problems, and barriers to care. *N Engl J Med.* 2004;351(1):13–22.

61. Kim PY, Thomas JL, Wilk JE, Castro CA, Hoge CW. Stigma, barriers to care, and use of mental health services among active duty and National Guard soldiers after combat. *Psychiatr Serv.* 2010;61(6):582–588.

62. Pietrzak RH, Johnson DC, Goldstein MB, Malley JC, Southwick SM. Perceived stigma and barriers to mental health care utilization among OEF-OIF veterans. *Psychiatr Serv.* 2009;60(8):1118–1122.

63. Vogt D. Mental health-related beliefs as a barrier to service use for military personnel and veterans: a review. *Psychiatr Serv.* 2011;62(2):135–142.

64. Greene-Shortridge TM, Britt TW, Castro CA. The stigma of mental health problems in the military. *Mil Med.* 2007;172(2):157–161.

65. Eisenberg D, Downs MF, Golberstein E, Zivin K. Stigma and help seeking for mental health among college students. *Med Care Res Rev.* 2009;66(5):522–541.

66. Dickstein BD, Vogt DS, Handa S, Litz BT. Targeting self-stigma in returning military personnel and veterans: a review of intervention strategies. *Mil Psychol.* 2010;22(2):224–236.

67. Martin N, Johnston V. A time for action: tackling stigma and discrimination. Available at: http://www.mentalhealthcommission.ca/SiteCollectionDocuments/Anti-Stigma/TimeforAction_Eng.pdf. Accessed September 10, 2012.

68. Corrigan P, Gelb B. Three programs that use mass approaches to challenge the stigma of mental illness. *Psychiatr Serv.* 2006;57(3):393–398.

69. Corrigan PW. Where is the evidence supporting public service announcements to eliminate mental illness stigma? *Psychiatr Serv.* 2012;63(1):79–82.

70. Pirkis J, Blood RW, Beautrais A, Burgess P, Skehan J. Media guidelines on the reporting of suicide. *Crisis.* 2006;27(2):82–87.

71. Stack S. Media coverage as a risk factor in suicide. *J Epidemiol Community Health.* 2003;57(4):238–240.

72. Gould M, Jamieson P, Romer D. Media contagion and suicide among the young. *Am Behav Sci.* 2003;46(9):1269–1284.

73. Stack S. Suicide in the media: a quantitative review of studies based on non-fictional stories. *Suicide Life Threat Behav.* 2005;35(2):121–133.

74. Stack S. Media coverage as a risk factor in suicide. *Inj Prev.* 2002;8(suppl 4):iv30–iv32.

75. Gould MS. Suicide and the media. *Ann N Y Acad Sci.* 2001;932:200–224.

76. Niederkrotenthaler T, Voracek M, Herberth A, et al. Role of media reports in completed and prevented suicide: Werther v. Papageno effects. *Br J Psychiatry.* 2010;197(3):234–243.

77. Recommendations for reporting on suicide. Available at: http://reportingonsuicide.org/. Accessed September 10, 2012.

78. Pirkis J, Dare A, Blood RW, et al. Changes in media reporting of suicide in Australia between 2000/01 and 2006/07. *Crisis.* 2009;30(1):25–33.

79. Niederkrotenthaler T, Sonneck G. Assessing the impact of media guidelines for reporting on suicides in Austria: interrupted time series analysis. *Aust N Z J Psychiatry.* 2007;41(5):419–428.

80. Suicide Prevention Resource Center. Safe and effective messaging for suicide prevention. Available at: http://www.sprc.org/sites/sprc.org/files/library/SafeMessagingrevised.pdf. Accessed September 10, 2012.

81. Borsari B, Carey KB. Descriptive and injunctive norms in college drinking: a meta-analytic integration. *J Stud Alcohol*. 2003;64(3):331–341.

82. Kline KN. A decade of research on health content in the media: the focus on health challenges and sociocultural context and attendant informational and ideological problems. *J Health Commun*. 2006;11(1):43–59.

83. Langford L, Gould MS, Norton K. Webinar: suicide narratives in the news media: what effect might they have and what can we do? Available at: http://sprc.org/training-institute/r2p-webinars/suicide-narratives-news-media-what-effect-might-they-have-and-what-1. Accessed September 10, 2012.

84. Collings SC, Kemp CG. Death knocks, professional practice, and the public good: the media experience of suicide reporting in New Zealand. *Soc Sci Med*. 2010;71(2):244–248.

85. Au JSKK, Yip PSFF, Chan CLWW, Law YW. Newspaper reporting of suicide cases in Hong Kong. *Crisis*. 2004;25(4):161–168.

PART VI

Field Action Reports

14

Implementation and Early Utilization of a Suicide Hotline for Veterans

Kerry L. Knox, MS, PhD, Janet Kemp, RN, PhD, Richard McKeon, PhD, and Ira R. Katz, MD, PhD

Suicide crisis lines have a respected history as a strategy for reducing deaths from suicide and suicidal behaviors. Until recently, however, evidence of the effectiveness of these crisis lines has been sparse. Studies published during the past decade suggest that crisis lines offer an alternative to populations who may not be willing to engage in treatment through traditional mental health settings. Given this promising evidence, in 2007, the Department of Veterans Affairs in collaboration with the Department of Health and Human Services' Substance Abuse and Mental Health Administration implemented a National Suicide Hotline that is staffed 24 hours a day, 7 days a week, by Veterans Affairs clinical staff. We report here on the implementation of this suicide hotline and our early observations of its utilization in a largely male population.

KEY FINDINGS

- Reducing deaths from suicide is an important priority for the VA. Beginning in 2006, the VA implemented several broadly sweeping initiatives to address the public health problem of veteran suicide.
- Successful engagement of veterans, especially men, through use of a suicide hotline, was determined by VA leadership to have the potential to inform system-level changes to facilitate help-seeking behaviors in veterans who are suicidal or in distress.
- We report on descriptive information available from 3 years of operation of the VA's hotline and discuss implications for future research.

Suicide has been the focus of national attention for more than a decade.[1-4] During this period, a heightened awareness of suicide in the military and in veterans has developed, largely in response to the wars in Afghanistan and Iraq. A Department of Defense task force has underscored the urgent need to address this public health problem in military and veteran populations[5]; the recently established National Action Alliance for Suicide Prevention[6] has incorporated a work group focused on veterans as a target population for prevention.

The Department of Veterans Affairs (VA) has been on the forefront of this groundswell and has implemented a comprehensive suicide prevention strategy. This strategy includes widescale enhancements for delivery of mental health care, the VA's National Suicide Hotline, a national network of VA suicide prevention teams, and targeted programs such as safety planning and follow-up for veterans identified as at risk for suicide through both inpatient and outpatient venues.

Historically, efforts have been expended to encourage suicidal individuals to call suicide crisis line telephone centers, without evidence that this approach decreases events of suicide.[7,8] Joiner et al.[9] noted that because crisis lines offer accessibility during multiple points along the path to suicidal behavior, they are uniquely poised to intervene in this pathway, including when individuals are in immediate danger of taking their own life. In a practical manner, these telephone services offer the opportunity to intervene during a suicidal crisis when no other help may be acceptable or available. Essentially, crisis lines have served as anonymous venues of contact with little or no longer-term follow-up, systematic referrals for case management, or treatment.

Recent evidence has emerged regarding the potential usefulness and effectiveness of suicide crisis lines. King et al.[10] demonstrated that in a small sample of adolescents, suicidality decreased after a call to a suicide crisis line. In studies funded by the Department of Health and Human Services' Substance Abuse and Mental Health Service Administration (SAMHSA), Kalafat et al.[11] and Gould et al.[12] provided data on the reduction in distress of callers to community suicide crisis lines at the end of a call and emphasized the need to conduct more rigorous suicide assessments. Mishara et al.[13,14] provided evidence that responder intervention styles play an important role in the outcome of the call. Despite these encouraging results, studies have reported that callers to suicide crisis lines are predominantly female and that positive effects during the course of the call are more likely to be detected in younger females.[10,12] In summary, suicide crisis lines in the general population thus far have been shown to be most effective for reaching a select population that is younger, female, and at a lower risk for self-harm.

The VA's population is largely male (representing predominantly Vietnam or returning veterans). Although evidence of the usefulness of suicide crisis lines existed at the time of implementation of VA's suicide hotline, whether a primarily male veteran population would call a hotline was unknown. The VA's suicide hotline is both similar to community suicide crisis lines and different in important ways. It is similar in that the hotline responds immediately to veterans in distress; it differs in that all hotline responders are trained clinicians who can access a veteran caller's electronic medical record regardless of the veteran's location, and records of the call can be immediately incorporated into the electronic medical record. Most importantly, a consenting veteran can be provided with an appropriate referral within the VA mental health care system.

IMPLEMENTATION OF THE DEPARTMENT OF VETERANS AFFAIRS SUICIDE HOTLINE

In July 2007, the VA partnered with the SAMHSA to become part of SAMHSA's National Suicide Prevention Lifeline Network (Lifeline; Box 1). The SAMSHA-funded network consists of more than 145 crisis centers nationwide.[15] The partnership between the VA and SAMHSA allows the VA to directly provide services to veterans anywhere in the country with the advantage of training and technological support from Lifeline, including backup services in times of high volume or line outage when calls can be taken by any 1 of Lifeline's 5 backup centers to the VA's suicide hotline. The program also adopted the National Suicide Prevention Lifeline Suicide Risk Assessment Standards described in detail by Joiner et al.[16] The VA's hotline has now been widely promoted through public awareness campaigns, for example, posters displayed on public transportation that convey the message that getting help is a sign of strength (Figure 1).

FINDINGS

Since the inception of the VA's suicide hotline, the percentage of veterans self-identifying as veterans has increased from 30% to just over 60% as of September 30, 2010; the volume of calls as of this time was 171 000. Seventy percent of callers were male veterans, and those who disclosed their age were between 40 and 69 years old. Approximately 4000 referrals were made to the VA's suicide prevention coordinators as of 2008; there were 16 000 referrals at the end of September 2010. In addition to these referrals, simultaneous referrals were made to diverse programs in the VA, including programs for returning veterans from the wars in Afghanistan and Iraq, programs for women, programs for homeless veterans, and substance abuse services. Community referrals were made for veterans not eligible for care within the VA.

CONCLUSIONS

These are the first data to demonstrate that a population consisting primarily of men is willing to call a suicide hotline and accept follow-up referrals; this finding is unprecedented in the history of suicide hotlines. It also demonstrates that men, especially men in the middle years of life who are at high risk for suicide,[17] can be engaged in an intervention that may result in longer-term treatment owing to intensive follow-up. Moreover, the VA's hotline consists of trained clinicians, whereas most community hotline responders have little if any training in crisis intervention.[18] Key to evaluating whether the VA's suicide crisis hotline is an effective component of the VA's overall comprehensive suicide prevention plan is to (1) describe whether calling the hotline diminishes distress, (2) determine the longer-term clinical outcomes of callers to the hotline, and (3) describe responder intervention behaviors and determine whether intervention styles impact changes in distress during the call and willingness to accept a referral to a VA suicide prevention coordinator. Although it will never be possible for us to know about veterans who do not call the hotline, the VA's electronic medical record allows tracking of longer-term clinical outcomes of callers to the hotline in a manner not possible in community suicide crisis lines. Therefore, future longitudinal analyses of the hotline data will permit us to identify the relation between risk and precipitating factors for subpopulations of veterans, their degree of suicidal

DEPARTMENT OF VETERANS AFFAIRS (VA) SUICIDE HOTLINE DELIVERY OF CARE

Callers to the National Suicide Prevention Lifeline receive the message that if they are a US veteran or are concerned about a US veteran, they should press "1," which then routes that caller to the VA's suicide hotline located at the Canandaigua VA Medical Center in Canandaigua, New York. Utilization of the existing 1-800-273-TALK number and the combined promotional efforts of the VA and the Substance Abuse and Mental Health Service Administration (SAMHSA) maximizes the likelihood that veterans at risk, or their friends and families, will hear about the veterans' suicide hotline.

An exclusive feature of the VA's suicide hotline is that concomitantly with the implementation of the hotline, the VA leadership mandated a Suicide Prevention Coordinators Program, which requires that every VA medical facility have a minimum of 1 full-time suicide prevention coordinator. Larger facilities now have teams comprising suicide prevention coordinators, suicide case managers, and administrative support. The VA's hotline responders provide referrals to these teams for follow-up of all veterans who call the suicide hotline and consent to be contacted. Thus, the hotline does not require veterans to initiate the process of accessing care through the usual means of entry to care, primarily through the VA's mental health system.

ideation or intent, and their previous or current use of mental health services in the VA. Future analysis will also provide critical information regarding outcomes in highly suicidal veterans or veterans suffering from mental distress resulting from, for example, depression, posttraumatic stress disorder, relationship problems, and substance use disorders.

ABOUT THE AUTHORS

Kerry L. Knox and Janet Kemp are with the Department of Veterans Affairs and the Center of Excellence for Suicide Prevention, Canandaigua VA Medical Center, Canandaigua, NY. Richard McKeon is with the Center for Mental Health Services, Substance Abuse and Mental Health Service Administration,

Rockville, MD. Ira R. Katz is with the Department of Veterans Affairs, Washington, DC.

HUMAN PARTICIPANT PROTECTION

Institutional review board approval was not needed because no research was conducted.

REFERENCES

1. *The Surgeon General's Call to Action to Prevent Suicide.* Washington, DC: US Department of Health and Human Services, Public Health Service; 1999.

2. *National Strategy for Suicide Prevention. Goals and Objectives for Action.* Rockville, MD: US Department of Health and Human Services, Public Health Service; 2001.

3. Committee on Pathophysiology and Prevention of Adolescent and Adult Suicide, Board on Neuroscience and Behavioral Health, Institute of Medicine. *Reducing Suicide. A National Imperative.* Washington, DC: National Academy Press; 2002.

4. Knox KL, Conwell Y, Caine ED. If suicide is a public health problem, what are we doing to prevent it? *Am J Public Health.* 2004;94(1):37–45.

5. Department of Defense Task Force on Suicide Prevention. *The Challenge and the Promise: Strengthening the Force, Preventing Suicide and Saving Lives.* Available at: http://www.health.mil/dhb/downloads/Suicide%20Prevention%20Task%20Force%20final%20report%208-23-10.pdf. Accessed September 16, 2011.

6. National Alliance for Suicide Prevention. Available at: http://actionallianceforsuicideprevention.org. Accessed September 16, 2011.

7. Leenaars AA, Lester D. The impact of suicide prevention centers on the suicide rate in the Canadian provinces. *Crisis.* 2004;25(2):65–68.

8. Mishara BL, Daigle M. Helplines and crisis intervention services: challenges for the future. In: Lester D, ed. *Suicide Prevention: Resources for the Miliennium.* Philadelphia, PA: Brunner-Routledge; 2000:153–171.
DA99B7369CB34B3D3651DFA357

9. Joiner TE, Walker RL, Rudd MD, Jobes DA. Scientizing and routinizing the assessment of suicidality in outpatient practice. *Prof Psychol Res Pr.* 1999;30(5):447–453.

10. King R, Nurcombe B, Beckman L, Hides L, Reid W. Telephone counseling for adolescent suicide prevention: changes in suicidality and mental state from beginning to end of a counseling session. *Suicide Life Threat Behav.* 2003;33(4):400–411.

11. Kalafat J, Gould MS, Munfakh JLHH, Leinman M. An evaluation of crisis hotline outcomes. Part I: Non-suicidal crisis callers. *Suicide Life Threat Behav.* 2007;37(3):322–337.

12. Gould MS, Kalafat J, Munfakh JLHH, Kleinman M. An evaluation of crisis hotline outcomes. Part II: Suicidal callers. *Suicide Life Threat Behav.* 2007;37(3):338–352.

13. Mishara BL, Chagnon F, Daigle M, et al. Which helper behaviors and intervention styles are related to better short-term outcomes in telephone crisis intervention? Results from a silent monitoring study of calls to the US 1-800 SUICIDE network. *Suicide Life Threat Behav.* 2007;37(3):308–321.

14. Mishara BL, Chagnon F, Daigle M, et al. Comparing models of helper behavior to actual practice in telephone crisis intervention: A silent monitoring study of calls to the US. 1-1800-SUICIDE network. *Suicide Life Threat Behav.* 2007;37(3):291–307.

15. National Suicide Prevention Lifeline. Available at: http://www.suicidepreventionlifeline.org. Accessed September 16, 2011.

16. Joiner T, Kalafat J, Draper J, et al. Established standards for the assessment of suicide risk among callers to the National Suicide Prevention Lifeline. *Suicide Life Threat Behav.* 2007;37(3):353–365.

17. Knox KL, Caine ED. Establishing Priorities for Reducing Suicide and Its Antecedents in the United States. *Am J Public Health.* 2005;95(11):1898–1903.

18. Daigle MS, Mishara BL. Intervention styles with suicidal callers at two suicide prevention centres. *Suicide Life Threat Behav.* 1995;25(2):261–275.

15

An Emergency Department-Based Brief Intervention for Veterans at Risk for Suicide (SAFE VET)

Kerry L. Knox, PhD, Barbara Stanley, PhD, Glenn W. Currier, MD, Lisa Brenner, PhD, Marjan Ghahramanlou-Holloway, PhD, and Gregory Brown, PhD

Reducing deaths from veteran suicide is a public health priority for veterans who receive their care from the Department of Veterans Affairs (VA) and those who receive services in community settings. Emergency departments frequently function as the primary or sole point of contact with the health care system for suicidal individuals; therefore, they represent an important venue in which to identify and treat veterans who are at risk for suicide. We describe the design, implementation and initial evaluation of a brief behavioral intervention for suicidal veterans seeking care at VA emergency departments. Initial findings of the feasibility and acceptability of the intervention suggest it may be transferable to diverse VA and non-VA settings, including community emergency departments and urgent care centers.

KEY FINDINGS

- An innovative project (SAFE VET) designed to help suicidal veterans in emergency departments in the Department of Veterans Affairs (VA) has been successfully implemented in 5 intervention sites.
- Using quality assurance data acceptability of the SAFE VET intervention was determined as percent of veterans willing to receive the intervention; information on follow-up mental health and other psychiatric services was also obtained.
- SAFE VET is a promising alternative and acceptable delivery of care system that augments the treatment of suicidal veterans in VA emergency

departments and helps ensure that they have appropriate follow-up care. If future research finds that this brief behavioral intervention is effective on key outcomes such as suicide attempts and engagement in care, the approach may be transferable to a wide variety of VA and non-VA settings, including community emergency departments and urgent care centers.

Reducing deaths from veteran suicide and decreasing the burden on individuals and families caused by suicidal behavior in veterans is an important priority for the Department of Veterans Affairs (VA). Emergency departments (EDs) frequently function as the primary or sole point of contact with the health care system for suicidal individuals.[1,2] This contact often occurs either immediately following a suicide attempt or when suicidal thoughts escalate and the individual feels in danger of acting on these thoughts. Moreover, the risk of suicide is very high following contact with acute psychiatric services,[3] and persistent challenges exist for providing continuity of care after discharge.[4,5] Therefore, EDs represent an important venue in which to identify and treat veterans who are at risk for suicide.

In response to a priority recommendation from a Blue Ribbon Panel on Veteran Suicide in 2008[6] VA leadership called for development and implementation of an ED-based intervention for suicidal veterans. The rationale for such an approach was based on the recognition that ED providers may prefer to hospitalize moderate risk patients because of limited availability and feasibility of interventions that can be provided in the ED. The Blue Ribbon panel recommended that the VA address this gap in services. We describe the design and implementation of an innovative brief behavioral intervention for suicidal veterans who seek care in VA hospital EDs. The overall vision of this VA initiative was to augment emergency mental health service delivery to (1) enhance identification of veterans at risk for suicide in VA hospital EDs, (2) provide a brief intervention to reduce risk, and (3) ensure that veterans receive appropriate and timely follow-up care. This clinical demonstration project became the Suicide Assessment and Follow-up Engagement: Veteran Emergency Treatment (SAFE VET) Project. Designed to mitigate suicidal thoughts and behaviors in veterans through a veteran-focused, clinical safety plan intervention conducted in EDs or Mental Health Urgent Care settings, SAFE VET includes an outreach protocol following discharge. The protocol includes facilitating the veteran's transition to outpatient mental health care, maintaining veteran safety during this transition through regular telephone contact and reviewing and revising the veteran's safety plan.

Prior to development of the SAFE VET project, Stanley and Brown[7] developed an innovative clinical approach to suicide risk reduction across clinical settings for the general population. Stanley and Brown's[7] initial strategy consisted of a brief behavioral intervention they called Safety Planning. Following the Blue Ribbon Panel recommendation, and in collaboration with VA clinicians, Stanley and Brown[8] then developed a modification of Safety Planning specifically tailored for the veteran population. The SAFE VET intervention is grounded on the tenets of Safety Planning, incorporating elements of 4 evidence-based suicide risk reduction strategies: (1) means restriction, (2) teaching brief problem-solving and coping skills (including distraction), (3) enhancing social support and identifying emergency contacts, and (4) motivational enhancement for further treatment. As a novel addition to Safety Planning, SAFE VET integrates intensive follow-up of veterans after discharge from the ED. Key to the delivery of the SAFE VET intervention was the creation of a new position in the VA, the acute services coordinator (ASC) who administers the veteran version of Safety Planning in the ED and makes all the follow-up contacts. The follow-up protocol involves both veterans and their families in implementation of the veteran's individualized safety plan, which is tailored to the veteran's distinctive warning signs, internal coping strategies, contacts of family members or friends, and contacts of professionals or agencies who can offer crisis assistance, including VA's Suicide Hotline (now known as the VA's Crisis Line).

SAFE VET primarily targets those veterans who are assessed as being at moderate risk for suicide and who often become hospitalized. SAFE VET allows for immediate reduction in distress and therefore can provide an alternative to hospitalization. However, identification of high risk veterans also is a critical component of the SAFE VET Project because veterans identified as high risk may be hospitalized, placed on a VA Suicide Prevention Coordinator's high-risk list, or referred for comprehensive outpatient follow-up. Regardless of level of risk, all veterans in the SAFE VET intervention receive VA's Crisis Line number. Figure 1 outlines the pathway of veterans seen in VA ED or Urgent Care who are determined to be at some level of risk for suicidal behaviors.

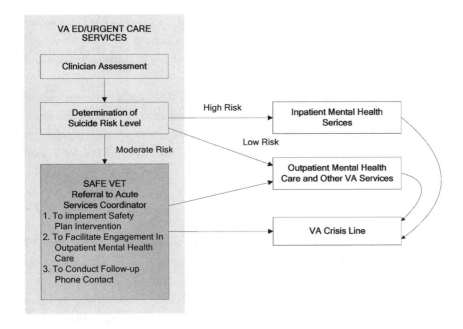

Figure 1. Pathways to care for veterans in Veterans Affairs (VA) emergency department (ED) or urgent care settings.

Note. SAFE VET = Suicide Assessment and Follow-up Engagement: Veteran Emergency Treatment.

EVALUATION

Because SAFE VET is a practical translation of science to service, VA leadership designated an executive committee to develop and oversee the project infrastructure, as well as to disseminate findings of the project. This committee is responsible for quality assurance and adherence of the SAFE VET protocol at each intervention site. In addition to the executive committee, clinical site leaders provide local guidance in their respective EDs. The initial evaluation of the project reported here uses quality assurance data to determine the acceptability of the intervention to veterans (as determined by willingness to receive the intervention) and the impact of intensive telephone contacts following the SAFE VET intervention in the ED (as determined by percentage of veterans who received either outpatient mental health services within 6 months or any psychiatric service within 14 days). As part of the follow-up protocol SAFE VET mainly targets transitioning veterans from the ED into outpatient mental health services, but it was also important to know whether SAFE VET veterans are getting any psychiatric services in the short-term.

Table 1 provides initial information on acceptability of the intervention and follow-up services use.

We also found a significant difference ($P < .001$) in the average number of outpatient mental health visits during the 6 months after the index ED SAFE VET intervention (mean = 9.2) compared with the average number of outpatient mental health visits before the index ED SAFE VET intervention (mean = 4.9).

CONCLUSIONS

Although there are other promising behavioral interventions for suicidal individuals, including the Collaborative Assessment and Management of Suicidality,[9] Cognitive Behavior Therapy,[10] and Dialectical Behavior Therapy,[11] Safety Planning should not be considered as substituting for these more intensive treatments. These interventions differ from Safety Planning in that the latter is readily accessible to patients and professionals, and in the context of a treatment trial conducted by Stanley et al., Safety Planning has been shown to be highly acceptable and feasible to implement.[10]

Table 1. Acceptability of the SAFE VET Intervention to Veterans and Follow-Up Mental Health Related Services Use

Measure	No., Mean ±SD, or No. (%)
Veterans referred to the SAFE VET Demonstration Project	471
Veterans who agreed to receive the SAFE VET intervention	438 (93)
Days between index ED visit and first follow-up	4.4 ±5.5
Follow-up calls made by acute services coordinators	6.2 ±4.4
Veterans who received ≥ 1 outpatient mental health follow-up visit 6 mo after SAFE VET intervention[a]	379 (80)
Percentage of SAFE VET veterans who received any psychiatric service within 14 d of ED discharge[b]	325 (69)

Note. ED = emergency department; SAFE VET = Suicide Assessment and Follow-up Engagement: Veteran Emergency Treatment.
[a]Excludes substance abuse services or admission to the ED and other VA services.
[b]Includes outpatient mental health, substance abuse services, or admission to the ED and other VA services.

Acceptance of the SAFE VET intervention has been extremely high from the perspective of the ED or urgent care mental health providers (see sidebar). Rather than placing a burden on ED clinical providers and overstressed inpatient units, the SAFE VET intervention provides a means of assisting these providers in addressing the needs of a significant subpopulation of veterans who are suicidal but not necessarily appropriate candidates for hospitalization. A key component of the SAFE VET intervention appears to be the intensive follow-up provided by the acute services coordinator (Table 1).

One limitation of the SAFE VET program has been that potentially critical connections between the VA acute services coordinators and community settings where veterans may receive care has yet to be fully realized. We do not have information regarding why 20% of the SAFE VET veterans did not receive any mental health services within 6 months of their index ED visit. It is possible that care was delivered in non-VA settings. Whether care was provided and unknown to us or was never provided would have been critical information to obtain for this demonstration project.

Long-term evaluation of the characteristics of follow-up care is a critical first step for demonstrating the effectiveness of the SAFE VET intervention in the VA. In the general population, the time between discharge from an ED and a follow-up visit to outpatient mental health care has persistently represented a challenge in terms of continuity of care. As shown in Table 1, 80% of SAFE VET veterans received 1 or more outpatient mental health services within 6 months, (including rescheduled visits). This is compared with the reported 10% to 40% of patients who are discharged from the ED in the general population who return for a follow-up visit or a rescheduled visit.[4,5,12]

Although implementation of the demonstration project and quality assurance data reported in this paper reveal that acceptability of the SAFE VET intervention has been high (93% of veterans agreed to receive the SAFE VET intervention; Table 1) and provide some promising information on follow-up services use (Table 1), a research study is needed to demonstrate the effectiveness of SAFE VET on key outcomes. Such a research study is now funded (A Brief Intervention to Reduce Suicide Risk in Military Service Members and Veterans; Award Number W81XWH-09-2-0129, Military Operational Medicine Research Program, Department of Defense) and will use a quasi-experimental design to compare the effectiveness of the SAFE VET intervention versus enhanced care on the following:

- the proportion of patients who attempt suicide within 6 months of the index ED visit,
- the severity of suicide ideation within 6 months after the index ED visit,
- the proportion of patients who attend more than 1 outpatient mental health or substance abuse treatment appointment within 30 days after the index ED visit,
- the degree of suicide-related coping strategies, and
- the motivation to attend treatment during the 6 month period.

"To understand the systemic effect of SAFE VET, I believe it is necessary to put oneself in the place of a frontline clinician in the emergency department who is seeing a patient with suicidal ideation. Such a clinician would be weighing multiple factors and priorities as they make the difficult decision to recommend discharge or admission. My initial impression was that when confronted with this choice, it seemed to be routine practice to suggest voluntary admission to almost every patient who presented with suicidal ideation regardless of the level of severity. Although this is a cautious approach, I wonder how such admissions affect a person who had never been psychiatrically hospitalized. I believe SAFE VET creates a third category of response that fits between discharge and admission. It allows the clinician to respond to the patient's at risk for suicide by implementing safety planning, and allowing the patient to leave the emergency department with some tangible plan for how they are going to cope, and people who they can contact. This seems to me to be a very appropriate response to patient's with non-acute suicidal ideation." (an acute services coordinator)

This future study will recruit up to 600 veterans for each condition and will include assessment at baseline (index ED visit) and 1, 3, and 6 months after the index ED visit to complete the follow-up research measures. If this future research finds that the SAFE VET intervention is effective on key outcomes such as suicide attempts, suicidal ideation, and engagement in care, the approach may be transferable to a wide variety of VA and non-VA settings, including community emergency departments and urgent care centers.

ABOUT THE AUTHORS

At the time of the study, Kerry L. Knox was with the Department of Veterans Affairs, VISN 2 Center of Excellence for Suicide Prevention, Rochester, NY. Barbara Stanley was with Columbia University, New York, NY. Glenn W.

Currier was with the University of Rochester Medical Center, Rochester, NY. Lisa Brenner was with the Department of Veterans Affairs, VISN 19 Mental Illness, Research, Education and Clinical Care, Denver, CO. Marjan Ghahramanlou-Holloway was with Uniformed Services University of the Health Sciences, Bethesda, MD. Gregory Brown was with the University of Pennsylvania, Philadelphia.

CONTRIBUTORS

K. L. Knox, B. Stanley, G. Currier and G. Brown jointly conceptualized and designed the project. G. Brown supervised data collection and data entry, and K. L. Knox supervised the data analysis. K. L. Knox took the lead on writing up the project; all authors contributed to the interpretation of the data and to writing and revising the article.

ACKNOWLEDGMENTS

The Suicide Assessment and Follow-up Engagement: Veteran Emergency Treatment (SAFE VET) project is supported by the Office of Mental Health Services, Department of Veteran Affairs.

Ira Katz, MD, PhD, provided valuable insight into the design of the project. The SAFE VET group consists of an executive committee (Kerry L. Knox, Gregory K. Brown, Glenn W. Currier, Barbara Stanley), site leads (Lisa Brenner, PhD, Joan Chips, LCSW, Joshua Hooberman, PhD, Christine Jackson, PhD, Mitchel Kling, MD, Keith Rogers, MD), and acute services coordinators (Patricia Alexander, PhD, Laura Blandy, PsyD, Aimee Coughlin, MSW, John Dennis, PhD, Michael Miello, PhD, Katherine Mostkoff, LCSW and Jarrod Reisweber, PsyD). We would like to acknowledge key individuals who facilitated implementation of SAFE VET and provided essential guidance: Lauren Denneson, PhD, Steven Dobscha,MD, Walter Matweychuk, PhD, Gerd Naydock, MSW, Keith Rogers, MD, Donald Tavakoli, MD, and Adam Wolkin, MD

HUMAN PARTICIPANT PROTECTION

Institutional review board approval was not required because no human participants were involved.

REFERENCES

1. Kurz A, Möller HJ. Help-seeking behavior and compliance of suicidal patients. *Psychiatr Prac.* 1984;11(1):6–13.

2. Taylor EA, Stansfeld SA. Children who poison themselves. I. A clinical comparison with psychiatric controls. *Br J Psychiatry.* 1984;145:127–132.

3. McCarthy JF, Valenstein M, Kim HM, Ilgen M, Zivin K, Blow FC. Suicide mortality among patients receiving care in the veterans health administration health system. *Am J Epidemiol.* 2009;169(8):1033–1038.

4. Boyer CA, McAlpine DD, Pottick KJ, Olfson M. Identifying risk factors and key strategies in linkage to outpatient psychiatric care. *Am J Psychiatry.* 2000;157(10):1592–1598.

5. Van Heeringen C, Jannes S, Buylaert W, Henderick H, De Bacquer D, Van Remoortel J. The management of non-compliance with referral to out-patient after-care among attempted suicide patients: a controlled intervention study. *Psychol Med.* 1995;25(5):963–970.

6. http://www.mentalhealth.va.gov/suicide_prevention/Blue_Ribbon_Report-FINAL_June-30-08.pdf. Accessed December 22, 2011.

7. Stanley B, Brown GK. Safety planning intervention: a brief intervention to mitigate suicide risk. *Cognit Behav Pract.* In press.

8. Stanley B, Brown GK. *Safety plan treatment manual to reduce suicide risk: veteran version.* Washington, DC: United States Department of Veteran Affairs; 2008.

9. Jobes DA. *Managing suicidal risk: A collaborative approach.* New York, NY: Guilford Press; 2006.

10. Stanley B, Brown GK, Brent DA, et al. Cognitive behavior therapy for suicide prevention (CBT-SP): treatment model, feasibility and acceptability. *J Am Acad Child Adoles Psychiatry.* 2009;48(10):1005–1013.

11. Linehan MM, Comtois KA, Murray AM, et al. Two-year randomized controlled trial and follow-up of dialectical behavior therapy vs therapy by experts for suicidal behaviors and borderline personality disorder. *Arch Gen Psychiatry.* 2006;63(7):757–766.

12. Currier GW, Fisher SG, Caine ED. Mobile crisis team intervention to enhance linkage of discharged suicidal emergency department patients to outpatient psychiatric services: a randomized controlled trial. *Acad Emerg Med.* 2010;17(1):36–43.

PART VII

Research and Practice

16

Prevalence and Characteristics of Suicide Ideation and Attempts Among Active Military and Veteran Participants in a National Health Survey

Robert M. Bossarte, PhD, Kerry L. Knox, PhD, Rebecca Piegari, MS, John Altieri, BS, Janet Kemp, RN, PhD, and Ira R. Katz, MD, PhD

The relationships between military service and suicide are not clear, and comparatively little is known about the characteristics and correlates of suicide ideation and attempts among those with history of military service. We used data from a national health survey to estimate the prevalence and correlates of suicidal behaviors among veterans and service members in 2 states. The prevalence of suicidal behaviors among Veterans was similar to previous estimates of ideation and attempts among adults in the US general population.

There is evidence of increased suicide risk among some veterans and active military. Previous research reported a 66% increase in suicide risk among veterans receiving services from the Veterans Health Administration (VHA),[1] and rates of suicide in some branches of the military have surpassed those of the general population.[2] Suicide among those with history of military service has been associated with psychiatric diagnoses,[3] active service,[4] and time since separation from military service.[5] However, the relationships between military service and suicide are not clear.[6] A study of suicide among older male veterans in the general population[7] and retrospective studies of veterans from previous conflicts[8] failed to identify general increases in risk. Less is known about the prevalence or characteristics of nonfatal suicidal behavior. One study of recent veterans reported a 12.5% prevalence of suicide ideation in the past 2 weeks; there were positive associations with depression and posttraumatic stress disorder (PTSD) and negative associations with the availability of social support.[9] The main objective of the present study was to identify the prevalence and correlates of nonfatal suicide among veterans and service members in the general population.

METHODS

Analyses were calculated using data from the 2010 Behavioral Risk Factor Surveillance System (BRFSS). BRFSS methodology has been previously described.[10] Briefly, BRFSS is an annual survey that utilizes a representative sample of noninstitutionalized US adults in US states and territories. Measures for this project were obtained from the core questionnaire and optional Veteran's Health Module (VHM) administered in 2 states (Nebraska and Tennessee). Optional modules contain questions asked in addition to the BRFSS core questionnaire and are selected by states on an annual basis. Among participating states, questions from the VHM were asked of participants reporting history of US military service, a measure included in the BRFSS core questionnaire. In 2010, the response rates in states participating in the VHM were 68.8% (Nebraska) and 54.6% (Tennessee).[11] Measures obtained from the core questionnaire included age, gender, race/ethnicity, marital status, self-rated health, history of active military service, and availability of emotional and social support. Measures obtained from the VHM included suicide ideation and suicide attempt during the past 12 months, service in combat or war zone, psychiatric diagnosis ("Has a doctor or other health professional ever told you that you have depression, anxiety, or PTSD?"), traumatic brain injury (TBI; "A TBI may result from a violent blow to the head or when an object pierces the skull and enters the brain tissue. Has a doctor or other health professional ever told you that you have suffered a TBI?"), and psychological or psychiatric counseling in the past 12 months. Outcome measures included suicide ideation ("Has there been a time in the past 12 months when you thought of taking your own life?") and suicide attempt ("During the past 12 months, did you attempt to commit suicide?"). The question about suicide attempts was limited to participants who endorsed thoughts of suicide in the past 12 months. Analyses were conducted in SAS version 9.2 (SAS Institute, Cary, North Carolina) and were weighted to adjust for nonresponse and sample selection.

RESULTS

A total of 2602 participants with history of military service completed the VHM. Among them, 3.8% (n = 66) reported suicide ideation and 0.4% (n = 8) reported a suicide attempt in the past 12 months (Table 1). An estimated 35.2% (95% confidence interval [CI] = 19.3, 51.2) of participants who reported mental health counseling received all or some of their care from the VHA. Veterans reporting suicide ideation were significantly more likely to be between 60 and 79 years of age, non-Hispanic Other, reported a psychiatric diagnosis or counseling, and reported lower levels of social support compared with those reporting no ideation. The prevalence of suicide ideation was highest among those who reported a diagnosis of depression, anxiety, or PTSD (17.4%; 95% CI = 7.9, 26.8). Recent service was also associated with differences in the prevalence of suicide ideation, with the highest proportion reported among those who had separated from active service between 1 and 12 months before survey participation (5.3%; 95% CI = 0.0, 11.4) compared with those actively serving (2.0%; 95% CI = 0.0, 5.4) or with more than 12 months since separation (3.7%; 95% CI = 1.7, 5.7). However, differences in the prevalence of suicide ideation related to recent service were not statistically significant. Results from regression analyses identified 2 measures significantly associated with suicide ideation (Table 2). Report of a psychiatric diagnosis was associated with an increased probability nearly 22 times that of those without similar reports, and social support was associated with an 82% decrease in the probability of suicide ideation in the past 12 months.

DISCUSSION

Results from this study supported previous reports of increased risk associated with psychiatric diagnoses[3] and the protective nature of social support.[9] There were no significant differences in suicide ideation associated with time since separation. Overall, the prevalence of suicide ideation and attempts identified in this study were similar to estimates of those outcomes in the US general population (3.7% and 0.5%, respectively).[12]

Table 1. Demographic and Risk Characteristics of Suicide Ideation and Attempts Among Active Military and Veteran Participants: Behavioral Risk Factor Surveillance System, 2010

	Full Sample (n = 2602), % (95% CI)	Suicide-IDE (n = 66), % (95% CI)	Suicide-NEG (n = 2536), % (95% CI)	Rao-Scott χ^2	P
Age 18–39 y	15.9 (10.2–21.5)	24.9 (0.0, 58.8)	15.5 (9.7, 21.3)	0.64	.42
Age 40–59 y	32.7 (27.9, 37.6)	53.4 (27.6, 79.3)	31.9 (27.0, 36.9)	3.09	.08
Age 60–79 y	41.6 (36.9, 46.3)	19.5 (3.3, 35.8)	42.4 (37.6, 47.3)	5.27	.02
Age ⩾ 80 y	9.8 (7.6, 12.1)	2.1 (0.0, 6.2)	10.2 (7.8, 12.5)	3.34	.07
Male	91.5 (88.8, 94.2)	73.3 (45.5, 100.0)	92.2 (89.7, 94.7)	5.19	.02
White, non-Hispanic	85.2 (80.4, 90.0)	70.8 (42.8, 98.9)	85.8 (80.9, 90.7)	1.89	.17
Black, non-Hispanic	7.1 (4.7, 9.5)	2.2 (0.0, 5.5)	7.3 (4.8, 9.7)	2.81	.09
Other, non-Hispanic	6.7 (2.2, 4.2)	25.7 (0.0, 54.3)	5.9 (1.4, 10.5)	5.10	.02
Hispanic	1.2 (0.4, 1.7)	1.2 (0.0, 3.2)	1.1 (0.4, 1.7)	0.04	.84
Married/cohabitating	75.1 (71.2, 78.9)	65.3 (42.2, 88.4)	75.5 (71.6, 79.4)	0.93	.33
Poor self-rated health	56.5 (53.3, 59.7)	72.9 (48.2, 97.7)	54.0 (48.8, 59.2)	1.99	.16
Active military	4.7 (1.9, 7.5)	2.4 (0.0, 6.7)	4.8 (1.9, 7.7)	0.61	.44
Veteran (service ≤ 12 mo)	12.5 (7.8, 17.2)	17.4 (0.0, 36.4)	12.3 (7.4, 17.1)	0.33	.56
Veteran (service > 12 mo)	82.8 (77.7, 88.0)	80.2 (60.7, 99.7)	82.9 (77.6, 88.2)	0.08	.78
Service in combat zone	43.5 (30.3, 48.8)	36.7 (11.3, 62.1)	43.8 (38.4, 49.2)	0.31	.58
Report of depression, anxiety, PTSD	16.5 (12.4, 20.5)	75.0 (52.4, 97.6)	14.1 (10.2, 18.1)	40.29	< .001
Traumatic brain injury	3.7 (1.3, 6.2)	8.9 (0.0, 20.1)	3.5 (1.0, 6.0)	1.84	.17
Mental health counseling/treatment	11.0 (7.4, 14.6)	52.1 (25.9, 78.1)	9.3 (5.8, 12.9)	26.42	< .001
Emotional/social support	81.7 (71.0, 86.4)	54.0 (28.1, 79.9)	82.8 (78.0, 87.6)	7.92	.005
Suicide ideation (past 12 mo)	3.8 (2.0, 5.6)	...	...	...	...
Suicide attempt (past 12 mo)	0.4 (0.0, 1.1)	...	...	...	...

Note. CI = confidence interval; IDE = ideation; NEG = negative; PTSD = posttraumatic stress disorder.

Table 2. Associations Between Risk Factors and Probability of Suicide Ideation and Attempts Among Active Military and Veteran Participants: Behavioral Risk Factor Surveillance System, 2010

Risk Factors	AOR (95% CI)
Age, y	
18–39 y (Ref)	1.0
40–59 y	1.5 (0.3, 7.1)
60–79 y	0.9 (0.2, 4.6)
≥80 y	0.6 (0.1, 5.5)
Gender	
Female (Ref)	1.0
Male	0.3 (0.1, 1.7)
Race/ethnicity	
White, Non-Hispanic (Ref)	1.0
Black, Non-Hispanic	0.4 (0.1, 2.6)
Other, Non-Hispanic	4.2 (0.7, 23.9)
Hispanic	3.1 (0.6, 17.7)
Mental health status	
No report of depression, anxiety, or PTSD (Ref)	1.0
Report of depression, anxiety, or PTSD	21.7 (5.6, 84.3)
Support status	
Never, rarely, or sometimes receive social and emotional support (Ref)	1.0
Usually or always receive social and emotional support	0.2 (0.1, 0.6)

Note. AOR = adjusted odds ratio; CI = confidence interval; PTSD = posttraumatic stress disorder.

There were several limitations that should be considered when interpreting results of this study. Estimates of suicide ideation or attempts, reports of military service (including combat), psychiatric diagnosis, TBI, and mental health treatment were based on self-reported data and were not validated. Data on dates of psychiatric diagnosis and suicide ideation or attempt were not available. Therefore, the order of these events could not be established. The optional module was limited to veterans in 2 states, and results might not be generalizable to the larger veteran or active service populations. The number of participants reporting suicide ideation was small, and this might have impacted the ability to identify statistically significant relationships with other measures. BRFSS contains self-reported data that were not validated using external sources. The prevalence of psychiatric disorders or TBI estimated using VHM data might not be consistent with estimates derived from clinical records or symptom assessment. Finally, the characteristics of BRFSS participants might not be similar to those who refused, were not selected, or were not eligible to participate.

Previous analyses of the relationships between military service and risk for suicide were primarily limited to studies of mortality and service-utilizing subpopulations and might not extend to nonfatal behaviors or veterans in the general population. The VHM was selected for use by 9 additional states in 2011. Future analyses should be conducted to confirm the relationships identified in this study.

ABOUT THE AUTHORS

Robert M. Bossarte, Kerry L. Knox, Rebecca Piegari and John Altieri are with the Veterans Integrated Service Network (VISN) 2 Center of Excellence for Suicide Prevention, Department of Veterans Affairs, Canandaigua, NY. Robert M. Bossarte and Kerry L. Knox are also with the Department of Psychiatry, University of Rochester, Rochester, NY. Janet Kemp is with the Office of Mental Health Services, Department of Veterans Affairs, Washington, DC. Ira R. Katz is with the Office of Mental Health Operations, Department of Veterans Affairs, Washington, DC.

ACKNOWLEDGMENTS

This work was supported by funding from the VISN 2 Center of Excellence for Suicide Prevention, Canandaigua, NY, and the Office of Mental Health Services, Department of Veterans Affairs, Washington, DC.

The authors would like to acknowledge the contributions of Alex Crosby, Marcia Valenstein, Mark Ilgen, John Crilly, and Glenn Currier for their participation in the development of the Veteran's Health Module.

HUMAN PARTICIPANT PROTECTION

Analysis of Behavioral Risk Factor Surveillance System data was approved by the Syracuse Veterans Affairs Medical Center Institutional Review Board.

REFERENCES

1. McCarthy JF, Valenstein M, Kim HM, Ilgen M, Zivin K, Blow FC. Suicide mortality among patients receiving care in the Veterans Health Adminstration Health System. *Am J Epidemiol.* 2009;169(8):1033–1038.

2. Kuehn BM. Military probes epidemic of suicide: mental health issues remain prevalent. *JAMA.* 2010;304(13):1427, 1429–1430.

3. Ilgen MA, Bohnert AS, Ignacio RV, et al. Psychiatric diagnoses and risk of suicide in veterans. *Arch Gen Psychiatry.* 2010;67(11):1152–1158.

4. Kang HK, Bullman TA. Risk of suicide among US veterans after returning from the Iraq and Afghanistan war zones. *JAMA.* 2008;300(6):652–653.

5. Kapur N, While D, Blatchley N, Bray I, Harrison K. Suicide after leaving the UK Armed Forces—a cohort study. *PLoS Med.* 2009;6(3):e26.

6. Bossarte RM, Claassen CA, Knox KL. Evaluating evidence of risk for suicide among veterans. *Mil Med.* 2010;175(10):703–704.

7. Miller M, Barber C, Azreal D, Calle E, Lawler E, Mukamal K. Suicide among US veterans: a prospective study of 500,000 middle-aged and elderly men. *Am J Epidemiol.* 2009;170(4):494–500.

8. Kang HK, Bullman TA. Is there an epidemic of suicides among current and former US military personnel? *Ann Epidemiol.* 2009;19(10):757–760.

9. Pietrzak RH, Goldstein MB, Malley JC, Rivers AJ, Johnson DC, Southwick SM. Risk and protective factors associated with suicidal ideation in veterans of Operations Enduring Freedom and Iraqi Freedom. *J Affect Disord.* 2010;123:102–107.

10. Centers for Disease Control and Prevention (CDC). *Behavioral Risk Factor Surveillance System: Operational and Users Guide.* Washington, DC: Department of Health and Human Services; 2006.

11. Centers for Disease Control and Prevention (CDC). Behavioral Risk Factor Surveillance System. Summary Data. *Qual Rep.* 2010. Version #1, Revised 05/02/ 2011.

12. National Survey on Drug Use and Health. *Suicidal Thoughts and Behaviors among Adults.* Rockville, MD: Substance Abuse and Mental Health Services Administration; 2009.

17

Characteristics of Suicides Among US Army Active Duty Personnel in 17 US States From 2005 to 2007

Joseph Logan, PhD, Nancy A. Skopp, PhD, Debra Karch, PhD, Mark A. Reger, PhD, and Gregory A. Gahm, PhD

Suicides are increasing among active duty US Army soldiers. To help focus prevention strategies, we characterized 56 US Army suicides that occurred from 2005 to 2007 in 17 US states using 2 large-scale surveillance systems. We found that intimate partner problems and military-related stress, particularly job stress, were common among decedents. Many decedents were also identified as having suicidal ideation, a sad or depressed mood, or a recent crisis before death. Focusing efforts to prevent these forms of stress might reduce suicides among soldiers.

In recent years, the suicide rate has increased among US Army active duty personnel.[1,2] The estimated suicide rate for this population nearly doubled from 2004 to 2008 (from 10.8 to 20.2 per 100 000).[1,2]

Mental health conditions, substance abuse problems, certain physical health problems (e.g., cancer, chronic pain), and financial, legal, and relationship problems are risk factors for suicide among civilian and military populations.[3–14] Building on this research, we used data from 2 large-scale surveillance systems to assess the frequency of these factors as well as other military-related stresses (e.g., recent combat exposure, job problems, disciplinary proceedings) among suicide decedents who were on active duty in the US Army and residing in the United States to determine the most prevalent circumstances preceding suicide for this population. A better understanding of the most common preceding circumstances among the number of known risk factors for suicide might help focus military suicide prevention initiatives.[15,16]

METHODS

We obtained data for active duty US Army suicide decedents who died during 2005 to 2007. Two large-scale surveillance systems, the National Violent Death Reporting System (NVDRS) and the Department of Defense Suicide Event Report (DoDSER) were linked to comprehensively characterize the decedents.

NVDRS uses coroner or medical examiner and toxicology reports, law enforcement records, and death certificates to provide details on suicides, such as decedent demographic information, mechanism or weapon information, and preceding health and stressful life-event circumstance information.[17] During the study, NVDRS collected data from 17 US states; therefore, case inclusion for this study was limited to suicide cases that had death certificates filed in one of those states. The 17 NVDRS states were Alaska, California, Colorado, Georgia, Kentucky, Maryland, Massachusetts, New Jersey, New Mexico, North Carolina, Oklahoma, Oregon, Rhode Island, South Carolina, Utah, Virginia, and Wisconsin. Data collected in NVDRS was statewide with the exception of California, which collected data in only 5 counties (Los Angeles, Riverside, San Francisco, Alameda, and Santa Clara). NVDRS has been described in detail elsewhere.[17,18]

DoDSER data provide details on suicides for all active duty service members. The DoDSER is part of a suicide surveillance program that standardizes retrospective suicide surveillance efforts across the US service branches. The DoDSER was first launched in 2008; however, the 2005–2007 data we used were collected from the Army Suicide Event Report (ASER), the predecessor to the DoDSER that collected data only for US Army suicide deaths. The DoDSER's web-based data collection process was modeled after the ASER and was developed by the National Center for Telehealth and Technology in collaboration with the Department of Defense's Suicide Prevention and Risk Reduction Committee's Suicide Prevention Program Managers representing all of the service branches. This system provides many details unavailable in NVDRS, such as the decedent's military background, family history, health service utilization, combat exposure, and military disciplinary history.[19] DoDSER data also provide details on circumstances preceding suicide. DoDSERs are completed by behavioral health providers within 60 days of the suicide; each report requires information from medical, mental health, and personnel records, any other relevant documents, and interviews with the decedent's coworkers, supervisors, friends, family members, and any other acquaintances or involved law enforcement and health professionals, as appropriate.[19]

The decedent population was initially identified in the DoDSER database. Cases were linked to NVDRS using incident variables (i.e., state and date of death) and decedent demographic variables (i.e., age, gender, race/ethnicity, marital status, veteran status, and occupation). No personal identifying information was linked into the final dataset. Fifty-nine decedents were identified in the DoDSER, and 56 (90%) cases were linked and thereby included in the study.

RESULTS

Table 1 shows that most decedents were males; of White, non-Hispanic race/ethnicity; less than 30 years old; married; and in the enlisted ranks. Approximately 46% of the decedents had children, and half of these decedents had children residing with them. Sixty-one percent of the decedents died in their personal residences, and 55% used a firearm in the incident. Over a third of the decedents left evidence suggesting their suicide was planned, and 21% left suicide notes, which also suggests premeditation.

Table 2 shows the prevalence of various health and stress-related circumstances preceding death. The most common circumstances were intimate partner problems (45%) and military-related stress (41%); current job problems and combat experiences were the most common military specific circumstances. Many decedents showed symptoms of mental health distress (e.g., 36% communicated their intent to self harm, 32% were identified as having a depressed mood) or had a recent crisis (32%). Twenty-three percent of the decedents received a mental health diagnosis. Alcohol was involved in over a quarter of the incidents. Alcohol and substance abuse, physical health, criminal and civil legal, and financial problems were also evident among some decedents.

Table 1. Demographic and Other Background Characteristics of Active Duty US Army Suicide Decedents and Characteristics of the Suicide Events: 2005–2007

Variable	No. (%)
Age, y	
18–24	21 (37.5)
25–29	14 (25.0)
30–39	13 (23.2)
40–49	6 (10.7)
50–59	...
Gender	
Male	53 (94.6)
Female	3 (5.4)
Race/ethnicity	
White, non-Hispanic	42 (75.0)
Black, non-Hispanic	9 (16.1)
American Indian/Alaskan Native	...
Asian/Pacific Islander	...
Hispanic	...
Marital status	
Married	34 (60.7)
Never married	16 (28.6)
Widowed, divorced, or separated	4 (7.1)
Single unspecified or unknown	...
Household and parental factors	
Decedent resided alone	17 (30.4)
Decedent had children	26 (46.4)
Children resided with decedent (% is calculated among decedents who had children)	13 (50.0)
US Army status	
Regular	43 (76.8)
Reserve	4 (7.1)
National Guard	8 (14.3)
Other	...
Duty status	
Active duty	45 (80.4)
Active Guard/Reserve	3 (5.4)
Active duty for training duty	4 (7.1)
Other	4 (7.1)
Pay grade	
E1–E2	6 (10.7)
E3	8 (14.3)
E4	16 (28.6)

(continued on next page)

Table 1. (*continued*)

Variable	No. (%)
E5	8 (14.3)
E6	6 (10.7)
E7	4 (7.1)
E8–E9	3 (5.4)
W1-5	...
O1-10	4 (7.1)
Location of death	
Personal residence	34 (60.7)
Residence of family or friend	6 (10.7)
Automobile (away from residence)	5 (8.9)
Other	11 (19.6)
Weapon/mechanism used	
Firearm	31 (55.4)
Poisoning	7 (12.5)
Hanging, strangulation	15 (26.8)
Other or unknown	3 (5.4)
Other event characteristics[a]	
Left evidence suggesting the event was planned	20 (35.7)
Left a suicide note	12 (21.4)

Note. E = enlisted ranks; O = commissioned officer ranks; W = warrant officer ranks. The Sample size was n = 56. Ellipses indicate that items with less than 3 counts (< 5% of the population) were suppressed to prevent potential identification of decedents.
[a]Categories are not mutually exclusive.

DISCUSSION

The range in rank distribution among suicide decedents reflected the general Army population,[20] and the decedent demographics were similar to other, mostly civilian, suicide populations.[21-23] The finding that intimate partner problems were the most common circumstances preceding suicide death was also similar to findings in other studies that described characteristics of a male suicide decedent population[21-23]; however, the proportion of decedents with preceding job problems was concerning. Among mostly male civilian suicide decedent populations during the same data years, only 12.3% to 12.6% of decedents had reported job problems.[21-23] Similar to other suicide populations, many decedents were identified as sad, depressed, or suicidal by family members, friends, coworkers, clinicians, and other acquaintances, which

Table 2. Health Related Characteristics of Active Duty US Army Suicide Decedents and Stressful Life-Event Circumstances Preceding Death: 2005–2007

Variable	No. (%)
Health–related factors	
Suicidal ideation—disclosed intent of self harm[a]	20 (35.7)
Current depressed mood	18 (32.1)
Substance use at time of incident	
Alcohol use[b]	16 (28.6)
Drug use[c] (% is calculated among those tested)	8 (30.8)
Current mental health problem	13 (23.2)
Diagnoses[d] (% is calculated among those who had current mental health problems)	
Depression/dysthymia	9 (69.2)
Posttraumatic stress disorder	3 (23.1)
Other	3 (23.1)
Unknown	...
Alcohol or other substance abuse problems	7 (12.5)
Current physical health problem[e]	4 (7.1)
Stressful life event factors[f]	
Recent intimate partner problems	25 (44.6)
Any military-related stressful circumstances[g]	23 (41.1)
Military specific circumstances[h] (% is calculated among those who had any military-related stress)	
Current job-related problems	14 (60.9)
Experienced combat in last deployment	9 (39.1)
Subject to administrative separation	5 (21.7)
Subject to AWOL proceedings	4 (17.4)
Subject to medical evaluation board	3 (13.0)
Subject to courts martial proceedings	...
Recent crisis (within 2 wk of death)	18 (32.1)
Subject to other civil criminal or Article 15 proceedings	8 (14.3)
Recent civil legal issues	8 (14.3)
Recently perpetrated interpersonal violence	5 (8.9)
Recent financial problems	4 (7.1)
Recent other relationship problems	...
Recently was a victim of interpersonal violence	...

Note. AWOL = absent-without-leave. The sample size was n = 56. Ellipses indicate that items with less than 3 counts (< 5% of the population) were suppressed to prevent potential identification of decedents.

[a]The decedent communicated potential for self harm. This variable excluded leaving a suicide note.

[b]Alcohol use was determined by toxicologic tests and whether there was evidence of use (e.g., witnesses or investigative reports that state the victim was seen drinking before the incident).
[c]Drug use was determined by toxicologic tests alone. Toxicologic tests were conducted for 26 decedents.
[d]Diagnostic categories are not mutually exclusive.
[e]Physical health problems refer to only medical problems perceived to have precipitated the suicide.
[f]Stressful life-event factors are not mutually exclusive.
[g]The variable "any military-related stressful circumstances" did not include those undergoing Article 15 proceedings as a circumstance because these decedents could have been actually undergoing civilian criminal proceedings based on how information for this variable is collected. However, over 90% of those who were identified as undergoing Article 15 proceedings also had other military-related stresses before death that were included in this variable; therefore, the proportion of decedents identified as having any military-related stressful circumstances was not largely underestimated.
[h]Categories are not mutually exclusive.

further shows the difficulty of knowing when and how to help someone in need of mental health services.[21-23]

These findings must be viewed cautiously. These results neither provided national representation nor representation of suicides that occurred overseas. Causality could not be inferred between the circumstances and the suicides, and all circumstance information was gleaned from previous reports and interviews, which might not reflect all information known about the incidents. Mental and medical health information was obtained from sources for NVDRS, which include coroner or medical examiners, family members, and friends of the victims. These informants might not have known all of the decedents' health information; therefore, some health conditions might have been underestimated.

This research used details from 2 federal surveillance systems to not only characterize US Army suicide incidents but also to help describe the most prevalent circumstances that commonly precede death. Future studies are planned to compare the characteristics of this population to those of soldiers who died by suicide overseas and civilian suicide decedents to further determine their unique suicide circumstances. The findings in this report suggest focusing military suicide prevention efforts toward building positive intimate partner relationships, increasing coping skills to handle job-related problems, increasing access to mental health or substance abuse treatment, and providing support for soldiers currently in treatment.

ABOUT THE AUTHORS

Joseph Logan and Debra Karch are affiliated with Centers for Disease Control and Prevention, National Center for Injury Prevention and Control, Division of Violence Prevention, Etiology and Surveillance Branch, Atlanta, GA. Nancy A. Skopp, Mark A. Reger, and Gregory A. Gahm are affiliated with the National Center for Telehealth and Technology, Tacoma, WA.

ACKNOWLEDGMENTS

We would like to thank all of the staff at the Centers for Disease Control and Prevention and the National Center for Telehealth and Technology who helped support this project, especially those who helped with the data linkage.

Note. The findings and conclusions in this manuscript are those of the authors and do not necessarily represent the views of the Centers for Disease Control and Prevention/the Agency for Toxic Substances and Disease Registry and National Center for Telehealth and Technology. Also, The opinions or assertions contained herein are the private views of the authors and are not to be construed as official or reflecting the views of the Department of the Army or the Department of Defense.

HUMAN PARTICIPANT PROTECTION

All appropriate institutional review board approvals were received for the data linkage. Approval was not necessary to conduct this study. No living human subjects were recruited for this study.

REFERENCES

1. Levin A. Dramatic increase found in soldier suicides. *Psychiatr News.* 2007;42(18):9.

2. Kuehn BM. Soldier suicide rates continue to rise: military, scientists work to stem the tide. *JAMA.* 2009;301(11):1111–1113.

3. Kung HC, Pearson JL, Liu X. Risk factors for male and female suicide decedents ages 15-64 in the United States. Results from the 1993 National Mortality Followback Survey. *Soc Psychiatry Psychiatr Epidemiol.* 2003;38(8):419–426.

4. Mościcki EK. Epidemiology of suicide. *Int Psychogeriatr.* 1995;7(2):137–148.

5. Miller M, Mogun H, Azrael D, Hempstead K, Solomon DH. Cancer and the risk of suicide in older Americans. *J Clin Oncol.* 2008;26(29):4720–4724.

6. Brådvik L, Berglund M. Depressive episodes with suicide attempts in severe depression: suicides and controls differ only in the later episodes of unipolar depression. *Arch Suicide Res.* 2010;14(4):363–367.

7. Brådvik L, Mattisson C, Bogren M, Nettelbladt P. Mental disorders in suicide and undetermined death in the Lundby Study. The contribution of severe depression and alcohol dependence. *Arch Suicide Res.* 2010;14(3):266–275.

8. Ilgen MA, Bohnert AS, Ignacio RV, et al. Psychiatric diagnoses and risk of suicide in veterans. *Arch Gen Psychiatry.* 2010;67(11):1152–1158.

9. CDC. Homicides and suicides—National Violent Death Reporting System, United States, 2003-2004. *MMWR Morb Motal Wkly Rep.* 2006;55(26):721–724.

10. Kõlves K, Värnik A, Schneider B, Fritze J, Allik J. Recent life events and suicide: a case-control study in Tallinn and Frankfurt. *Soc Sci Med.* 2006;62(11):2887–2896.

11. Stack S, Wasserman I. Economic strain and suicide risk: a qualitative analysis. *Suicide Life Threat Behav.* 2007;37(1):103–112.

12. Jakupcak M, Cook J, Imel Z, Fontana A, Rosenheck R, McFall M. Posttraumatic stress disorder as a risk factor for suicidal ideation in Iraq and Afghanistan War veterans. *J Trauma Stress.* 2009;22(4):303–306.

13. Mahon MJ, Tobin JP, Cusack DA, Kelleher C, Malone KM. Suicide among regular-duty military personnel: a retrospective case-control study of occupation-specific risk factors for workplace suicide. *Am J Psychiatry.* 2005;162(9):1688–1696.

14. Pietrzak RH, Goldstein MB, Malley JC, Rivers AJ, Johnson DC, Southwick SM. Risk and protective factors associated with suicidal ideation in veterans of Operations Enduring Freedom and Iraqi Freedom. *J Affect Disord.* 2010;123(1-3):102–107.

15. Bagley SC, Munjas B, Shekelle P. A systematic review of suicide prevention programs for military or veterans. *Suicide Life Threat Behav.* 2010;40(3):257–265.

16. Ramchand R, Acosta J, Burns RM, Jaycox LH, Pernin CG. The war within: preventing suicide in the US military. Santa Monica, CA: RAND Corporation. Available at http://www.rand.org/pubs/monographs/MG953. Accessed July 25, 2011.

17. Paulozzi LJ, Mercy J, Frazier L Jr, Annest JL. CDC's National Violent Death Reporting System: background and methodology. *Inj Prev.* 2004;10(1):47–52.

18. CDC. National Violent Death Reporting System (NVDRS) Coding Manual Version 3; National Center for Injury Prevention and Control, Centers for Disease Control and Prevention, Atlanta, GA; 2008. Available at: http://www.cdc.gov/violenceprevention/pdf/NVDRS_Coding_Manual_Version_3-a.pdf. Accessed February 10, 2011.

19. Army Behavioral Health Technology Office. *Suicide Risk Management & Surveillance Office. Army Suicide Event Report (ASER) CY 2007.* Tacoma, WA: Madigan Army Medical Center; 2007:98431.

20. Department of Defense. Demographics 2009: Profile of the military community. Office of the Deputy Under Secretary of Defense Military and Family Policy. Available at: http://www.militaryhomefront.dod.mil/portal/page/mhf/MHF/MHF_DETAIL_0?current_id=20.20.60.70.0.0.0.0.0. Accessed on July 25, 2011.

21. Karch DL, Dahlberg LL, Patel N. Surveillance for violent deaths—National Violent Death Reporting System, 16 States, 2007. *MMWR Surveill Summ.* 2010;59(4):1–50.

22. Karch DL, Dahlberg LL, Patel N, et al. Surveillance for violent deaths—National Violent Death Reporting System, 16 States, 2006. *MMWR Surveill Summ.* 2009;58(1):1–44.

23. Karch DL, Lubell KM, Friday J, Patel N, Williams DD. Surveillance for violent deaths—National Violent Death Reporting System, 16 states, 2005. *MMWR Surveill Summ.* 2008;57(3):1–45.

18

Suicidal Ideation Among Sexual Minority Veterans: Results From the 2005–2010 Massachusetts Behavioral Risk Factor Surveillance Survey

John R. Blosnich, PhD, Robert M. Bossarte, PhD, and Vincent M. B. Silenzio, MD

Suicide is a public health problem disproportionately associated with some demographic characteristics (e.g., sexual orientation, veteran status). Analyses of the Massachusetts Behavioral Risk Factor Surveillance Survey data revealed that more lesbian, gay, and bisexual (i.e., sexual minority) veterans reported suicidal ideation compared with heterosexual veterans. Decreased social and emotional support contributed to explaining the association between sexual minority status and suicidal ideation. More research is needed about suicide risk among sexual minority veterans; they might be a population for outreach and intervention by the Veterans Health Administration.

In 2008, over 400 000 people engaged in suicidal behavior, with suicide ranking as the tenth leading cause of death.[1] Although the etiologies of suicide-related morbidity and mortality are complex, research documented that lesbian, gay, and bisexual (i.e., sexual minority) populations bore a disproportionate burden of suicidal ideation and behavior.[2] Although excess risk for suicide was identified among veterans who received services from the Veterans Health Administration[3] or experienced active duty in Iraq or Afghanistan,[4] the literature was unclear about whether veteran status might be universally associated with elevated suicide risk.[5] Gates[6] estimated that there were nearly 1 million gay and lesbian veterans; however, currently, there is little—if any—literature about sexual minority veterans' health. This report aimed (1) to document the prevalence of sexual minority status among veterans in a representative statewide sample and (2) to compare mental health indicators and suicidal ideation by sexual minority status.

METHODS

Data were combined from the 2005 to 2010 Massachusetts Behavioral Risk Factor Surveillance Survey (BRFSS), which used random samples of noninstitutionalized adults ($>$ 18 years) within the state.[7] The analytic sample was limited to respondents randomly selected for a state-added module that assessed suicidal ideation ("During the past 12 months, did you ever seriously consider attempting suicide?"). Sexual orientation was assessed with a state-added question: "Do you consider yourself to be: heterosexual or straight; homosexual or gay or lesbian; bisexual; or other?" Veteran status was ascertained with a standardized item ("Have you ever served on active duty in the United States Armed Forces, either in the regular military or in a National Guard or military reserve unit? Active duty does not include training for the Reserves or National Guard, but DOES include activation, for example, for the Persian Gulf War."). Veterans were defined as indicating "Yes, on active duty during the last 12 months, but not now," or "Yes, on active duty in the past, but not during the last 12 months."

Group differences were examined with the χ^2 test of independence and the Fisher exact test for small sample sizes, and outcomes were tested with logistic regression models adjusted for demographic characteristics, social and emotional support ("How often do you get the social and emotional support you need?"), poor mental health ("Now thinking about your mental health, which includes stress, depression, and problems with emotions, for how many days during the past 30 days was your mental health not good?"), and perceived health status ("Would you say that in general your health is...; see Table 1). Maximum likelihood estimation was used to replace missing data for measures other than sexual orientation and suicidal ideation. The Syracuse Veterans Affairs (VA) Medical Center Institutional Review Board approved this project. All analyses were conducted using SAS version 9.2 (SAS Institute, Cary, North Carolina).

RESULTS

Concordant with previous findings, veteran status was proportionally higher among sexual minority women than heterosexual women.[6] Sexual minority veterans had significantly less availability of social and emotional support and higher prevalence of suicidal ideation. Sexual minority status was significantly associated with suicidal ideation in a model adjusted only by demographic covariates (data not shown); however, the addition of poor mental health and availability of social and emotional support variables attenuated the association (Table 1).

DISCUSSION

Among the entire sample, veteran suicidal ideation (3.76%) did not differ significantly from findings in other studies of veterans[8] or the US general population.[9] However, our results suggested that sexual minority veterans had a higher burden of suicidal ideation, which was concordant with other studies comparing outcomes by sexual orientation.[2] Moreover, although sexual minority veterans had higher odds of suicidal ideation, the difference was explained by poor mental health and lower social and emotional support. This finding lent evidence that sexual orientation, in itself, was not a risk factor for poor health outcomes or risk behaviors.[10,11] It also demonstrated that, in explaining the excess burden of suicidal ideation among sexual minority veterans, a key factor might be perceived social isolation, of which 1 hypothesized source could be marginalization because of homophobia and heterosexism.

Several limitations must be noted. Although a probability-based sample, the number of sexual minority respondents reporting suicidal ideation was small, and estimates were unweighted, limiting generalizability. Causation could not be inferred from this cross-sectional data. Underreporting was a likely issue given the stigma surrounding both sexual orientation and suicidal behavior. Omitted variable bias might have resulted because potentially key variables explaining suicide risk among veteran populations—namely, substance use—were not included in the analyses. Lastly, the self-identified veteran status limited the abilities to verify history of military service and to discern characteristics germane to suicidal behavior among veterans (e.g., period of service).[12]

To our knowledge, this report was one of the first to document the prevalence of and mental health indicators among sexual minority veterans.

Table 1. Demographics and Mental Health Indicators and Odds of Past 12 Months Suicidal Ideation Among Veterans, by Sexual Orientation: Massachusetts Behavioral Risk Factor Surveillance Survey, 2005–2010

Variables	Bivariate Comparisons		Multivariate Analysis: Suicidal Ideation AOR (95% CI)
	Sexual Minority, No. (%)	Heterosexual,[a] No. (%)	
Demographics			
Sexual orientation	61 (3.59)	1639 (96.41)	2.40 (0.92, 6.28)
Sex			
Males	49* (80.33)	1482 (90.42)	0.59 (0.29, 1.25)
Females[b]	12* (19.67)	157 (9.58)	...
Age, y			
18–39[b]	6 (9.84)	177 (10.80)	...
40–64	42 (68.85)	977 (59.61)	1.01 (0.36, 2.79)
> 64	13 (21.31)	485 (29.59)	0.73 (0.23, 2.30)
Race[c]			
Non-White[b]	2 (3.38)	173 (10.56)	...
White	59 (96.72)	1465 (89.44)	1.18 (0.48, 2.89)
Partnership status			
Married/cohabitating	19* (31.15)	952 (58.12)	0.57 (0.32, 1.03)
Single/divorced/ separated/widowed[b]	41* (68.85)	686 (41.88)	...
Mental health indicators			
Poor mental health			
> 15 d/30 d	10 (16.39)	180 (10.98)	...
< 15 d/30 d[b]	51 (83.61)	1459 (89.02)	5.66* (3.10, 10.35)
Perceived health status			
Excellent/very good/good	47 (77.05)	1360 (82.98)	0.48* (0.26, 0.88)
Fair/poor[b]	14 (22.95)	279 (17.02)	...
Availability of social/emotional support			
Always/usually	41* (67.21)	1337 (81.57)	0.34* (0.19, 0.62)
Rarely/never[b]	20* (32.79)	302 (18.43)	...
Outcome: suicidal ideation	7 (11.48)*	57 (3.48)	...

Note. AOR = adjusted odds ratios; CI = confidence interval.

[a]Reference group for comparisons between sexual orientation groups (i.e., heterosexual vs. sexual minority).

[b]Reference categories for multivariate analyses.

[c]Dichotomized into White versus non-White (i.e., Black/African American, Asian, Native Hawaiian/Other Pacific Islander, American Indian or Alaska Native, other race).

*$P < .05$.

Further research is needed to confirm elevated prevalence of suicidal ideation among sexual minority veterans and to clarify the underlying mechanisms of this disparity, which may be targeted to reduce the burden of suicide and related outcomes in this population.

ABOUT THE AUTHORS

John R. Blosnich and Robert M. Bossarte are with the Veterans Integrated Services Network 2 Center of Excellence for Suicide Prevention, Canandaigua VA Medical Center, Canandaigua, NY, and Department of Psychiatry, Center for the Study and Prevention of Suicide, University of Rochester, Rochester, NY. Vincent M. B. Silenzio is with the Department of Psychiatry, Center for the Study and Prevention of Suicide, University of Rochester, Rochester.

CONTRIBUTORS

J.R. Blosnich suggested the study and composed the first draft of the article. R.M. Bossarte oversaw data acquisition and conducted analyses and contributed to writing all parts of the article. V.M.B. Silenzio contributed to the Introduction and Discussion and reviewed drafts of the article.

ACKNOWLEDGMENTS

The authors thank the Massachusetts State Department of Public Health for use of state BRFSS datasets. The authors also thank John Altieri and Eric Silver with the Center of Excellence for Suicide Prevention at the Veterans Administration Medical Center at Canandaigua for their assistance in procuring and coding the data.

HUMAN PARTICIPANT PROTECTION

The Syracuse Veterans Administration Medical Center Institutional Review Board approved this study.

REFERENCES

1. Centers for Disease Control and Prevention. Injury prevention & control: data & statistics (WISQARS). Available at: http://www.cdc.gov/injury/wisqars/index.html. Accessed September 1 2011.

2. King M, Semlyen J, Tai S, Killaspy H, Osborn D, Popelyuk D, et al. A systematic review of mental disorder, suicide, and deliberate self harm in lesbian, gay and bisexual people. *BMC Psychiatry.* 2008;8(1):70.

3. McCarthy JF, Valenstein M, Kim HM, Ilgen M, Zivin K, Blow FC. Suicide mortality among patients receiving care in the Veterans Health Administration Health System. *Am J Epidemiol.* 2009;169(8):1033–1038.

4. Kang HK, Bullman TA. Risk of suicide among US Veterans after returning from the Iraq or Afghanistan War Zones. *JAMA.* 2008;300(6):652–653.

5. Miller M, Barber C, Asrael D, Calle EE, Lawler E, Mukamal KJ. Suicide among US veterans: a prospective study of 500,000 middle-ages and elderly men. *Am J Epidemiol.* 2009;170(4):494–500.

6. Gates G. *Gay Men and Lesbians in the US military: Estimates from Census 2000.* Washington, DC: The Urban Institute; 2004.

7. Massachusetts Office of Health and Human Services. Behavioral Risk Factor Surveillance, Methodology. Available at: http://www.mass.gov/eohhs/consumer/community-health/brfss/methodology.html. Accessed September 21, 2011.

8. Bossarte RM, Knox KL, Piegari R, Altieri J, Kemp J, Katz IR. Prevalence and characteristics of suicide ideation and attempts among active military and veteran participants in a national health survey. *Am J Public Health.* 2012;102(Suppl 1):S38–S40.

9. Substance Abuse and Mental Health Services Administration, Office of Applied Studies. *The NSDUH Report: Suicidal thoughts and behaviors among adults.* Rockville, MD: Substance Abuse and Mental Health Services Administration; 2009.

10. Stall R, Friedman M, Catania J. Interacting epidemics and gay men's health: a theory of syndemic production among urban gay men. In: Wolitski R, Stall R, Valdiserri R, eds. *Unequal Opportunity: Health Disparities Affecting Gay and Bisexual Men in the United States.* New York, NY: Oxford University Press; 2008:251–274.

11. Meyer IH. Prejudice, social stress, and mental health in lesbian, gay, and bisexual populations: conceptual issues and research evidence. *Psychol Bull.* 2003;129(5):674–697.

12. Bruce ML. Suicide risk and prevention in veteran populations. *Ann N Y Acad Sci.* 2010;1208:98–103.

19

Evaluation of a Family-Centered Prevention Intervention for Military Children and Families Facing Wartime Deployments

Patricia Lester, MD, William R. Saltzman, PhD, Kirsten Woodward, LCSW, Dorie Glover, PhD, Gregory A. Leskin, PhD, Brenda Bursch, PhD, Robert Pynoos, MD, and William Beardslee, MD

Objectives. We evaluated the Families OverComing Under Stress program, which provides resiliency training designed to enhance family psychological health in US military families affected by combat- and deployment-related stress.

Methods. We performed a secondary analysis of Families OverComing Under Stress program evaluation data that was collected between July 2008 and February 2010 at 11 military installations in the United States and Japan. We present data at baseline for 488 unique families (742 parents and 873 children) and pre–post outcomes for 331 families.

Results. Family members reported high levels of satisfaction with the program and positive impact on parent–child indicators. Psychological distress levels were elevated for service members, civilian parents, and children at program entry compared with community norms. Change scores showed significant improvements across all measures for service member and civilian parents and their children ($P < .001$).

Conclusions. Evaluation data provided preliminary support for a strength-based, trauma-informed military family prevention program to promote resiliency and mitigate the impact of wartime deployment stress.

More than 1.7 million children in the United States have a parent serving in the military. Since September 11, 2001, approximately 900 000 children have had a parent who deployed multiple times as part of Operation Iraqi Freedom or Operation Enduring Freedom. For a decade, children and their parents have negotiated repeated separations and subsequent family reunions in the context of wartime risk. Recent studies have begun to document the psychological health impact of wartime deployments on service members, spouses, and children, suggesting that greater attention should be paid to the implementation and evaluation of selective prevention strategies that target at-risk families and promote resilience across the military community.[1-4]

Deployed service members are often exposed to a landscape of chronic stressors, potential traumatic events, and harsh environmental risk factors during combat duty. Among those service members returning from deployment to Iraq, 16% to 17% meet criteria for depression, posttraumatic stress disorder (PTSD), or generalized anxiety.[5] Repeated deployments or exposure to adverse conditions have been associated with higher rates of combat-related psychological health problems, traumatic brain injury, substance abuse, and marital conflict.[6-15]

Extended separations in the context of combat deployment may also affect psychological health for the at-home spouse and children. Recent evidence suggests that distress levels of at-home family members increase as the number of deployment months increases.[16] Military children may also be vulnerable to emotional and behavior disruptions, including heightened anxiety and academic difficulties.[1,17-21] Consistent with the larger literature on child distress,[22] psychological symptoms in military parents predict child adjustment problems.[16,23,24] Additionally, the cumulative length of parental deployments correlates with increased risk for depression and behavioral disruptions in school-aged children[16] and with increased distress in adolescents.[24]

Interventions that target families facing adversity and build on family strengths to reduce psychological distress have been shown to have a positive effect on parent and child adjustment and to provide sustained benefits.[25] In randomized controlled trials involving families in challenging circumstances (i.e., parental medical illness, parental depression), targeted family interventions that strengthen parent–child relationships, promote effective parenting practices, and increase family understanding have consistently demonstrated positive outcomes in child development and psychological health over time.[25-28] Effective coping skills, particularly those that address traumatic stress reactions, are associated with enhanced stress management,[29-31] and effective caregiver–child relationships support the development of child adaptive skills such as emotional and behavioral regulation.[32,33]

The FOCUS (Families OverComing Under Stress) project for military families emerged from foundational research on a previously described family-centered preventive intervention model and then was adapted and manualized by a University of California, Los Angeles (UCLA)–Harvard intervention development team at Marine Corps Base, Camp Pendleton.[34,35] The program was subsequently implemented as a large-scale demonstration program for the US Marine Corps and US Navy, funded by the US Navy's Bureau of Medicine and Surgery. Importantly, potential barriers to accessing mental health services have been addressed by a FOCUS implementation emphasis on being strength and skills based, practical, and easily accessible and applicable for military families. Implementation also includes strong military leadership involvement and community partnership to ensure active outreach and family engagement.

FOCUS provides education and skills training for military parents and children. Training is designed to enhance coping with deployment-related experiences, including possible combat-related psychological or physical injury in the service member. Through a structured narrative approach, family members share their unique perspectives of deployment-related experiences, thereby enhancing understanding, bridging communication, and increasing family cohesion and support. This process mobilizes theoretically and empirically supported family resiliency processes.[36,37] FOCUS also integrates the US Navy and US Marine Corps stress continuum model,[38] which categorizes deployment stress into 4 color zones—green, yellow, orange, and red—reflecting an increasing level of risk for psychological distress, injury, and disorder and providing a framework to guide risk identification and referral. Details regarding the FOCUS program foundation, model, and implementation are described elsewhere.[34,39]

We hypothesized that parents completing the program would report improved understanding of deployment and combat stress, improved family skills (emotional regulation, communication, family goal setting, management of stress reminders and triggers) and intrafamilial support, satisfaction with the program, and a likelihood of recommending the program to others. We also hypothesized that families who completed the program would experience improved individual psychological health outcomes and improved family functioning. To our knowledge, this is the first systematic program evaluation examining the effectiveness of a trauma-informed, selective prevention program for military families experiencing wartime deployments.

METHODS

We conducted the evaluation as part of the FOCUS service delivery project funded by the US Navy's Bureau of Medicine and Surgery. We performed a secondary analysis of de-identified data originally collected (July 2008–February 2010) to customize delivery and improve program quality. The program-level data we have presented is from 11 US Marine Corps and US Navy installations located in California (4 sites); North Carolina; Hawaii; Okinawa, Japan; Virginia (2 sites); Mississippi; and Washington State.

FOCUS family resiliency training is delivered to individual families in 8 sessions scheduled according to the family's convenience. Parent and family sessions last 90 minutes and child sessions last 30–60 minutes, depending on the child's developmental level. Although standardized and manualized to ensure that each family learns core FOCUS skills, the intervention allows flexibility and customization to address specific family goals and needs. FOCUS providers (called resiliency trainers) are master- or doctoral-level specialists in child and family mental health. They complete extensive web-based and in-person initial training from UCLA-based supervisors and then participate in weekly reviews of the intervention delivery with their team and with supervisors. UCLA staff also provide ongoing training, intervention materials, emergency support, and technical assistance. Centralized management of the program ensures adherence to program fidelity, coordinated military partnerships, and ongoing quality improvement processes.

An innovative Internet-based "cloud-computing" management system (described in Lester et al.[34]) is used for quality control and to track implementation. The web-based, real-time assessment provides immediate feedback, enabling families to receive appropriate psychoeducational materials, a customized intervention protocol, and timely service referrals if needed. The assessment protocol includes standardized psychological health and coping measures that children, parents, and FOCUS providers complete. We obtained community norms for comparison and cutoffs for clinically significant symptoms from instrument-specific published sources (e.g., a scoring manual, meta-analyses, or similar peer-reviewed data). For measures with psychometrically established properties, we have reported Cronbach α for this sample. Cronbach α is a measure of the internal consistency (reliability) of responses on a questionnaire. Values that fall between 0.70 and 1.0 are acceptable.

Demographics and Descriptive Assessments

Parents answer general demographic and deployment history questions at intake. Active duty parents then complete the PTSD Checklist-Military,[40] a 17-item self-report measure to assess the severity of PTSD symptoms in the past month. Non–active duty parents complete the PTSD Checklist-Civilian.[40] Both the PTSD Checklist-Military and the PTSD Checklist-Civilian are administered at entry to guide program delivery (e.g., to identify need for referral or skills to target in intervention); we include them here to provide a description of population risk. A score of ≥ 30 is considered clinically significant for screening purposes in primary care settings.[41,42]

Parent and Family Outcome and Process Assessments

Parent emotional distress was used to assess psychological distress symptoms. Brief Symptom Inventory (BSI) 18[43] is an abbreviated version of the widely used BSI,[44] a self-report inventory with extensively published psychometric data and community norms by gender. Parents complete the BSI at program entry and at 1 and 4 to 6 months postintervention. Cronbach α for this sample was excellent (0.91). We have reported details for global severity and prevalence of clinically significant symptoms of anxiety and depression. BSI norms are gender specific, and both genders were represented in non–active duty and active duty groups. Thus, all pre–post analyses of the BSI included gender as a covariate. To determine family adjustment, parents complete the McMaster Family Assessment Device (FAD),[45] used to assess problem solving, communication, roles, affective responsiveness, affective involvement, behavior control, and general functioning. The FAD is administered at program entry and exit. For this sample, Cronbach α was excellent (0.92). An FAD general functioning score ≥ 2 is considered unhealthy functioning.[45]

The FOCUS resiliency trainer completes a Global Assessment of Functioning (GAF) rating for each family member at entry, midpoint, and exit. GAF is a numeric scale (0–100) of overall current functioning that can be used with adults and children. Scores are characterized as follows: moderate to severe impairment (0–50); variable or single area difficulty (51–70); and slight or no impairment across all areas of home, school, and peers (71–100).

Upon completing FOCUS, parents are asked to rate their perception of change. Adapted from a previous prevention trial,[47] this 29-item scale assesses the parents' perception of improvement regarding 6 core intervention domains, including communication, problem solving, emotional regulation, managing trauma reminders, goal setting, and overall family support. Ratings anchors are 1 = less than before, 4 = same as before, and 7 = much more than before. Cronbach α was excellent (0.96).

At the time of program completion, parents are asked to rate their overall satisfaction with their family's participation in the program on the basis of how harmful or helpful the program was (1 = very harmful to 7 = very helpful), the parent's satisfaction with the program (1 = very dissatisfied to 7 = very satisfied), and whether the parent would recommend this program to another family (1 = definitely not recommend to 7 = definitely recommend).

Child Outcome Assessments

Child psychological adjustment at baseline and follow-up was assessed using the Strengths and Difficulties Questionnaire–Parent Report (SDQ),[48] a widely used instrument with subscales for conduct problems, emotional symptoms, and prosocial behavior as well as a summary score of total difficulties. Normative data are available for both genders and for individuals aged 4 to 18 years. For simplicity, we have reported details for the total score and prevalence of clinically significant conduct problems and prosocial behaviors for the age groups specified in the SDQ manual.

Child coping was assessed using the Kidcope measure,[49] a self-report checklist to assess the use of various types of coping strategies in youths. Children aged 7 to 18 years complete the coping measure at baseline and program exit. Cronbach α was acceptable (0.73).

We analyzed continuous intake data (e.g., comparing those with and those without post data on severity of distress) using analysis of variance. We analyzed categorical intake data (e.g., prevalence of clinically significant distress) with the χ^2 test. We analyzed pre–post change score continuous data using the single-sample t test, comparing data to the null hypothesis (no change) or to community norms when available, using the paired sample t test, or using the mixed model linear models when comparing groups. We analyzed pre–post categorical data with the χ^2 and the McNemar tests. We addressed violations of normality or homogeneity of variance assumptions with nonparametric tests (e.g., the Mann–Whitney U test) that confirm results by providing a more conservative analysis without such assumptions.

RESULTS

There were 488 families (742 parents) enrolled in FOCUS family resiliency training from July 2008 through February 2010. Participants were self-referred (51.2%) or referred by providers (42.6%), including military medical, mental health, social services, chaplain, or school staff, with 6.2% indicating another referral source such as a military volunteer or a friend. The mean number of active duty parent deployments since the birth of the family's first child was 4.51 (SD = 4.78). Of 488 families, 331 (67.8%) completed the intervention; 89 (18.2%) were unable to complete it because of relocation or deployment, 42 (8.6%) reported the family was too busy to complete the program, 13 (2.7%) reported they no longer needed services, and 13 (2.7%) had not completed the program for unspecified "other" reasons.

Non–active duty and active duty parents enrolled in the program did not differ from each other on self-reported family functioning (FAD) or BSI distress levels, and both groups were significantly more distressed than were community norms. Non–active duty (mean = 1.93; SD = 0.54) and active duty (mean = 2.02; SD = 0.51) parents reported less healthy family functioning compared with community norms (mean = 1.84; SD = 0.43; t_{741} = 6.32; $P < .001$). On the global severity index of the BSI, both non–active duty (mean = 10.82; SD = 10.60) and active duty (mean = 7.89; SD = 9.20) parents had elevated distress relative to gender-specific community norms (females: mean = 8; t_{471} = 5.67; $P < .001$; males: mean = 5; t_{268} = 4.87; $P < .001$). Notably, 33.7% (n = 150) of non–active duty parents were above the cutoff of 30 for elevated posttraumatic stress symptoms at intake compared with 23.3% (n = 69) of active duty parents.

SDQ scores for boys enrolled in the program (mean = 13.54; SD = 6.9) were significantly higher than were those of normative data (mean = 7.63; SD = 5.9; t_{486} = 18.86; $P < .001$), as were scores for girls enrolled in the program (mean = 11.11; SD = 6.3 vs norms mean = 6.56; SD = 5.2; t_{378} = 4.55; $P < .001$).

There were no substantive differences in parent or child outcomes as a function of military branch, thus results are from combined data.

Characteristics of Participating Families

We have reported pre- and postintervention data from 331 families representing 466 parents (300 non–active duty and 166 active duty), with pre- and postassessment for at least 1 parent and 493 children from those families. The BSI was not part of the original follow-up assessment (it was added after the program's initial implementation for service delivery needs), and thus matched data for the BSI are available for only 287 parents (221 non–active duty and 66 active duty).

Non–active duty primary caretakers were predominantly female (97.2%). Of the 166 active duty caretakers, 27 (16.3%) were female. Most parents (95.6%) were married. The mean age of parents was 34.39 (SD = 6.04), with no difference between non–active duty and active duty parents. Posttraumatic stress symptoms were assessed once, soon after intake, showing elevations (PTSD Checklist $\geq$ 30) among 94 (31.3%) of non–active duty and 35 (21.2%) of active duty parents and no difference between families who completed intervention versus those who did not.

Reflecting the age demographics of the child population within the military at large, there were more children aged 3 to 7 years (61.1%) than aged 8 to 10 years (19.0%) or aged 11 years and older (19.9%). There were more boys (55.1%) than girls (44.9%).

Families and parents who completed the intervention were more likely to be self-referred, less distressed on the BSI and FAD, and older than noncompleters. Children who completed the intervention did not differ from those who did not at intake on the SDQ.

Implementation Process Outcomes

Perception of change and parent satisfaction ratings (from 0 to 7) were completed by 363 parents. Mean values ranged from 5.52 (SD = 0.79) for improvements in emotional regulation to 6.05 (SD = 0.95) for improvements in understanding combat stress and parent–child stress reactions, indicating a high degree of perceived change. Parent satisfaction mean ratings were also high, with 6.51 (SD = 0.69) for overall helpfulness to their family; a satisfaction with the program rating of 6.58 (SD = 0.62); and a willingness to recommend the program to another family rating of 6.70 (SD = 0.60). Ratings were similar for active duty and non–active duty parents.

Intervention Effects

Parental distress, family functioning, and global functioning levels at intake and postintervention are shown in Table 1. There were no significant time × group effects on any outcome.

Change scores showed significant improvements across all measures for non–active duty parents and active duty parents ($P < .001$). BSI-assessed parental distress and FAD-assessed unhealthy family functioning were significantly reduced, and post scores were at or better than normative data. The provider GAF rating for global functioning was significantly improved after intervention, despite mean intake scores indicating minimal impairment at the outset. Figure 1 illustrates the percentage of parents with clinically meaningful impairments in family functioning and anxiety and depression symptoms at intake and postintervention. Both non–active duty families and active duty families demonstrated significant decreases in prevalence of impairment and distress symptoms from pre- to postintervention (all P values $< .001$).

The SDQ total difficulties score and the prosocial behaviors subscale, by age and gender, are in Table 2. At intake, girls and boys in every age group were rated as significantly less adjusted than were comparative gender- and age-specific norms ($P < .001$). Change scores indicate significant reductions in the total difficulties score for boys and girls across all age groups ($P < .001$) and significant improvements in prosocial behaviors ($P < .05$ to $P < .001$). Figure 2 shows the prevalence of clinically significant conduct problems, emotional symptoms, and total difficulties at intake and postintervention. Reductions in the prevalence of children with clinically significant symptoms over time were all significant ($P < .001$).

Children aged 7 years and older who completed a self-report of coping at intervention intake and exit (Kidcope; n = 298) evidenced significant increases in the use of positive coping strategies. McNemar tests indicated improvements in emotional regulation, problem solving, cognitive restructuring, and increased use of social support (all P values significant at $P < .001$).

DISCUSSION

Increased attention has been paid to identifying the psychological health needs of service members and their families and to identifying and responding to

Table 1. Changes in Parental Distress, Family Functioning, and Global Functioning at Intake and Postintervention: Families OverComing Under Stress, United States and Japan, July 2008–February 2010

	Non-Active Duty, Mean (SD)		Normative Data, Mean (SD)		Active Duty, Mean (SD)		Time Effect (95% CI)	Group Effect (95% CI)
	Intake	Post	Female	Male	Intake	Post		
BSI global severity index	0.56 (0.56)	0.29 (0.33)	0.35 (0.37)	0.25 (0.24)	0.47 (0.53)	0.21 (0.38)	0.27*** (0.21, 0.33)	0.09[a] (0.01, 0.18)
BSI anxiety	0.65 (0.67)	0.37 (0.43)	0.44 (0.54)	0.26 (0.31)	0.52 (0.59)	0.28 (0.41)	0.27*** (0.20, 0.35)	0.10[a] (0.01, 0.21)
BSI depression	0.69 (0.73)	0.32 (0.47)	0.36 (0.56)	0.21 (0.33)	0.60 (0.68)	0.18 (0.32)	0.38*** (0.30, 0.47)	0.13** (0.03, 0.23)
Family Assessment Device, general functioning[b]	1.89 (0.54)	1.73 (0.43)	1.84 (0.43)	1.84 (0.43)	2.00 (0.49)	1.82 (0.46)	0.68*** (0.13, 0.20)	0.09* (0.01, 0.18)
Global Assessment of Functioning	72.54 (10.78)	78.13 (9.53)	...	...	74.46 (11.54)	79.46 (9.43)	−5.40*** (−6.05, −4.75)	1.43[a] (0.36, 3.21)

Note. BSI = brief symptom inventory; CI = confidence interval. Family and global functioning increase and distress declines over time. BSI was analyzed with gender as covariate.

[a] Not significant.

[b] A Family Assessment Device score ≥ 2 refers to unhealthy functioning.

*P < .05; **P < .01; ***P < .001.

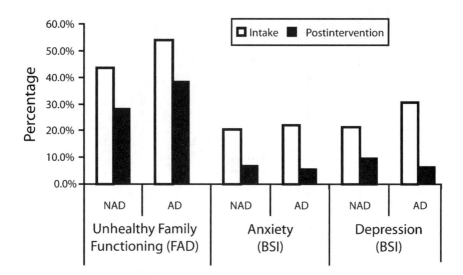

Figure 1. Reduction in prevalence of parental symptoms by phase (intake or postintervention): Families OverComing Under Stress, United States and Japan, July 2008–February 2010.

Note. BSI = Brief Symptom Inventory[43]; FAD = McMaster Family Assessment Device.[41] All non-active duty (NAD) and active duty (AD) pre–post changes are significant ($P < .001$). Unhealthy functioning is indicated by a FAD score ≥ 2; only percentages > 2 are shown. We used BSI manual gender-specific clinically significant symptoms cutoffs; The figure shows percentages greater than the cutoff.

gaps in the continuum of preventive care for military families.[27,50] This has led to the proliferation of expanded and new programs and resources to address the needs of military families. Despite the expansion of family services provided by the public and private sectors, there has been limited systematic evaluation of these programs to guide national screening and prevention efforts. Our evaluation provides both implementation process and effectiveness findings that demonstrate the acceptability, feasibility, and effectiveness of strength-based, family-centered skills training designed to promote resilience and mitigate wartime deployment distress in military families.

The implementation and process outcomes provide preliminary evidence that recipients of FOCUS perceive that the program addresses relevant issues facing them during deployment and reintegration transitions. Consistent with the implementation of FOCUS as a selective prevention program, families entering the program may be proactively seeking to enhance coping in the face

Table 2. Changes in Child Adjustment on the Strengths and Difficulties Questionnaire at Intake and Postintervention: Families OverComing Under Stress, United States and Japan, July 2008–February 2010

Age, y	Girls (n = 216)			Boys (n = 277), Mean (SD)			Time Effect (95% CI)	Gender Effect (95% CI)
	Intake, Mean (SD)	Post, Mean (SD)	Norms, Mean (SD)	Intake, Mean (SD)	Post, Mean (SD)	Norms, Mean (SD)		
Total difficulties								
3–7[a]	11.59 (5.65)	8.25 (5.20)	6.8 (5.1)	13.54 (6.93)	9.71 (5.70)	7.9 (5.5)	3.59*** (2.98, 4.20)	1.62** (0.43, 2.80)
8–10[b]	11.00 (7.23)	7.41 (5.52)	6.4 (5.1)	13.47 (6.78)	9.98 (6.57)	7.9 (6.4)	3.54*** (2.51, 4.57)	2.55* (0.22, 4.88)
≥ 11[c]	11.63 (6.97)	7.59 (5.72)	6.5 (5.5)	14.55 (6.59)	10.25 (6.27)	7.1 (5.8)	4.17*** (3.03, 5.32)	2.75* (0.43, 5.06)
Prosocial behavior								
3–7[a]	8.13 (1.97)	8.86 (1.55)	8.6 (1.7)	7.21 (2.01)	8.28 (1.78)	8.2 (2.0)	−0.89*** (−0.69, −1.10)	−0.68*** (−0.32, −1.04)
8–10[b]	8.32 (1.90)	8.80 (1.76)	9.0 (1.5)	7.61 (2.15)	8.19 (1.75)	8.6 (1.8)	−0.52** (−0.17, −0.88)	−0.64[d] (0.02, −1.29)
≥ 11[c]	8.24 (1.90)	9.12 (1.36)	8.9 (1.6)	7.55 (2.06)	8.07 (2.02)	8.5 (1.9)	−0.65*** (−0.30, −1.00)	−0.93** (−0.29, −1.57)

Note. CI = confidence interval; NS = not significant. Time × gender effects were not significant and are not shown. Total difficulties decline and prosocial behavior increases.

[a] Sample size is n = 295: 131 girls and 164 boys.

[b] Sample size is n = 101: 44 girls and 57 boys.

[c] Sample size is n = 97: 41 girls and 56 boys.

[d] Not significant.

$*P < .05$; $**P < .01$; $***P < .001$.

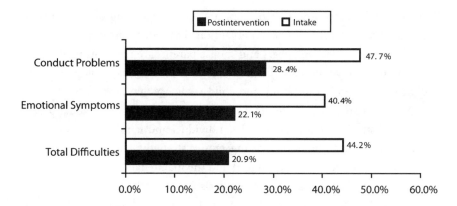

Figure 2. Reduction in prevalence of child symptoms by phase (intake or postintervention): Families OverComing Under Stress, United States and Japan, July 2008–February 2010.

Note. The single-sample *t*-test against null hypothesis (no change) was significant (*P* < .001) for all scales. Subscales are from the Strengths and Difficulties Questionnaire.[46] Per the manual, the cutoff for "normal," conduct problems: 2; emotional symptoms: 3; total difficulties: 13. Percentages greater than normal are shown.

of increased challenges or may already be experiencing deployment distress. About one third of individuals entering the program were also referred to other social support and mental health providers, indicating the potential for selective prevention as a gateway to other services when needed.

Consistent with recent studies of military families who experienced wartime deployments, parents and children entering FOCUS were more likely to report symptoms of psychological distress than were nonmilitary gender-matched peers.[2,16,24] Notably, non–active duty spouses were as vulnerable to distress, including posttraumatic stress symptoms, as were their active duty partners. Military family experts have noted that the stress demands of civilian spouses may equal or even surpass their active duty partners because they lack the support of being embedded in a cohesive unit, they frequently lack clear information on the risk status of their loved one, and they are unable to act instrumentally on his or her behalf.[51] Child distress was common at program entry, underscoring the relevance of providing selective preventive services that may provide early mitigation of child psychological distress.[25]

As anticipated, both parents and children participating in FOCUS demonstrated significant improvement in emotional and behavioral adjustment.

Further, children's prosocial behaviors and positive coping skills increased from initiation of training to postintervention. The reductions in psychological distress for both service members and spouse parents are noteworthy given the brevity of the intervention and the importance of parental psychological health and effective parenting to family and child resilience and adaptation.[2,36,52]

FOCUS enhances family resilience processes and targets individual parent and child distress. The model provides individual and family level training in resiliency skills and builds on existing family strengths and increases family cohesion, communication, and support and the maintenance of consistent care routines in the home—all core characteristics of resilient families.[36,53] On standardized assessment, we found that family adjustment improved significantly. We hypothesized that reduced parental distress and improved family adjustment would support positive child adaptation. Significant postintervention reductions in emotional and behavioral problems for boys and girls in all age groups support this hypothesis.

This evaluation also provides initial information regarding the challenges of implementing family prevention services for a mobile military population. Of the approximately 30% of families who initiated services but did not complete the intervention, more than half (18.2%) did not complete because of work-related relocations or deployments. Despite this "artificially inflated" attrition rate, almost 70% of families enrolled completed the FOCUS intervention, representing service completion rates much higher than those of community child mental health services (25%–60%; for review, see Greeno et al.[54]). The evaluation also indicates that more distressed parents may have had greater difficulty completing the program, suggesting that higher risk families may require greater outreach and engagement, processes to bridge services during relocations, or improved identification and support for referral.

We conducted this service program evaluation on an existing data set, and it is limited by the lack of a control group. We have addressed the absence of a control group in several ways. We conducted analysis of change scores, verifying that reductions in symptoms occurred among those parents and children who were above and below clinical cutoffs at baseline. Reductions in the prevalence of clinically significant distress after intervention also suggest meaningful improvement. Both parents and children gave satisfaction ratings, and parents also rated the degree of perceived change around the core family domains, which were the intended targets for intervention change. Children also self-reported on specific ways of coping with a self-selected problem, indicating the process by which mental health symptoms may have improved. Also, clinician ratings of change augmented participant self-report measures. Although child developmental processes could have contributed to the positive outcomes, the brief nature of the intervention makes it unlikely that nonintervention changes could account for such rapid improvement across all age groups. An "attention-control" group in future evaluation studies may help to verify the active ingredients of positive intervention change.

Despite its limitations, this evaluation provides preliminary evidence that FOCUS for military families is feasible, is well tolerated, and can lead to significant benefits for parents, children, and families. Future examination of implementation challenges and program evaluation of FOCUS services in other service branches and for geographically dispersed populations, such as the National Guard and Reservists, will be important to provide information about program generalizability for other military branches.

ABOUT THE AUTHORS

Patricia Lester, William R. Saltzman, Dorie Glover, Gregory A. Leskin, Brenda Bursch, and Robert Pynoos are with the Semel Institute for Neuroscience and Human Behavior, University of California, Los Angeles. Kirsten Woodward is with the United States Bureau of Navy Medicine and Surgery, Washington, DC. William Beardslee is with Children's Hospital Boston and Harvard Medical School, Boston, MA.

CONTRIBUTORS

P. Lester, W.R. Saltzman, R. Pynoos, and W. Beardslee codeveloped the family preventive intervention program. P. Lester and W. Saltzman codeveloped the implementation design and program evaluation methodology. K. Woodward contributed to the program evaluation and implementation for the Navy and Marine Corps. D. Glover, G.A. Leskin, and B. Bursch contributed to the program evaluation methodology design. D. Glover was the primary analyst on this study. G.A. Leskin and B. Bursch contributed to data analysis. R. Pynoos and W. Beardslee contributed to the program design and implementation and data interpretation. All authors contributed to the writing of the article.

ACKNOWLEDGMENTS

The US Department of the Navy, Bureau of Medicine and Surgery (contract No. N00189-09-C-Z057) and the Frederick R. Weisman Philanthropic Foundation and Discretionary Trust supported Families OverComing Under Stress.

HUMAN PARTICIPANT PROTECTION

The University of California, Los Angeles institutional review board approved this evaluation.

REFERENCES

1. Lincoln A, Swift E, Shorteno-Fraser M. Psychological adjustment and treatment of children and families with parents deployed in military combat. *J Clin Psychol.* 2008;64(8):984–992.

2. Palmer C. A theory of risk and resilience factors in military families. *Mil Psychol.* 2008;20(3):205–217.

3. Waldrep DA, Cozza SJ, Chun RS. The impact of deployment on the military family. In: The National Center for Post Traumatic Stress Disorder, ed. *The Iraq War Clinician Guide.* 2nd ed. Washington, DC: Department of Veterans Affairs; 2004:83–86.

4. National Research Council, Institute of Medicine. *Preventing Mental, Emotional, and Behavioral Disorders Among Young People: Progress and Possibilities.* Washington, DC: National Academies Press; 1994.

5. Hoge CW, Castro CA, Messer SC, McGurk D, Cotting DI, Koffman RL. Combat duty in Iraq and Afghanistan, mental health problems, and barriers to care. *N Engl J Med.* 2004;351(1):13–22.

6. Baker DG, Heppner P, Niloofar A, et al. Trauma exposure, branch of service, and physical injury in relation to mental health among U.S. veterans returning from Iraq and Afghanistan. *Mil Med.* 2009;174(8):773–778.

7. Erbes C, Westermeyer J, Engdahl B, Johnsen E. Post-traumatic stress disorder and service utilization in a sample of service members from Iraq and Afghanistan. *Mil Med.* 2007;72(4):359–363.

8. Gibbs DA, Martin SL, Kupper LL, Johnson RE. Child maltreatment in enlisted soldiers' families during combat-related deployments. *JAMA.* 2007;298(5):528–535.

9. Hoge CW, McGurk D, Thomas JL, Cox AL, Engel CC, Castro CA. Mild traumatic brain injury in U.S. soldiers returning from Iraq. *N Engl J Med.* 2008;358(5):453–463.

10. Lew HL, Poole JH, Guillory SB, Salerno RM, Leskin G, Sigford BJ. Persistent problems after traumatic brain injury: the need for long-term follow-up and coordinated care. *J Rehabil Res Dev.* 2006;43(2):vii–x.

11. McCarroll JE, Fan Z, Newby JH, Ursano RJ. Trends in US army child maltreatment reports: 1990–2004. *Child Abuse Rev.* 2008;17(2):108–118.

12. Okie S. Traumatic brain injury in the war zone. *N Engl J Med.* 2005;352(20): 2043–2047.

13. Rentz ED, Marshall SW, Loomis D, Casteel C, Martin SL, Gibbs DA. Effects of deployment on the occurrence of child maltreatment in military and nonmilitary families. *Am J Epidemiol.* 2007;165(10):1199–1206.

14. Seal KH, Metzler TJ, Gima KS, Bertenthal D, Maguen S, Marmar CR. Trends and risk factors for mental health diagnoses among Iraq and Afghanistan veterans using Department of Veterans Affairs health care, 2002–2008. *Am J Public Health.* 2009;99(9):1651–1658.

15. Vasterling JJ, Proctor SP, Friedman MJ, et al. PTSD symptom increases in Iraq-deployed soldiers: comparison with nondeployed soldiers and associations with baseline symptoms, deployment experiences, and postdeployment stress. *J Trauma Stress.* 2010;23(1):41–51.

16. Lester P, Peterson K, Reeves J, et al. The long war and parental combat deployment: effects on military children and at-home spouses. *J Am Acad Child Adolesc Psychiatry.* 2010;49(4):310–320.

17. Flake EM, Davis BE, Johnson PL, Middleton LS. The psychosocial effects of deployment on military children. *J Dev Behav Pediatr.* 2009;30(4):271–278.

18. Chandra A, Burns RM, Tanielian TL, et al. *Understanding the Impact of Deployment on Children and Families: Findings From a Pilot Study of Operation Purple Camp Participants.* Santa Monica, CA: RAND; 2008.

19. Chartrand MM, Frank DA, White LF, Shope TR. Effect of parents' wartime deployment on the behavior of young children in military families. *Arch Pediatr Adolesc Med.* 2008;162(11):1009–1014.

20. Rosen LN, Teitelbaum JM, Westhuis DJ. Children's reactions to the Desert Storm deployment: initial findings from a survey of army families. *Mil Med.* 1993;158(7):465–469.

21. Huebner AJ, Mancini JA, Wilcox RM, Grass SR, Grass GA. Parental deployment and youth in military families: exploring uncertainty and ambiguous loss. *Fam Relat.* 2007;56(2):112–122.

22. Rutter M, Quinton D. Parental psychiatric disorder: effects on children. *Psychol Med.* 1984;14(4):853–880.

23. Cozza SJ, Chun RS, Polo JA. Military families and children during operation Iraqi Freedom. *Psychiatr Q.* 2005;76(4):371–378.

24. Chandra A, Lara-Cinisomo S, Jaycox LH, et al. Children on the homefront: the experience of children from military families. *Pediatrics.* 2009;125(1):16–25.

25. National Research Council and Institute of Medicine. *Depression in Parents, Parenting, and Children: Opportunities to Improve Identification, Treatment and Prevention.* Washington, DC: National Academies Press; 2009.

26. Beardslee WR, Avery MW, Ayoub C, Watts CL. Family connections: helping Early Head Start/Head Start staff and parents address mental health challenges. *Zero to Three.* 2009;29(6):34–42.

27. Rotheram-Borus MJ, Lee MB, Gwadz M, Draimin B. An intervention for parents with AIDS and their adolescent children. *Am J Public Health.* 2001;91(8):1294–1302.

28. Lester P, Rotheram-Borus MJ, Elia C, Elkavich A, Rice E. TALK: teens and adults learning to communicate. In: LeCroy CW, ed. *Evidence-Based Treatment Manuals for Children and Adolescents.* New York: Oxford University Press; 2008:170–285.

29. Compas BE, Phares V, Ledoux N. Stress and coping preventive interventions with children and adolescents. In: Bond LA, Compas BE, eds. *Primary Prevention and Promotion in the Schools.* Beverly Hills, CA: Sage; 1989:60–89.

30. Patterson JM, McCubbin HI. Adolescent coping style and behaviors: conceptualization and measurement. *J Adolesc.* 1987;10(2):163–186.

31. Layne CM, Saltzman WR, Poppleton L, et al. Effectiveness of a school-based psychotherapy program for war-exposed adolescents: a randomized controlled trial. *J Am Acad Child Adolesc Psychiatry.* 2008;47(9):1048–1062.

32. Spoth RL, Kavanagh K, Dishion T. Family-centered preventive intervention science: toward benefits to larger populations of children, youth, and families. *Prev Sci.* 2002;3(3):145–152.

33. Sroufe LA. Attachment and development: a prospective, longitudinal study from birth to adulthood. *Attach Hum Dev.* 2005;7(4):349–367.

34. Lester P, Leskin G, Woodward K, et al. Wartime deployment and military children: applying prevention science to enhance family resilience. In: MacDermid Wadsworth S, Riggs D, eds. *Risk and Resilience in U.S. Military Families.* New York: Springer; 2010:149–173.

35. Saltzman WR, Lester P, Pynoos R, et al. *FOCUS for Military Families: Individual Family Resiliency Training Manual.* 2nd ed; 2009 [unpublished manual].

36. Walsh F. *Strengthening Family Resilience.* 2nd ed. New York: Guilford Press; 2006.

37. MacDermid SM, Samper R, Schwarz R, Nishida J, Nyaronga D. *Understanding and Promoting Resilience in Military Families.* West Lafayette, IN: Military Family Research Institute, Purdue University; 2008.

38. Nash WP. U.S. Marine Corps and Navy combat and operational stress continuum model: a tool for leaders. In: Ritchie EC, ed. *Combat and Operational Behavioral Health.* Washington, DC: Borden Institute Textbook of Military Psychiatry; 2011:107–119.

39. Lester P, Mogil C, Saltzman W, et al. Families OverComing Under Stress: implementing family-centered prevention for military families facing wartime deployments and combat operational stress. *Mil Med.* 2011;176(1):19–25.

40. Weathers FW, Litz BT, Herman DS, Huska JA, Keane TM. *The PTSD Checklist (PCL): Reliability, Validity, and Diagnostic Utility.* Presented at the Ninth Annual Meeting of ISTSS; October 1993; San Antonio, TX.

41. Walker EA, Newman E, Dobie DJ, Ciechanowski P, Katon W. Validation of the PTSD Checklist in an HMO sample of women. *Gen Hosp Psychiatry.* 2002;24(6):375–380.

42. Bliese PD, Wright KM, Adler AB, Cabrera O, Castro CA, Hoge CW. Validating the primary care posttraumatic stress disorder screen and the posttraumatic stress disorder checklist with soldiers returning from combat. *J Consult Clin Psychol.* 2008;76(2):272–281.

43. Derogatis LR. *Brief Symptom Inventory 18 (BSI-18): Administration, Scoring, and Procedures Manual.* Minneapolis: National Computer Systems Pearson, Inc; 2001.

44. Derogatis LR. *Brief Symptom Inventory (BSI): Administration, Scoring, and Procedures Manual.* 3rd ed. Minneapolis: National Computer Systems Pearson, Inc; 1993.

45. Ryan CE, Epstein NB, Keitner GI, Miller IW, Bishop DS. *Evaluation and Treating Families: The McMaster Approach.* New York: Routledge; 2005.

46. *Diagnostic and Statistical Manual of Mental Disorders.* Rev 4th ed. Washington, DC: American Psychiatric Association; 2000.

47. Beardslee WR, Gladstone TRGG, Wright EJ, Cooper AB. A family-based approach to the prevention of depressive symptoms in children at risk: evidence of parental and child change. *Pediatrics.* 2003;112:e119–e131.

48. Goodman R, Ford T, Simmons H, Gatward R, Meltzer H. Using the Strengths and Difficulties Questionnaire (SDQ) to screen for child psychiatric disorders in a community sample. *Br J Psychiatry.* 2000;177:534–539.

49. Spirito A, Stark LJ, Williams C. Development of a brief coping checklist for use with pediatric populations. *J Pediatr Psychol.* 1988;13(4):555–574.

50. Department of Defense Task Force on Mental Health. *An Achievable Vision: Report of the Department of Defense Task Force on Mental Health.* Falls Church, VA: Defense Health Board; 2007.

51. Nash W. *Combat Operational Stress Control: The Family Dynamic.* Presented at a Professional Development Training Course of the Department of the Navy; 2009; Washington, DC.

52. Gewirtz A, Forgatch M, Wieling E. Parenting practices as potential mechanisms for child adjustment following mass trauma. *J Marital Fam Ther*. 2008;34(2):177–192.

53. Walsh F. A family resilience framework: innovative practice applications. *Fam Relat*. 2002;51(2):130–137.

54. Greeno CG, Anderson CM, Stork E, Kelleher KJ, Shear K, Mike G. Treatment after assessment in a community children's mental health clinic. *Psychiatr Serv*. 2002;53(5):624–626.

20

Effect of Dwell Time on the Mental Health of US Military Personnel With Multiple Combat Tours

Andrew J. MacGregor, PhD, MPH, Peggy P. Han, MPH, Amber L. Dougherty, MPH, and Michael R. Galarneau, MS

Objective. We investigated the association of the length of time spent at home between deployments, or dwell time, with posttraumatic stress disorder (PTSD) and other mental health disorders.

Methods. We included US Marine Corps personnel identified from military deployment records who deployed to Operation Iraqi Freedom once (n = 49 328) or twice (n = 16 376). New-onset mental health diagnoses from military medical databases were included. We calculated the ratio of dwell-to-deployment time (DDR) as the length of time between deployments divided by the length of the first deployment.

Results. Marines with 2 deployments had higher rates of PTSD than did those with 1 deployment (2.1% versus 1.2%; $P < .001$). A DDR representing longer dwell times at home relative to first deployment length was associated with reduced odds of PTSD (odds ratio [OR] = 0.47; 95% confidence interval [CI] = 0.32, 0.70), PTSD with other mental health disorder (OR = 0.56; 95% CI = 0.33, 0.94), and other mental health disorders (OR = 0.62; 95% CI = 0.51, 0.75).

Conclusions. Longer dwell times may reduce postdeployment risk of PTSD and other mental health disorders. Future research should focus on the role of dwell time in adverse health outcomes.

Military deployment has long been recognized as a stressor because it removes individuals from the comfort of home and can strain relationships with spouses and other family members.[1,2] The number of combat deployments increases during times of military conflict, as was the case in the years following the events of September 11, 2001. With the initiation of Operation

Enduring Freedom (OEF) in October 2001 and Operation Iraqi Freedom (OIF) in March 2003, the pace of military operations increased markedly and many service members experienced multiple deployments to the combat zone.[3] The cumulative health-related effects of multiple combat deployments are not well understood and are an emerging public health problem.

Multiple studies have identified an increase in mental health morbidity following a single deployment.[4-7] Research on the mental health effects of multiple deployments, however, is limited. In 2007, the Mental Health Advisory Team (MHAT) found that soldiers on their third or fourth deployment in support of OIF had a significantly higher risk of mental health and work-related problems than did soldiers on their first or second deployment.[8] Other studies have also identified increases in mental health symptoms, particularly symptoms of posttraumatic stress disorder (PTSD), among personnel preparing for and after their second OIF deployment.[9,10] One study of British military personnel found that a higher prevalence of mental health symptoms was associated with deployment length but not with frequency of deployments.[11] The most recent MHAT report was the first to provide evidence suggesting a protective effect of dwell time (or the period of time at home between deployments) on self-reported adverse mental health symptoms, though actual medical utilization was not examined.[12]

Dwell time and multiple deployments have also been the subject of recent media reports. Secretary of Defense Robert Gates and Senator Jim Webb recently called for establishing minimum requirements for time at home between deployments.[13,14] A variety of factors can influence the determination of a service member's dwell time, including current operational needs and unit rotation schedule. In our study, we aimed to identify new-onset mental health diagnoses among US Marines with 1 and 2 OIF deployments. Among those with 2 OIF deployments, we examined the association of dwell time with PTSD and other mental health disorders. We hypothesized that increased dwell time relative to first deployment length would be associated with lower rates of adverse mental health outcomes.

METHODS

We used electronic military deployment records from the Defense Manpower Data Center (DMDC) to identify the study population. US Marine Corps personnel with 1 and 2 OIF deployments, identified as deployment to Iraq or Kuwait between January 2003 and December 2007, were included in the analysis. For the purposes of our study, we defined a deployment as lasting between 1 and 18 months. The study population was further restricted to those with deployments between 4 and 8 months, which encapsulated the interquartile range of all deployed personnel. A total of 65 704 deployed personnel met this criterion (representing 71% of all deployments). Exclusion criteria were Reserve or National Guard status (because of the potential for differential access to medical care), personnel with any deployment to a non-OIF location, women (because of the small sample size), and those with previous mental health diagnoses before the first or second deployment identified from inpatient and outpatient medical databases. This study was approved by the institutional review board at the Naval Health Research Center, San Diego, California.

Measures

We calculated length of deployment from DMDC records as the difference between the start and end dates of deployment. For those with 2 deployments, we calculated dwell time by subtracting the start date of the second deployment from the end date of the first deployment. We then calculated the dwell-to-deployment time ratio (DDR) as the length of time between deployments divided by length of the first deployment and categorized this variable into the following 3 ratios: less than 1:1, 1:1, or 2:1. The less than 1:1 ratio represents a shorter dwell time or time spent at home than deployed, 1:1 represents as much dwell time as deployed, and the 2:1 ratio represents longer dwell times (at least 2 times longer) relative to the length of the first deployment. We conducted an additional analysis by using the continuous form of DDR.

We identified provider-diagnosed mental health disorders from inpatient and outpatient military medical databases. The observation period for those with 1 or 2 deployments was the duration of deployment plus 1 year. A mental health disorder was indicated by the presence of an inpatient or outpatient *International Classification of Diseases, Ninth Revision, Clinical Modification* (*ICD-9-CM*)[15] code in the range of 290 to 319. Outcome was categorized into PTSD (*ICD-9-CM* 309.81) and other mental health disorder (all other mental health disorder *ICD-9-CM* codes, excluding 305.1, tobacco addiction), and the PTSD group was further dichotomized into PTSD only and PTSD with other mental health disorder. The other mental health disorder category included mood disorders (*ICD-9-CM* 296, 300.4, 301.13, 311), anxiety disorders (*ICD-9-CM* 300.00–300.02, 300.21–300.29, 300.3, 308.3, 308.9), adjustment disorders (*ICD-9-CM* 309.0–309.9, excluding 309.81, PTSD), substance-abuse disorders (*ICD-9-CM* 291, 292.0–292.1, 292.3–292.9, 303, 304, 305.0, 305.2–305.7, 305.9), and other (other *ICD-9-CM* codes between 290 and 319 not previously listed). For those with 2 deployments, we used inpatient medical databases to identify those with a hospitalization during their first deployment, because this could affect dwell time.

We abstracted age and military rank from DMDC records. Age was assessed as a continuous variable and rank was categorized into junior enlisted (E1–E5), senior enlisted (E6–E9), and officer or warrant officer. For those with 2 deployments, age and military rank at the time of second deployment were used in the analysis.

Statistical Analysis

We performed descriptive analysis for characteristics of personnel with 1 and 2 deployments. Crude rates of PTSD and other mental health disorders were calculated, stratified by number of deployments, and compared with chi-square testing. Dwell time was analyzed with DDR calculated in both its continuous and categorical form. The distributions of DDR and other deployment-specific variables were compared by using Wilcoxon testing across outcome groups. Rates of PTSD and other mental health disorders were compared across different DDR categories, and Mantel–Haenszel testing was used to assess for trend. We conducted polychotomous logistic regression to evaluate the odds of PTSD and other mental health disorders with adjustment for covariates, and we evaluated a separate model excluding personnel with a hospitalization during their first deployment.

RESULTS

The study population consisted of 49 328 Marines deployed once and 16 376 deployed twice to OIF. Descriptive information for the study population is listed in Table 1. For those with 2 deployments, median days of both the first and second deployment (203 and 205 days, respectively) were similar to the median deployment length for those with 1 deployment (203 days). The distribution of

Table 1. Demographic Characteristics of US Marines with 1 and 2 Deployments to Operation Iraqi Freedom (N = 65 704): 2003–2007

Characteristic	1 Deployment (n = 49 328)	2 Deployments (n = 16 376)
Age, y, median (range)[a]	22 (17–57)	22 (19–53)
Military rank, no. (%)[a]		
E1–E5	40 762 (82.6)	13 363 (81.6)
E6–E9	4923 (10.0)	1818 (11.1)
Officer or warrant officer	3643 (7.4)	1195 (7.3)
Time, d, median (range)		
First deployment	203 (120–240)	203 (120–240)
Second deployment	...	205 (120–240)
Dwell-to-deployment ratio, median (range)	...	1.7 (0.1–11.8)
Dwell-to-deployment ratio, no. (%)		
< 1:1	...	3270 (20.0)
1:1	...	8041 (49.1)
2:1	...	5065 (30.9)

[a]For those with 2 deployments, age and military rank at the beginning of the second deployment were used.

DDR was heavily skewed to the right, with a median of 1.7 (interquartile range = 1.2–2.3), approaching the DDR category of 2:1 with longer dwell times relative to first deployment length. Overall, 80% of those with 2 deployments were home for at least as long as the length of their first deployment.

Rates of mental health disorders are detailed in Table 2. The overall rate of PTSD and other mental health disorders was 1.5% and 6.1%, respectively, with higher rates of PTSD among personnel with 2 deployments compared with those with 1 deployment (2.1% versus 1.2%) and, conversely, higher rates of other mental health disorders among those with 1 deployment compared with 2 (6.3% versus 5.7%). A breakdown of the other mental health disorder category indicates substance abuse disorder as the most common subcategory, with higher rates among those with 1 deployment than among those with 2 (2.4% versus 1.7%). Similarly, mood disorders were slightly higher among those with 1 deployment.

For those with 2 deployments, we calculated the distribution of DDR and other deployment-specific variables stratified by outcome category (PTSD diagnosis only, other mental health disorder, PTSD with other mental health

Table 2. Percentage of New-Onset Mental Health Disorders Among US Marines With 1 and 2 Deployments to Operation Iraqi Freedom: 2003–2007

Disorder[a]	1 Deployment (n = 49 328), No. (%)	2 Deployments (n = 16 376), No. (%)	P
Posttraumatic stress disorder (PTSD)	609 (1.2)	347 (2.1)	< .001
PTSD only	333 (0.7)	225 (1.4)	< .001
PTSD with other mental health disorder	276 (0.6)	122 (0.7)	.01
Other mental health disorder	3094 (6.3)	936 (5.7)	.01
Mood disorder	535 (1.1)	136 (0.8)	.01
Substance abuse disorder	1177 (2.4)	284 (1.7)	< .001
Adjustment disorder	604 (1.2)	227 (1.4)	.11
Anxiety disorder	434 (0.9)	161 (1.0)	.23
Other	838 (1.7)	243 (1.5)	.06

[a]Diagnostic categories were not mutually exclusive; patients could be counted in more than one category.

disorder, and no mental health disorder). The details of these distributions are shown in Table 3. Median DDR differed significantly across outcome groups ($P < .001$); those with PTSD only and PTSD with other mental health disorder had the lowest DDR (1.5), demonstrating shorter dwell times relative to first deployment length, and those with no mental health disorder had the highest DDR (1.7), or longer dwell times at home relative to time spent on first deployment. Those with no mental health disorder also had the highest first and third quartile values for DDR, as shown by the interquartile range (1.3–2.3). The results were similar for the continuous form of dwell time; those with PTSD only and PTSD with other mental health disorder had the lowest median dwell times (296 and 298 days, respectively), and those with no mental health disorder had the highest median dwell time (342 days). Length of first deployment differed significantly across outcome groups ($P = .007$).

A summary of the DDR and mental health analysis is presented in Table 4. A high DDR of 2:1, representing a longer dwell time relative to first deployment length, was associated with a significantly lower rate of PTSD diagnosis only (0.9% versus 1.8%) and PTSD with other mental health disorder (0.5% versus 1.0%) when compared with a low DDR or shorter dwell time ratio of less than 1:1. Rates of other mental health disorders were also significantly lower among those with a high DDR (2:1, 4.3%) versus a low DDR (less than

Table 3. Distributions of Deployment-Specific Variables Stratified by Outcome Category Among US Marines with 2 OIF Deployments: 2003-2007

Deployment Variable	PTSD Only (n = 225)	PTSD With Other Mental Health Disorder (n = 122)	Other Mental Health Disorder (n = 936)	No Mental Health Disorder (n = 15 093)	P^a
DDR					< .001
Median (range)	1.5 (0.6-9.5)	1.5 (0.4-3.8)	1.6 (0.1-11.2)	1.7 (0.1-11.8)	
Interquartile range	1.0-1.9	0.9-1.9	1.0-1.9	1.3-2.3	
1st deployment time					.007
Median (range)	207 (120-240)	206 (120-238)	205 (120-240)	203 (120-240)	
Interquartile range	185-212	188-212	182-211	175-212	
2nd deployment time					.053
Median (range)	206 (132-240)	206 (124-228)	205 (120-240)	205 (120-240)	
Interquartile range	202-212	201-209	198-210	195-210	
Dwell time					< .001
Median (range)	296 (132-1172)	298 (100-770)	314 (29-1360)	342 (24-1425)	
Interquartile range	206-367	206-370	206-367	220-412	

Note. The sample size was n = 16 376. DDR = dwell-to-deployment ratio; OIF = Operation Iraqi Freedom; PTSD = posttraumatic stress disorder.
[a]Wilcoxon test for difference across medians.

Table 4. Mental Health Diagnoses Among US Marines with 2 OIF Deployments by Dwell-To-Deployment Time Ratio (DDR): 2003–2007

DDR[a]	Total (n = 16 376)	PTSD Only		PTSD With Other Mental Health Disorder		Other Mental Health Disorder	
		No. (%)[b]	OR (95% CI)[c]	No. (%)[d]	OR (95% CI)[c]	No. (%)[b]	OR (95% CI)[c]
< 1:1 (Ref)	3 270	60 (1.8)	1.00	32 (1.0)	1.00	233 (7.1)	1.00
1:1	8 041	122 (1.5)	0.83 (0.60, 1.13)	64 (0.8)	0.82 (0.53, 1.25)	485 (6.0)	0.84 (0.72, 0.99)
2:1	5 065	43 (0.9)	0.47 (0.32, 0.70)	26 (0.5)	0.56 (0.33, 0.94)	218 (4.3)	0.62 (0.51, 0.75)

Note. CI = confidence interval; OR = odds ratio; PTSD = posttraumatic stress disorder.

[a]Defined as the period of time at home between deployments divided by the length of first deployment.

[b]Mantel-Haenszel test for trend: $P < .001$.

[c]ORs and 95% CIs were calculated by using polychotomous logistic regression with adjustment for age and military rank.

[d]Mantel-Haenszel test for trend: $P = .01$.

1:1, 7.1%). The Mantel–Haenszel test indicated a significant trend across DDR categories for PTSD only ($P < .001$), PTSD with other mental health disorder ($P = .01$), and other mental health disorder ($P < .001$). After adjustment for age and military rank in the polychotomous logistic regression, a DDR of at least 2:1 was strongly associated with reduced odds of PTSD only (OR = 0.47; 95% CI = 0.32, 0.70), PTSD with other mental health disorder (OR = 0.56; 95% CI = 0.33, 0.94), and other mental health disorders (OR = 0.62; 95% CI = 0.51, 0.75) when compared with the low DDR category (less than 1:1). DDR was also analyzed as a continuous variable where longer dwell time at home relative to first deployment length was associated with reduced odds of PTSD only (OR = 0.80; 95% CI = 0.70, 0.93), PTSD with other mental health disorder (OR = 0.75; 95% CI = 0.61, 0.93), and other mental health disorder (OR = 0.87; 95% CI = 0.82, 0.93). The results did not change after the exclusion of personnel with a hospitalization during their first deployment (n = 36). In addition, a separate adjustment for age at first deployment did not affect the results.

DISCUSSION

This study provides the first preliminary evidence linking dwell time spent at home to subsequent postdeployment mental health diagnoses. There has been much discussion on setting a dwell time policy, that is, a standard length of time military members must be home before consideration for their next deployment. Although further research is needed to elucidate the potential protective effect of dwell time, the results of the present study advance the discussion on the utility and potential effectiveness of regulating dwell time.

The rates of PTSD and other mental health disorders that we reported were consistent with previous research, as was the finding that only PTSD rates were elevated in personnel with 2 deployments. Larson et al. found similar rates among deployed US Marines, although when compared with a nondeployed control group, only PTSD was significantly higher.[16] Those authors identified the "healthy warrior effect" as a possible explanation, that is, the overall healthier status of personnel who deploy compared with those who do not, and the results of the present study suggest an extension of that effect to personnel with 2 deployments compared with 1.[16,17] It is possible that disorders perceived as more serious, such as depression and bipolar disorder, become disqualifying conditions and therefore prevent the service member from subsequent deployments. As such, those with multiple deployments may represent a more resilient population. This may be supported by the marginally significant finding in the present study of lower rates of other mental health disorders among personnel with 2 deployments.

The primary findings of our study suggest that longer dwell times are associated with lower odds of mental health diagnoses, which is consistent with a stress–exhaustion model in which the cumulative effects of multiple deployments eventually lead to higher mental health morbidity.[18] This effect has been shown in multiple studies of OIF combat populations.[8-10] The opposite relationship, however, has been identified following multiple peacekeeping deployments.[1] Two recent studies identified a correlation between multiple deployments and increased mental health symptom reporting, but did not address the effect of dwell time.[9,10] Although the theory behind the stress–exhaustion model is based on stressor duration, lack of an adequate dwell time may prevent the service member from fully recovering from the first deployment, which suggests that a mental "reset" period is needed before subsequent deployment. This is supported by the most recent MHAT survey among US Army personnel, in which it was found that increased dwell time resulted in a steady decline in self-reported mental health problems.[12]

Future studies on dwell time should focus on characterization of the dwell time variable. For the purposes of our study, we placed dwell time over first deployment length to create a unitless measure of DDR. This ratio measure was skewed and subsequently categorized to reflect time at home relative to first deployment length. This methodology was a strength of our study because it used the current political language to characterize dwell time, thus making it more applicable to future policy decisions. For example, Senator Jim Webb's dwell time proposal called for the establishment of a 1:1 DDR for all military personnel.[13] Alternatively, Secretary of Defense Robert Gates called for the establishment of an immediate 1:1 DDR for specific units (e.g., brigade combat teams with typically high levels of combat exposure), with an eventual progression to a DDR of 2:1.[14] It is possible, however, that there are other ways of exploring the relationship between dwell time and postdeployment mental health, including examining different inflection points, as well as more complex interactions with deployment length.

Other strengths of our study include the use of electronic deployment records that allowed for a large and robust study sample. At least one previous study found a high correlation between self-reported deployment dates and DMDC electronic records.[19] The use of electronic deployment records also allowed us to exclude personnel with previous non-OIF deployments, which removed potential confounding or mediating effects of other combat tours with differing deployment experiences (e.g., OEF) and noncombat tours (e.g., peacekeeping missions).

The limitations of the present study include the use of electronic medical databases for ascertainment of mental health diagnosis. This methodology likely resulted in an underestimate of mental health morbidity because stigma often prevents military personnel from presenting for care. Thus, mild cases of mental health disorder may be underrepresented. In addition, unmeasured variables may have affected the results of the study. Combat exposure, a mediator of the relationship between deployment and mental health, was not measured.[20,21] Many life and work-related experiences during a service member's dwell time, such as advances in rank, onset or dissolution of personal relationships, and changes in financial status, may also mediate the relationship between dwell time and mental health.

In conclusion, increased dwell time relative to first deployment length was associated with reduced odds of both PTSD and other mental health disorders. Combined with operational and logistical considerations, the findings of the present study may be useful in guiding future policy decisions on multiple deployments and dwell time. These results also highlight the importance of further research on dwell time, especially because multiple deployments are likely to continue for the foreseeable future. Future studies should incorporate self-report measures of mental health status, attempt to document specific dwell time experiences, examine effects on military attrition, and extend the population to those with 3 or more deployments. Furthermore, more extreme deployment lengths should be assessed. Many personnel experiencing multiple deployments will eventually transition to civilian life. As such, the cumulative health effects of multiple deployments present an emerging public health problem for the military, as well as for the general population. For present and future military conflicts, dwell time policies should focus on evidence-based decision making and work toward amelioration of the overall health of the US Armed Forces.

ABOUT THE AUTHORS

Andrew J. MacGregor, Peggy P. Han, Amber L. Dougherty, and Michael R. Galarneau are with the Department of Medical Modeling, Simulation, and Mission Support, Naval Health Research Center, San Diego, CA.

CONTRIBUTORS

A. J. MacGregor led the study conception and design, analyses and interpretation of data, drafting of the article, and approval of the final version. P. P. Han contributed to the data analyses, revision of the article, and approval of the final version. A. L. Dougherty contributed to the study design, interpretation of data, revision of the article, and approval of the final version. M. R. Galarneau assisted with study conception, revision of the article, and approval of the final version.

ACKNOWLEDGMENTS

This work was supported by the US Navy Bureau of Medicine and Surgery under the Wounded, Ill, and Injured/Psychological Health/Traumatic Brain Injury program.

We thank Troy Holbrook for her assistance with revision of the article. We also thank Science Applications International Corporation, Inc., for its contributions to this work.

Note. The views and opinions expressed herein are those of the authors and do not necessarily reflect the official policy or position of the Department of the Navy, Department of Defense, or the US Government.

HUMAN PARTICIPANT PROTECTION

This research was conducted in compliance with all applicable federal regulations governing the protection of human subjects in research and was approved by the institutional review board, Naval Health Research Center, San Diego, CA (protocol no. NHRC.2003.0025).

REFERENCES

1. Adler AB, Huffman AH, Bliese PD, Castro CA. The impact of deployment length and experience on the well-being of male and female soldiers. *J Occup Health Psychol.* 2005;10(2):121–137.

2. Castro CA, Adler AB. OPTEMPO: effect on soldier and unit readiness. *Parameters.* 1999;29:86–95. Available at: http://www.carlisle.army.mil/USAWC/parameters/Articles/99autumn/castro.htm. Accessed June 15, 2009.

3. Bender B. Repeat tours of combat-zone duty put strains on families, Pentagon. *Boston Globe.* November 26, 2004. Available at: http://www.boston.com/news/world/articles/2004/11/26/repeat_tours_of_combat_zone_duty_put_strains_on_families_pentagon. Accessed June 15, 2009.

4. Ozer EJ, Weiss DS. Who develops posttraumatic stress disorder? *Curr Dir Psychol Sci.* 2004;13(4):169–172.

5. Health status of Vietnam veterans. I. Psychosocial characteristics. The Centers for Disease Control and Prevention Vietnam Experience Study. *JAMA.* 1988;259(18):2701–2707.

6. Stimpson NJ, Thomas HV, Weightman AL, Dunstan F, Lewis G. Psychiatric disorder in veterans of the Persian Gulf War of 1991. *Br J Psychiatry.* 2003;182:391–403.

7. Hoge CW, Auchterlonie JL, Milliken CS. Mental health problems, use of mental health services, and attrition from military service after returning from deployment to Iraq or Afghanistan. *JAMA.* 2006;295(9):1023–1032.

8. Office of the Surgeon Multi-National Force-Iraq, Office of the Command Surgeon, and Office of the Surgeon General United States Army Medical Command. Mental Health Advisory Team (MHAT) V Operation Iraqi Freedom 06-08: Iraq; Operation Enduring Freedom 8: Afghanistan. 14 February 2008. Available at: http://www.armymedicine.army.mil/reports/mhat/mhat_v/Redacted1-MHATV-4-FEB-2008-Overview.pdf. Accessed June 15, 2009.

9. Reger MA, Gahm GA, Swanson RD, Duma SJ. Association between number of deployments to Iraq and mental health screening outcomes in US Army soldiers. *J Clin Psychiatry.* 2009;70(9):1266–1272.

10. Polusny MA, Erbes CR, Arbisi PA, et al. Impact of prior Operation Enduring Freedom/Operation Iraqi Freedom combat duty on mental health in a predeployment cohort of National Guard soldiers. *Mil Med.* 2009;174(4):353–357.

11. Rona RJ, Fear NT, Hull L, Greenberg N, Earnshaw M, Hotopf M. Mental health consequences of overstretch in the UK armed forces: first phase of a cohort study. *BMJ.* 2007;335(7620):603–607.

12. Office of the Surgeon Multi-National Force-Iraq, Office of the Command Surgeon, and Office of the Surgeon General United States Army Medical Command. Mental Health Advisory Team (MHAT) VI Operation Iraqi Freedom 07-09: Iraq. 8 May 2009. Available at: http://www.armymedicine.army.mil/reports/mhat/mhat_vi/mhat-vi.cfm. Accessed March 15, 2009.

13. Maze R. Webb wants to put dwell-time rule into law. *Army Times.* December 2, 2008. Available at: http://www.armytimes.com/news/2008/12/military_webb_dwelltime_120108w. Accessed June 15, 2009.

14. McMichael WH. Gates details plans for deployment, dwell time. *Air Force Times.* January 29, 2009. Available at: http://www.airforcetimes.com/news/2009/01/military_gates_012709w. Accessed June 15, 2009.

15. *International Classification of Diseases, Ninth Revision, Clinical Modification.* Hyattsville, MD: National Center for Health Statistics; 1980. DHHS publication PHS 80-1260.

16. Larson GE, Highfill-McRoy RM, Booth-Kewley S. Psychiatric diagnoses in historic and contemporary military cohorts: combat deployment and the healthy warrior effect. *Am J Epidemiol.* 2008;167(11):1269–1276.

17. Haley RW. Point: bias from the "healthy-warrior effect" and unequal follow-up in three government studies of health effects of the Gulf War. *Am J Epidemiol.* 1998;148(4):315–323.

18. Lazarus RS, Folkman S. *Stress, appraisal, and coping.* New York, NY: Springer; 1984.

19. Smith B, Wingard DL, Ryan MA, Macera CA, Patterson TL, Slymen DJ. US military deployment during 2001–2006: comparison of subjective and objective data sources in a large prospective health study. *Ann Epidemiol.* 2007;17(12):976–982.

20. Rona RJ, Hooper R, Jones M, et al. The contribution of prior psychological symptoms and combat exposure to post Iraq deployment mental health screening in the UK military. *J Trauma Stress.* 2009;22(1):11–19.

21. Smith TC, Ryan MA, Wingard DL, Slymen DJ, Sallis JF, Kritz-Silverstein D. New onset and persistent symptoms of post-traumatic stress disorder self reported after deployment and combat exposures: prospective population based US military cohort study. *BMJ.* 2008;336(7640):366–371.

21

Use of the Air Force Post-Deployment Health Reassessment for the Identification of Depression and Posttraumatic Stress Disorder: Public Health Implications for Suicide Prevention

Michael D. McCarthy, PhD, Sanna J. Thompson, PhD, and Kerry L. Knox, PhD, MS

Objectives. Military members are required to complete the Post-Deployment Health Assessment on return from deployment and the Post-Deployment Health Reassessment (PHDRA) 90 to 180 days later, and we assessed the PDHRA's sensitivity and specificity in identifying posttraumatic stress disorder (PTSD) and depression after a military deployment among US Air Force personnel.

Methods. We computed the PDHRA's sensitivity and specificity for depression and PTSD and developed a structural model to suggest possible improvements to it.

Results. For depression, sensitivity and specificity were 0.704 and 0.651, respectively; for PTSD, they were 0.774 and 0.650, respectively. Several variables produced significant direct effects on depression and trauma, suggesting that modifications could increase its sensitivity and specificity.

Conclusions. The PDHRA was moderately effective in identifying airmen with depression and PTSD. It identified behavioral health concerns in many airmen who did not develop a diagnostic mental health condition. Its low level of specificity may result in reduced barriers to care and increased support services, key components of a public health approach to suicide prevention, for airmen experiencing subacute levels of distress after deployment, which may, in part, account for lower suicide rates among airmen after deployment.

The conflicts in Iraq and Afghanistan represent the longest wartime engagement in US military history.[1] Their impact on military members is only beginning to be understood, and the effects are likely to reverberate for decades. Because of the protracted nature of these conflicts, military members and veterans may have increased mental health needs.[2] As of 2009, 1.6 million US military members had deployed in support of Operation Enduring Freedom (Afghanistan) and Operation Iraqi Freedom. Of these, an estimated 300 000 have returned with a mental health condition, such as depression or posttraumatic stress disorder (PTSD).[3] Exposure to violent combat is often a precursor to emotional dysfunction, most notably an increased risk of PTSD and depression,[4-6] that may lead to suicidal behavior, including suicide attempts and ideation. The relatively high rates of depression and PTSD and the marked increase in military suicide rates from 2005 to 2009 have made mental health issues the source of significant concern for the military.[6-8]

In response to the physical and emotional hazards of deployment and the increasing frequency of suicides among military members that some believe are a consequence of prolonged and repeated deployments,[6,7,9,10] the US Department of Defense established a robust program to screen and track deployment-related physical and psychiatric illnesses.[11,12] Thus, all military members are currently required to complete the Post-Deployment Health Assessment, which is part of a broader military health monitoring system, immediately on their return from deployment. A nearly identical screening tool, the Post-Deployment Health Reassessment (PDHRA), is administered 90 to 180 days later.[13] Additional screening may occur at the discretion of medical providers or military members' commanders.[14]

The PDHRA has been used since 2005 to assess the health of military members in the months after a deployment.[14] It was augmented in 2008 by broadening questions about traumatic brain injury (TBI) and alcohol misuse.[15]

Although significant resources have been dedicated to identifying postdeployment health and mental health issues, the efficacy of the screening and assessment instruments has not been established.[16,17] Postdeployment assessments were developed by consensus in professional working groups and rapidly deployed in response to a congressional mandate.[16] No scaling or testing of the assessments was or has been conducted before or since implementation;[16] therefore, their reliability and validity have not been established. Specifically, whether the PDHRA is an effective tool for identifying military members at risk for developing mental health concerns after a deployment is not known.

To address this gap, we evaluated the PDHRA's effectiveness in identifying military members at risk for depression and PTSD and identified ways to improve its sensitivity and specificity. In addition, we assessed the relationship between deployment and other factors associated with depression and PTSD to further understand factors that might increase the risk of negative outcomes, including suicide, after a deployment.

METHODS

We used a comprehensive population sampling strategy. All active, reserve, and National Guard airmen (n = 58 242) who completed the PDHRA between January 1, 2008, and December 31, 2008, were included in this study. Because of the study's large sample size, we used a rigorous standard for statistical significance, $P < .001$, to avoid capitalization on chance. Study participants were aged 17 years or older because of Department of Defense regulations.[18] Study participants included all pay grades from Airman Basic (E-1) to Major General (O-8).

The PDHRA is a Web-based, 3-page, self-report questionnaire that includes questions on demographic characteristics, general health, physical symptoms, and environmental exposures and mental health items that may be deployment related.[13] It is the primary tool used by the military medical system to identify individuals who have physical or behavioral health concerns after a deployment. The PDHRA is also the last in a series of formal screenings that the Department of Defense uses to identify service members who are experiencing distress after a deployment.[13] When completed, the PDHRA becomes part of the military member's medical record[14] and is integrated into the Defense Medical Surveillance System database.[13] Consequently, the PDHRA's effectiveness in identifying service members who may be at elevated risk for PTSD or depression is central to maintaining a healthy military population and decreasing the risk for suicide.

PDHRA managers are responsible for triaging all positive PDHRAs at their military base. The criteria for a positive PDHRA are defined in a comprehensive algorithm available in the *Post-Deployment Health Reassessment User's Guide.*[14] Contact with airmen whose responses on the PDHRA indicate areas of concern may occur by telephone or immediate referral to a medical provider. The PDHRA manager or other medical provider typically calls the military member to discuss the results of his or her PDHRA and explores the need for follow-up. An airman's primary care physician and the physician's support staff have access to the airman's PDHRA results, which provide clinically relevant information for use in determining treatment needs. In addition to the PDHRA's primary questions, specific question sets were developed to assess for certain behavioral health disorders, such as PTSD and depression. Thus, airmen who screen positive for behavioral health concerns are offered the opportunity to complete the PTSD Checklist–Military Version (PCL-M), which assesses for trauma symptoms, and the Patient Health Questionnaire–9 (PHQ-9), which assesses for depression.[14] The results of the PCL-M and PHQ-9 are also available to medical personnel and used to evaluate specific mental health concerns.

The data used in the current analysis were drawn from the M-2 military public health database of PDHRA results, housed at Brooks City-Base, San Antonio, Texas. The M-2 is a comprehensive database that includes all diagnostic data for all Air Force members. A data request was submitted for diagnostic data on all airmen. The primary dependent variables for this study were the *International Classification of Diseases, Ninth Revision (ICD-9)*[19] codes that identified a diagnosis of depression or PTSD and acute stress disorder. We used the *ICD-9* codes for PTSD and acute stress disorder to create the endogenous variable trauma diagnosis, and we used the *ICD-9* codes for dysthymic disorder, major depressive disorder, depressive episode, and depression not otherwise specified to create the endogenous variable depression diagnosis (Figure 1). All trauma-related or depressive diagnoses were assigned by a physician, a licensed psychologist, or a licensed clinical social worker after an evaluation that determined that the airman met the criteria for these conditions.

We developed structural models using a 3-step process. All PDHRA questions related to behavioral health concerns according to the user's manual were entered into a theoretically derived confirmatory factor analysis. Factors

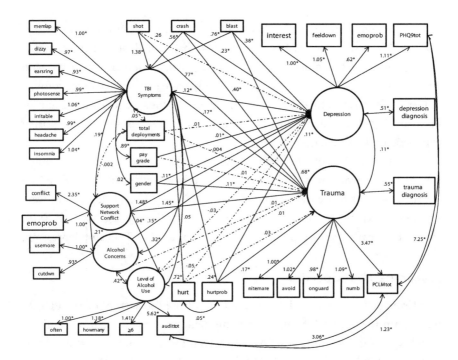

Figure 1. Post-Deployment Health Reassessment structural model for 58 242 airmen taken from the M-2 military public health database: Brooks City-Base, San Antonio, TX, January 1–December 31, 2008.

Note. PCL-M = PTSD Checklist–Military Version; PHQ-9 = Patient Health Questionnaire–9; TBI = traumatic brain injury. *Indicates $P < .001$

were then modeled on the basis of their hypothesized relationship to the endogenous variables (Figure 1). We then used the Wald χ^2 test and Lagrange multiplier test to identify the best-fitting structural model.[20] We conducted all statistical analyses using Mplus Version 5 software.[21]

RESULTS

Most of the sample were enlisted airmen (n = 48 290), and the largest group represented was staff sergeants (E-5; n = 15 139). The officer corps made up about 17% of the sample (n = 9817), compared with 18.6% of the total Air Force.[20] Although women make up 19% of the total Air Force,[22] 15% of this study's sample (n = 8859) were female.

The average respondent in this study had deployed twice (mean = 1.98; SD = 1.76), and many (17.8%; n = 10 344) had not deployed to a combat zone but were sent to more forward locations, such as Germany, to assist with combat operations. Many airmen in this study were exposed to direct combat. For example, many (13.4%; n = 7823) reported exposure to an explosion or blast during their deployment, whereas only 3% (n = 1757) reported experiencing a vehicular crash.

Although 16.5% of the sample noted 1 or more traumatic combat experiences, participants had a very low prevalence of diagnosed PTSD (0.3%; n = 160) or depression (0.6%; n = 338). PTSD and depression were significantly correlated in this sample (r = 0.346; P < .001), but only 0.1% (n = 81) of participants were diagnosed with comorbid PTSD and depression.

Psychometric Properties

The Cronbach's α for the PDHRA question set used to screen for the PCL-M was within the acceptable range for nomothetic research (α = 0.76), and the Cronbach α for the question set used to screen for the PHQ-9 (α = 0.83) was high enough to serve as a guide for clinical decision-making.[23–25]

The PHQ-9's internal consistency was excellent (α = 0.98). Its mean for this sample (mean = 2.10; SD = 9.37) was within 1 standard deviation of the clinical range of 5, which suggests mild concerns, and 10, which suggests moderate concerns;[26] this score suggests that PDHRA depression screening items identify participants who may benefit most from early intervention.[27] Similarly, the PCL-M's internal consistency was excellent (α = 0.99). The mean score of airmen completing the PCL-M was more than 3 standard deviations below the PCL-M's clinical cutoff level of 50 (mean = 6.91; SD = 14.08);[28] this score suggests that PDHRA trauma-related screening items are too inclusive.

In this sample, depression diagnoses were significantly more common among individuals with PDHRA scores that were positive for behavioral health concerns than among those with PDHRA scores suggesting few behavioral health concerns ($\chi^2_{1, \, n \, = \, 58 \, 242}$ = 186.43; P < .001). One of 85 individuals with positive PDHRA scores eventually received a diagnosis of depression, compared with 1 of 378 individuals with negative PDHRA scores. This finding translates to airmen with positive PDHRA scores being more than 4 times as likely to be diagnosed with depression than airmen with PDHRA scores that do not indicate behavioral health concerns.

PTSD diagnoses were also significantly more common among individuals with PDHRA scores positive for behavioral health concerns than among those with negative PDHRA scores ($\chi^2_{1,\ n\ =\ 58\ 242}$ = 108.81; $P \leq .001$). Among airmen with positive PDHRA scores, 1 of 171 eventually received a diagnosis of PTSD, compared with only 1 of 922 airmen with negative PDHRA scores. Thus, airmen with PDHRA scores that indicated behavioral health concerns were more than 5 times as likely to be diagnosed with PTSD than were airmen with negative PDHRA scores.

Specificity and Sensitivity for Depression and Posttraumatic Stress Disorder

The 2 most common ways to assess the clinical value of a test are to determine its sensitivity and specificity.[29] Sensitivity is the proportion, for a given condition, of actualpositives that are correctly identified; specificity is the proportion of actual negatives that are correctly identified.[30,31] Specificity is related to the Type I error of a measure, with higher specificity suggesting a low Type I error rate, or fewer false positives. Sensitivity is related to the Type II error of a measure, with higher sensitivity suggesting a low Type II error rate, or fewer false negatives.[32-34]

In this study, the PDHRA's sensitivity for depression was 0.704 (n = 238), and its specificity was 0.651 (n = 37 713); its specificity for PTSD was 0.744 (n = 119), and its sensitivity was 0.650 (n = 37 772). The PDHRA's lack of sensitivity for depression was 0.296 (n = 100), and its lack of specificity was 0.349 (n = 20 191); its lack of sensitivity for PTSD was 0.256 (n = 41), and its lack of specificity was 0.350 (n = 20 310).

Structural Equation Modeling Analysis

We analyzed a structural equation model to determine the contribution made by each PDHRA item to identify airmen at risk for experiencing trauma-related or depressive symptoms. The PDHRA structural model assessed the relationship between answers on the PDHRA and the later development of a diagnosis of depression or PTSD. The analysis suggested a good-fitting model (Figure 1). The χ^2 test of model fit was significant ($\chi^2_{160,\ n\ =\ 58\ 242}$ = 6530.03;

$P \le .001$). Other fit indices suggested a good- to excellent-fitting model: comparative fit index = 0.94; Tucker-Lewis index = 0.97; root-mean-square error of approximation = 0.03.[20] The latent variable depression produced a large, positive direct effect (b = 0.51; $P \le .001$) on the variable depression diagnosis, and the latent variable trauma produced a large direct effect (b = 0.55; $P \le .001$) on the variable trauma diagnosis.

The largest direct effects were produced by the latent variable support network conflict. Support network conflict produced a large, positive, statistically significant effect on depression (b = 1.48; $P \le .001$) and trauma (b = 1.45; $P \le .001$). Other variables produced statistically significant direct effects on depression and trauma: Being shot (b = 0.77; $P \le .001$) and being exposed to a blast (b = 0.68; $P \le .001$) had a large, positive direct effect on trauma. Being involved in a vehicle crash also had a moderate, positive direct effect on depression (b = 0.38; $P \le .001$) and trauma (b = 0.40; $P \le .001$). TBI symptoms had a small, positive direct effect on depression (b = 0.12; $P \le .001$) and trauma (b = 0.17; $P \le .001$). We found no statistically significant relationship between the number of deployments and depression (b = −0.01; $P = .017$) or trauma (b = −0.004; $P = .479$).

The structural model accounted for 22.2% ($r^2 = 0.222$) of the variance in depression diagnosis and 26.2% ($r^2 = 0.262$) of the variance in trauma diagnosis. It accounted for 64.5% ($r^2 = 0.645$) of the variance in the latent variable depression, and 61.3% ($r^2 = 0.613$) of the variance in the latent variable trauma.

DISCUSSION

We should consider several limitations. First, the PDHRA is based on self-report and may therefore be subject to the usual biases associated with these types of data. Second, the data used in this study were retrospective; if the PDHRA's psychometric characteristics are improved, the relationships modeled in this study may not be replicable. Suggestions for enhancing the PDHRA are discussed later in this section.

The PDHRA appears to be a moderately effective clinical screening tool with this sample of airmen. Individuals whose PDHRA scores were positive for behavioral health concerns were significantly more likely to develop a diagnosis of PTSD or depression than individuals whose PDHRA scores did not indicate behavioral health concerns. The PDHRA's sensitivity for both depression and PTSD did not reach the 0.85 threshold set forth in this study (depression = 0.71; PTSD = 0.74),[35] which was surprising given that it was designed to be overly inclusive of behavioral health concerns. Airmen who were diagnosed with depression or PTSD but for whom the PDHRA did not indicate behavioral health concerns may not have been directed or referred for services to address their mental health needs. Although the PDHRA's sensitivity is inadequate for diagnostic purposes, it seems to provide medical and mental health professionals with a screening tool that is useful for identifying most individuals who are at risk for depressive and trauma-related disorders after a deployment.

The PDHRA's lower than expected sensitivity may have resulted partially because some individuals were diagnosed with depression or PTSD that was the result of factors that occurred after their PDHRA screening and had little connection to their deployment. If this pattern was present in a very small segment of the overall sample, it would account for most of the false negative results. Future research controlling for life stressors that occur after PDHRA completion would more accurately describe its sensitivity.

Because the PDHRA was designed to be an overly inclusive screening tool,[16] its low specificity was not surprising. However, its poor specificity may have resulted in many airmen who did not have acute levels of psychiatric distress being provided supportive services by medical and mental health providers. This process may have promoted help-seeking behaviors and facilitated the delivery of preventive medical interventions.[36,37] Recent research with veterans of Operation Iraqi Freedom and Operation Enduring Freedom has found high utilization of mental health services.[11] In short, after a deployment, those who need care appear to be receiving it, which may contrast with the experience of military members who have non–deployment-related depression or trauma. Prior studies have documented significant stigma associated with seeking care for mental health issues within military cohorts.[36]

In addition, mental health screening during the military accession process and during annual physical health assessments is much less robust than postdeployment,[38,39] which may help explain the elevated risk of suicide among airmen who have not deployed.[40,41] Although the postdeployment screening process may be protective, our findings suggest several areas in which the PDHRA's accuracy could be improved.

Support Networks

The latent variable support network conflict produced by far the largest effects on both depression and trauma in both PDHRA measurement models. The importance of support networks in enhancing resilience after traumatic exposure in combat veterans is well established in the literature.[42,43] On the PDHRA, support network conflict encompasses family, social, and occupational support networks. Social support, family functioning, and occupational satisfaction are each important components of a support network. Combat veterans who have high levels of social support are at less risk for depression, trauma-related problems, and suicide after a combat experience than peers who have inadequate social resources.[42,44] Closeness to family members also enhances military members' resilience after traumatic combat-related experiences,[44] as do homecoming ceremonies.[6] Because the PDHRA measures these 3 separate aspects of a support network with only 2 questions, it may undervalue and under-assess the role of support networks. The inclusion of a more robust assessment of support network functioning may provide critical clinical information about the presence or lack of the resiliency-enhancing systems available to military members after a deployment. A small set of screening questions for each of the constructs of social support, family functioning, and occupational satisfaction could be included in the PDHRA with minimal impact on the its length. For example, adding a question that directly asks whether the respondent had an important relationship end or change significantly during or since the deployment may be of value. These screening questions could then be supplemented with standardized measures of these constructs, similar to the use of the PCL-M and PHQ-9.

Gender

Previous research has identified a higher prevalence of depression and PTSD among women.[46,47] Being female was associated with marginally higher levels of trauma and depression. For military health care providers to be aware of the additional risk female airmen face during and after a deployment may be of value. In its present form, the PDHRA does not include gender as a behavioral health risk factor.[14] Developing gender-specific thresholds for various behavioral health items on the PDHRA may improve its sensitivity. The PDHRA does not include gender-specific cutoffs for variables measuring alcohol-related problems.[14] Expanding the use of these cutoffs to other constructs may be of value. Modifications to the PDHRA may help clarify gender-related risks associated with trauma and depression. Developing gender-specific clinical thresholds for depression and trauma screening questions may improve its sensitivity.

Traumatic Brain Injury Symptoms

The TBI symptoms factor produced significant effects on both trauma and depression. Another potential limitation is that the PDHRA does not currently include TBI symptoms items to identify behavioral health concerns. The variables that make up the TBI symptoms factor are used in the PDHRA to identify physical concerns. Medical providers must be informed that the TBI symptoms items may be indicative of both physical concerns and behavioral health concerns.

Previous research has suggested that military members may be at greater risk for injury after a deployment,[48] and increasing suicide rates among service members have recently been speculated to be a consequence of repeated deployments. However, current research has demonstrated a strong, negative correlation between the number of deployments and suicide among airmen ($r = -0.994$; $P = .006$).[41,49] These findings may, in part, be explained by the healthy warrior effect. Previous research identified a disproportionate loss of psychologically unfit personnel during early military training.[50-52] Consequently, military members who are able to serve long enough to deploy 1 or more times appear to have a certain level of resilience that increases over time. Noteworthy is the work of psychopathologist Henry A. Murray, who found in a 1948 study of returning veterans that combat experience did not always result in negative outcomes. Indeed, veterans with considerable trauma exposure were among the strongest and most resilient.[53]

Our findings suggest an additional hypothesis for the low suicide rate among military deployers. The PDHRA process provides airmen who have only minor behavioral health concerns and do not have an acute level of psychiatric distress with supportive services from medical and mental health providers. This process may remove barriers to care for airmen experiencing more common precipitants of suicide among military members such as relationship problems, legal problems, or financial hardship[9] and may prevent minor symptoms and issues that are unrelated or indirectly related to combat from escalating.[11,37]

In summary, early detection and treatment of an array of common precipitants of suicide, such as addressing relationship, financial, and legal problems, are key components of a public health model of suicide prevention.[54] Although war is usually regarded as a serious stressor for military troops, some individuals may perceive it in a very positive and challenging way.[55] Individuals who have more support safety nets are not only protected from the potentially damaging impact of stressful events but also appear to experience fewer negative events.[56] This study lends important support to this observation. Moreover, early access to care for mental health and psychosocial problems, which may be facilitated by the PDHRA process, appears to play an important part in mitigating psychosocial risk factors for suicide. Taken together, our findings contribute to the overall observation of the expected effects of a public health–focused intervention, albeit brought about through a clinically focused assessment. To our knowledge, this study is the first demonstration of a screening and assessment instrument, the PDHRA, used in a military population that, because of its low specificity, meets one of the key tenets of a public health approach to suicide prevention. It underscores the need, from a population-based point of view, to assess for the presence of a mental health concern rather than the severity of the diagnosis. Most important, the observation of an inverse relationship between deployment and suicide among airmen is critical, given the abundance of media attention paid to this topic. We provide the first evidence of how an instrument designed to be a clinical triage tool resulted in effects that would be desirable in any program using a public health approach to suicide prevention. As such, it may provide future guidance in developing interventions and programs for reducing deaths from suicide in both military and veteran populations.

ABOUT THE AUTHORS

Michael D. McCarthy is with the Air Force Medical Support Agency, Arlington, VA. Sanna J. Thompson is with the School of Social Work, University of Texas at Austin. Kerry L. Knox is with the School of Medicine and Dentistry, University of Rochester, Rochester, New York.

CONTRIBUTORS

M. D. McCarthy developed all models, conducted all statistical analyses, and contributed to the interpretation of the study's findings. S. J. Thompson served as editor of the article and contributed significantly to the study's conceptualization. K. L. Knox contributed significant sections to the article's Discussion section. All authors contributed substantially to the writing of the article.

ACKNOWLEDGMENTS

Appreciation is expressed to Roberta Greene, Laura Baugh, and Bree McCarthy for their helpful comments on earlier versions of this article.

HUMAN PARTICIPANT PROTECTION

This study was approved by exempt status on August 12, 2010, by the institutional review board at the University of Texas at Austin.

REFERENCES

1. Salter C. Why is Afghanistan important? *Geogr Teach.* 2010;7(1):16–21.

2. Seal KH, Bertenthal D, Miner CR, Sen S, Marmar C. Bringing the war back home: mental health disorders among 103 788 US veterans returning from Iraq and Afghanistan seen at Department of Veterans Affairs facilities. *Arch Intern Med.* 2007;167(5):476–482.

3. RAND. *Invisible Wounds of War: Summary and Recommendations for Addressing Psychological and Cognitive Injuries.* Santa Monica, CA: Rand Center for Military Health Policy Research; 2008.

4. Lapierre CB, Schwegler AF, LaBauve BJ. Posttraumatic stress and depression symptoms in soldiers returning from combat operations in Iraq and Afghanistan. *J Trauma Stress.* 2007;20(6):933–943.

5. Shalev AY, Freedman S, Peri T, et al. Prospective study of posttraumatic stress disorder and depression following trauma. *Am J Psychiatry.* 1998;155(5):630–637.

6. Lynch MD, Foley-Peres KR, Sullivan SS. Piers Harris and Coopersmith Measure of Self-Esteem: a comparative analysis. *Educ Res Q.* 2008;32(2):49–68.

7. Braswell H, Kushner HI. Suicide, social integration, and masculinity in the US military. *Soc Sci Med.* 2011;Epub ahead of print.

8. Kuehn BM. Soldier suicide rates continue to rise. *JAMA.* 2009;301(11):1111–1113.

9. Bryan CJ, Cukrowicz KC. Associations between types of combat violence and the acquired capability for suicide. *Suicide Life Threat Behav.* 2011;41(2):126–136.

10. Kang HK, Bullman TA. Risk of suicide among US veterans after returning from the Iraq or Afghanistan war zones. *JAMA.* 2008;300(6):652–653.

11. Hoge CW, Auchterlonie JL, Milliken CS. Mental health problems, use of mental health services, and attrition from military service after returning from deployment to Iraq or Afghanistan. *JAMA.* 2006;295(9):1023–1032.

12. Trump DH, Mazzuchi JF, Riddle J, Hyams KC, Balough B. Force health protection: 10 years of lessons learned by the Department of Defense. *Mil Med.* 2002;167(3):179–185.

13. Milliken CS, Auchterlonie JL, Hoge CW. Longitudinal assessment of mental health problems among active and reserve component soldiers returning from the Iraq War. *JAMA.* 2007;298(18):2141–2148.

14. Population Health Support Division, Air Force Modernization Directorates, & Office of the USAF Surgeon General. *Post-Deployment Health Reassessment: Application User's Guide.* San Antonio, TX: Author; 2008.

15. Loftus T. *Implementation of Revised DD Forms 2796 and 2900.* Washington, DC: Department of the Air Force, Headquarters United States Air Force; 2008.

16. Ozanian A. *Development of the Post-Deployment Health Reassessment.* Edwards Air Force Base, CA: US Department of the Air Force; 2010.

17. Gates R. *Fiscal Year 2009 Department of Defense Budget.* Washington, DC: US Department of Defense; 2009.

18. Chu D. *Qualification Standards for Enlistment, Appointment, and Induction.* Washington, DC: US Department of Defense; 2007. Department of Defense Instruction 1304.26.

19. *International Classification of Diseases, Ninth Revision, Clinical Modification.* Hyattsville, MD: National Center for Health Statistics; 1980. DHHS publication PHS 80-1260.

20. Kline R. *Principles and Practices of Structural Equation Modeling.* 2nd ed. New York, NY: Guilford Press; 2005.

21. Muthén L, Muthén B. *Mplus User's Guide.* 5th ed. Los Angeles, CA: Muthén & Muthén; 2007.

22. Military demographics. Air Force Demographics. Available at: https://www.my.af.mil/raw/asp/SecBroker/

22

Mental and Physical Health Status and Alcohol and Drug Use Following Return From Deployment to Iraq or Afghanistan

Susan V. Eisen, PhD, Mark R. Schultz, PhD, Dawne Vogt, PhD, Mark E. Glickman, PhD, A. Rani Elwy, PhD, Mari-Lynn Drainoni, PhD, Princess E. Osei-Bonsu, MSPH, PhD, and James Martin, PhD

Objectives. We examined (1) mental and physical health symptoms and functioning in US veterans within 1 year of returning from deployment, and (2) differences by gender, service component (Active, National Guard, other Reserve), service branch (Army, Navy, Air Force, Marines), and deployment operation (Operation Enduring Freedom/Operation Iraqi Freedom [OEF/OIF]).

Methods. We surveyed a national sample of 596 OEF/OIF veterans, oversampling women to make up 50% of the total, and National Guard and Reserve components to each make up 25%. Weights were applied to account for stratification and nonresponse bias.

Results. Mental health functioning was significantly worse compared with the general population; 13.9% screened positive for probable posttraumatic stress disorder, 39% for probable alcohol abuse, and 3% for probable drug abuse. Men reported more alcohol and drug use than did women, but there were no gender differences in posttraumatic stress disorder or other mental health domains. OIF veterans reported more depression or functioning problems and alcohol and drug use than did OEF veterans. Army and Marine veterans reported worse mental and physical health than did Air Force or Navy veterans.

Conclusions. Continuing identification of veterans at risk for mental health and substance use problems is important for evidence-based interventions intended to increase resilience and enhance treatment.

The mental and physical health of veterans returning from war zone deployment is of substantial concern to the public as well as military leaders and civilian policymakers.[1] Although most veterans return from deployment without suffering long-term consequences, a significant number experience serious psychological harm. Recent research on the Gulf War and Operation Enduring Freedom/Operation Iraqi Freedom (OEF/OIF) veterans confirmed increased risk for mental health problems, including posttraumatic stress disorder (PTSD), depression, suicidality, neuropsychological deficits, and alcohol and drug use.[2–7] These disorders have implications for individual and unit readiness; physical, social, and emotional health of veterans and their families; and the Veterans Health Administration and other health care systems in which veterans obtain services.[4,7,8] Mental health problems are also often compounded by problems with physical health.[9] Recent conflicts resulted in over 46 000 soldiers wounded in action, some with serious and debilitating conditions, such as chronic pain, traumatic brain injury, and high risk for cardiovascular disease.[10–13]

The objectives of our study were to examine (1) mental and physical health symptoms and functioning, including posttraumatic stress symptoms (PTSS), and alcohol and drug use in a national sample of veterans within 1 year of returning from deployment in Afghanistan or Iraq; and (2) differences in mental and physical health and alcohol and drug use by gender, service component (Active, National Guard, other Reserve), service branch (Army, Navy, Air Force, Marines), and deployment operation (OIF or OEF). Examination of differences in mental health, alcohol use, and drug use is important for identifying those at high risk so that evidence-based interventions to prevent and treat serious disorders can be implemented when indicated. Gender, service component, branch, and deployment operation are of interest because previous research identified differences in mental health, alcohol use, and drug use as a function of these factors. Continued assessment of these issues is valuable, because as the focus and scope of military engagement changes over time, the sequelae of deployment may also change, resulting in different subgroups emerging as high risk.

Previous research suggested that women were at higher risk for mental health conditions including depression, anxiety, and PTSD after traumatic exposure, whereas men were at higher risk for substance use disorders.[14–19] Based on these findings, we hypothesized that women would report more symptoms of depression and PTSD but less alcohol and drug use than men. Previous research found National Guard and Reservists to be at higher risk for mental health, alcohol use, and drug use disorders than Active component personnel.[20-23] Consequently, we hypothesized more mental health, alcohol use, and drug use problems among National Guard and Reservists than among Active component members. Several studies identified Army or Marine veterans as at higher risk for PTSD, depression, or alcohol misuse compared with Navy or Air Force veterans.[16,22,24-27] Based on these findings, we hypothesized higher levels of PTSD, other mental health symptoms, alcohol use, and drug use among Army and Marines compared with Navy and Air Force veterans. Significantly more mental health symptoms were reported among OIF (Iraq) veterans compared with OEF (Afghanistan) veterans,[2,4,11,28] leading us to hypothesize more mental health symptoms and greater substance use among OIF than OEF veterans.

METHODS

We used an observational research design in which a national random sample of US OEF/OIF veterans was surveyed within 12 months of returning from deployment. Surveys were mailed in November 2008, and data collection, which included repeat mailings and reminder phone calls, was completed by the end of 2009. We allowed up to 1 year for receipt of completed surveys.

Sampling Plan

The sample was stratified by service component (50% Active, 25% National Guard, and 25% other Reserve) and gender, with oversampling of women to make up 50% of the total within each service component. Two thousand OEF/OIF veterans, meeting these stratification specifications and who returned from deployment between 3 and 12 months previously, were obtained from the Defense Manpower Data Center (DMDC). The DMDC is the Department of Defense central repository for personnel data, maintaining 230 secure and protected databases, websites, and programs.[29] A total of 167 individuals were determined to be ineligible because they had a military address outside the United States (n = 102), were redeployed (n = 52), or indicated that they had not been deployed in OEF/OIF (n = 13). Of the 1833 eligible individuals, we confirmed that 1043 received the survey materials, and we obtained completed surveys from 598, although 2 surveys were received too late to include in the data analysis. Likely reasons for not receiving the survey included high mobility of the sample, many of whom were still on active duty and might have been deployed elsewhere, moved, or changed telephone numbers. Survey respondents came from every state except Wyoming, as well as the District of Columbia, Puerto Rico, and the US Virgin Islands.

Procedure

Prenotification letters and an "opt-out" postcard were sent to all eligible service members to inform them about the study. Anyone who returned the opt-out postcard within 2 weeks was not recontacted. Two weeks after the prenotification mailing, each eligible veteran was sent a cover letter, an information sheet detailing all elements of informed consent, the survey, and a preaddressed, postage paid return envelope. A modified Dillman method was used to enhance response rates.[30] If completed surveys were not returned within 2 weeks, a reminder letter was sent. Up to 6 reminder telephone calls were made, followed by a repeat mailing to remaining nonrespondents. To further maximize response rates, an Internal Revenue Service (IRS) address search, available via a VA Environmental Epidemiology Service interagency agreement with the IRS, was initiated to obtain updated addresses for individuals who could not be reached by mail or phone. This procedure was approved by the institutional review board. Those who returned a completed survey received a $30 gift card.

Measures

Established, reliable. and valid self-report instruments were used to assess mental and physical health symptoms and functioning, including PTSS, alcohol use, and drug use. Demographic characteristics including race and Hispanic ethnicity, length of deployment, service component, service branch, and deployment operation (OEF/OIF) were obtained from the DMDC. Additional demographic and descriptive information were obtained using self-reported questions used in previous VA research studies.[31,32] Race/ethnicity was obtained for descriptive purposes and is presented in Table 1 based on self-report.

Mental and physical health, alcohol use, and drug use.

Mental and physical health functioning, alcohol use, and drug use were assessed with the Veterans Rand-12 (VR-12),[33,34] Behavior and Symptom

Identification Scale (BASIS-24),[35] PTSD Checklist Military Version (PCL-M),[36] Alcohol Use Disorders Identification Test (AUDIT-C),[37] and Drug Abuse Screening Test (DAST).[38]

The VR-12 is a brief version of the Veterans RAND-36, assessing 2 broad domains of mental and physical health functioning (Mental Component Score [MCS] and Physical Component Score [PCS]).[34,39] The VR- and Short Form-12 are among the most widely used functional status measures in the world and have been shown to be highly reliable and valid. The reliability estimate for the PCS-12 was 0.80, and for the MCS-12 was 0.76.

The PCL-M is a 17-item instrument derived from PTSD diagnostic criteria to assess PTSS severity among veterans. High test–retest and internal consistency reliability and good concurrent validity have been reported.[40] The BASIS-24 is a multidimensional mental health assessment instrument. We used 5 of the 6 BASIS-24 subscales: depression and functioning, interpersonal relationships, emotional lability, psychotic symptoms, and substance use. A sixth subscale assessing self-harm was excluded because it was deemed inappropriate for use in a mailed survey in which risk of self-harm could not be followed up locally. Reliability of the subscales ranges from 0.77 to 0.91 with good concurrent and discriminant validity.[35] BASIS-24 was validated in a national sample of more than 5800 recipients of mental health or substance abuse services, and was also used in other VA mental health studies.[31,32,35]

The AUDIT-C is a brief version of the 10-item AUDIT, a self-report measure designed to identify individuals experiencing problems with alcohol. AUDIT-C identified 90% of patients with alcohol abuse or dependence and 98% of patients with heavy drinking.[37] The DAST-10 is a 10-item instrument designed to identify illegal drug use problems. It has high internal consistency reliability ($\alpha = 0.94$), test–retest reliability (intraclass correlation coefficient = 0.71), and has been found to discriminate between outpatients with and without drug use disorders.[38]

Data Analysis

Sample weights.

Two survey respondent weightings were applied to enhance the representativeness of the sample to the larger OEF/OIF cohort. First, we computed sampling weights for the original sample of 2000 across each of the 6 strata from which service members were sampled (all combinations of men and

Table 1. Sample Characteristics for Health Status, Alcohol and Drug Use Following Return from Deployment to Iraq or Afghanistan: United States, 2008–2009

Variables[a]	No. (%) or Mean ±SD
Gender	
Male	253 (42.4)
Female	343 (57.6)
Age, y	
18–24	117 (19.6)
25–29	127 (21.3)
30–39	180 (30.2)
≥ 40	172 (28.9)
Race[a]	
White	448 (75.2)
African-American	107 (18.0)
Asian	20 (3.4)
American Indian/Alaskan native	20 (3.4)
Native Hawaiian/Pacific Islander	10 (1.7)
Hispanic	70 (11.8)
Education	
High school grad/GED/vocational school	94 (15.8)
Some college/associates degree	287 (48.2)
Bachelors degree	137 (23.0)
Post-bachelors degree	74 (12.4)
Marital status	
Single (never married)	174 (29.2)
Married/with partner	326 (54.7)
Separated	16 (2.7)
Divorced	79 (13.3)
Widowed	1 (< 1)
Employment status[b]	
Working for pay	495 (83.1)
Working as volunteer	31 (5.2)
Student	84 (14.1)
Homemaker	24 (4.0)
Not working but actively looking for work	66 (11.1)
Not working and not looking	8 (1.3)
Retired	6 (1.0)
Unable to work	10 (1.7)
Time in military, y	
< 1	0 (0)
1–2	32 (5.4)

(continued on next page)

Table 1. (*continued*)

Variables[a]	No. (%) or Mean ±SD
3–4	91 (15.3)
5–10	187 (31.4)
>10 y	285 (47.8)
Most recent deployment operation	
OIF (Iraq)	401 (67.3)
OEF (Afghanistan)	181 (30.4)
Other	11 (1.8)
Service component	
Active	249 (41.8)
National Guard	170 (28.5)
Other Reserve	177 (29.7)
Branch of service	
Army	344 (57.7)
Navy	101 (16.9)
Air Force	125 (21.0)
Marines	25 (4.2)
Total no. of deployments at time of survey	
1	333 (55.7)
2	165 (27.7)
3	57 (9.6)
≥ 4	40 (6.7)
Length of most recent deployment, d	
≤ 90	110 (18.5)
91–180	82 (13.8)
181–365	274 (46.0)
> 365	123 (20.6)
Current military status	
Enrolled	511 (85.7)
Discharged	73 (12.2)
Mental/physical health	
PTSS (PCL-M)[c]	31.06 ±14.00
MCS (VR-12 mental health)[d]	40.56 ±7.91
PCS (VR-12 physical health)[d]	49.51 ±9.63
Depression/functioning (BASIS-24)[e]	0.95 ±0.80
Interpersonal relations (BASIS-24)[e]	1.17 ±0.78
Emotional lability (BASIS-24)[e]	1.52 ±0.97
Psychotic symptoms (BASIS-24)[e]	0.56 ±9.81
Overall score (BASIS-24)[e]	1.03 ±0.68
Alcohol/drug use	

(*continued on next page*)

Table 1. (*continued*)

Variables[a]	No. (%) or Mean $\pm$ SD
Substance abuse (BASIS-24)[e]	0.45 $\pm$ 0.69
Alcohol Use (AUDIT-C)[f]	3.92 $\pm$ 2.84
Drug Use (DAST)[g]	0.41 $\pm$ 0.81

Note. AUDIT-C = Alcohol Use Disorders Identification Test; BASIS-24 = Behavior and Symptom Identification Scale; DAST = Drug Abuse Screening Test; GED = General Equivalency Diploma; MCS = Mental Component Score; OEF/OIF = Operation Enduring Freedom/Operation Iraqi Freedom; PCL-M = PTSD Checklist Military Version; PCS = Physical Component Score; PTSD = posttraumatic stress disorder; PTSS = posttraumatic stress symptoms; VR-12 = Veterans Rand-12. The sample size was n = 596.
Missing values for each variable ranges between 0 and 12.
Percentage exceeds 100% because multiple categories may be endorsed.
PCL-M scores range from 1 to 68; higher scores indicate greater symptom severity.
MCS and PCS mean (SD) = 50 (10). Their ranges are unbounded. Higher scores indicate better mental health.
BASIS-24 scores range from 0 to 4; higher scores indicate greater symptom or problem severity or frequency.
AUDIT-C scores range from 0 to 12; higher scores indicate greater risk of alcohol abuse.
DAST-10 scores range from 0 to 10; higher scores indicate greater risk of drug abuse.

women with Active Component, National Guard, and other Reserve). Second, we computed weights to account for survey nonresponse. This was done by performing a logistic regression on the initial sample of 2000 with "returned survey" (0/1) as the dependent variable, and age, gender, race, and service component as independent variables to estimate a probability of returning the survey for each person in the sample. The reciprocal of these probabilities were the values of the second set of weights. The final set of weights was the product of an individual's sampling weight and the nonresponse weight. These weights were used in the calculation of mental health and substance use scores.

Data analysis.

We used the t test to assess differences in mental health and substance use by gender, and by deployment operation (OEF/OIF). Analysis of variance was used to assess differences by component and branch of service. All analyses incorporated sampling and nonresponse weights as previously described. In addition, for the PCL-M, AUDIT-C, and DAST-10, we used previously established cut scores to compare probable PTSD, alcohol, and drug use between gender, component, service, and deployment operation. Results based on cut scores are reported in the text but not in tables. Significance level adjustments for multiple testing were not performed, as these adjustments are not recommended for studies in which multiple hypotheses are tested.[41-43]

RESULTS

To identify differences between survey respondents and nonrespondents, we used descriptive data obtained from the DMDC to compare demographic and deployment characteristics of the 596 survey respondents with those of the 1237 nonrespondents. Survey respondents were more likely than were nonrespondents to be women ($\chi^2 = 15.8$; $P < .001$), older (t $= -8.48$; $P < .001$), National Guard or Other Reserve ($\chi^2 = 10.7$; $P = .005$), and from the Air Force or Navy ($\chi^2 = 16.9$; $P = .001$) than from the Army or Marine Corps. There were no differences in response rate as a function of race, Hispanic ethnicity, or length of previous deployment.

Sample Characteristics

Table 1 presents demographic and deployment characteristics of the 596 survey respondents. Fifty-eight percent were female; average age was 33.9 years; and 75% were White, 18% were African American, and 12% were Latino. Reflecting the oversampling of National Guard and other Reserve personnel, 58% were from these groups. Two thirds of the sample were deployed most recently to Iraq. The majority (87.5%) were still in the military.

Mental and Physical Health, Alcohol Use, and Drug Use

Addressing our first study objective, mean mental and physical health, alcohol use, and drug use scores are presented for the full sample in Table 1. The mean (SD) MCS score on the VR-12 was 40.56 (7.91), more than 1 SD below the general population mean of 50, whereas the mean (SD) PCS score was 49.51 (9.63), which was close to the general population mean.[44] The mean (SD) PCL-M score was 31.06 (14.00); 13.9% of the sample met the established threshold score of 50, indicating a likely diagnosis of PTSD.[45] Mean BASIS-24 subscale and overall scores ranged from 0.56 to 1.52 and were consistently worse than BASIS-24 scores obtained from a national, nonclinical community sample, but better than scores reported for both veteran and nonveteran samples receiving outpatient mental health treatment (T. Idiculla, PhD, unpublished data, 2011).[31,32,46] Using the VA-established AUDIT-C threshold for probable alcohol use disorder (≥ 5 for both genders),[19] 39.2% of the total sample screened positive for probable alcohol use disorder. Regarding drug abuse, 2.9% screened positive for drug abuse on the DAST-10.

Gender differences.

Contrary to our hypothesis that women would report higher levels of depression and PTSS, there were no statistically significant gender differences on any of the mental health or PTSS measures (Table 2). However, our hypothesis regarding

Table 2. Gender Differences in Mental and Physical Health Status, Alcohol and Drug Use: United States, 2008–2009

Variables	Men (n = 253), Mean (SD)	Women (n = 343), Mean (SD)	t	P
Mental/physical health				
PTSS (PCL-M)[a]	31.17 (14.04)	29.97 (13.54)	1.04	≤ .297
Depression/functioning (BASIS-24)[b]	0.95 (0.80)	0.95 (0.85)	0.01	≤ .989
Interpersonal relations (BASIS-24)[b]	1.18 (0.78)	1.11 (0.79)	1.08	≤ .282
Emotional lability (BASIS-24)[b]	1.51 (0.97)	1.60 (1.00)	−1.09	≤ .275
Psychotic symptoms (BASIS-24)[b]	0.57 (0.82)	0.45 (0.69)	1.89	≤ .06
BASIS-24 overall score[b]	1.03 (0.68)	1.00 (0.69)	0.55	≤ .582
MCS (VR-12 mental health)[c]	40.55 (7.78)	40.67 (9.11)	−0.16	≤ .87
PCS (VR-12 physical health)[c]	49.50 (9.64)	49.57 (9.55)	−0.08	≤ .937
Alcohol/drug use				
Alcohol Use (AUDIT-C)[d]	4.06 (2.86)	2.54 (2.27)	6.99	≤ .001
Substance abuse (BASIS-24)[b]	0.47 (0.70)	0.24 (0.42)	4.74	≤ .001
Drug Use (DAST)[e]	0.42 (0.82)	0.30 (0.63)	2.01	≤ .045

Note. AUDIT-C = Alcohol Use Disorders Identification Test; BASIS-24 = Behavior and Symptom Identification Scale; DAST = Drug Abuse Screening Test; MCS = Mental Component Score; PCL-M = PTSD Checklist Military Version; PCS = Physical Component Score; PTSD = posttraumatic stress disorder; PTSS = posttraumatic stress symptoms; VR-12 = Veterans Rand-12.
PCL-M scores range from 1 to 68; higher scores indicate greater symptom severity.
BASIS-24 Scores range from 0–4; higher scores indicate greater symptom or problem severity or frequency.
MCS and PCS mean (SD) = 50 (10). Their ranges are unbounded. Higher scores indicate better mental health.
AUDIT-C scores range from 0–12; higher scores indicate greater risk of alcohol abuse.
DAST-10 scores range from 0–10; higher scores indicate greater risk of drug abuse.

substance use was largely supported in that men reported higher mean AUDIT-C, DAST, and BASIS-24 substance use scores than women. Using the AUDIT-C cut score (≥ 5) indicating probable alcohol abuse, significantly more men (41.4%) than women (17.0%) screened positive ($\chi^2 = 12.3; P < .001$), although there was no significant gender difference in the proportion of respondents who screened positive for drug abuse (3% of men and 2% of women).

Deployment operation (OEF/OIF) differences.

In partial support of our hypothesis, OIF veterans reported significantly more difficulty in the areas of depression or functioning, overall mental health, and alcohol or drug use than did OEF veterans, as reflected in higher mean BASIS-24 scores in these areas, as well as higher mean levels of alcohol use on the AUDIT-C and more positive screens for drug use (4% OIF vs < 1% OEF; $\chi^2_1 = 5.29; P = .02$; Table 3).

Component differences.

The hypothesis regarding poorer mental health and increased substance use among National Guard/Reservists versus Active Component was not supported. There were no significant differences among the components on any of the measures using mean scores or cut points for PTSD, alcohol use, or drug use (data not shown).

Service branch differences.

Supporting hypotheses regarding service branch differences, results indicated statistically significant differences on all of the measures (Table 4). Post hoc t tests indicated that Army and Marine veterans differed most from Air Force veterans, with statistically significant differences on 8 of the 11 measures. Army and Marine veterans indicated significantly poorer mental health functioning, including more PTSS, depression, and anxiety symptoms, higher alcohol and drug use, and more problematic relationships than did Air Force veterans. Army veterans indicated significantly higher emotional liability and psychotic symptoms than did Air Force veterans. Twenty-five percent of Marines and 15% of Army respondents screened positive for probable PTSD compared with 9.5% of Air Force and 5.9% of Navy veterans. Forty-seven percent of Army respondents and 45% of Marines screened positive for alcohol use compared with 26% of both Air Force and Navy respondents ($\chi^2_3 = 24.91$;

Table 3. Differences in Mental and Physical Health Status, Alcohol and Drug Use by Deployment Operation: United States, 2008–2009

	Iraq (OIF; n = 401), Mean (SD)	Afghanistan (OEF; n = 181), Mean (SD)	t	P
Mental/physical health				
PTSS (PTSD checklist)	31.69 (14.28)	30.54 (13.70)	0.89	≤ .371
Depression/functioning (BASIS-24)[a]	1.01 (0.84)	0.82 (0.74)	2.72	≤ .007
Interpersonal relations (BASIS-24)[a]	1.21 (0.80)	1.07 (0.74)	1.93	≤ .054
Emotional lability (BASIS-24)[a]	1.57 (1.00)	1.42 (0.96)	1.68	≤ .093
Psychotic symptoms (BASIS-24)[a]	0.54 (0.76)	0.60 (0.93)	−0.70	≤ .484
BASIS-24 overall score[a]	1.07 (0.69)	0.93 (0.67)	2.37	≤ .018
MCS (VR-12 mental health)[b]	40.69 (8.05)	40.24 (7.82)	0.63	≤ .529
PCS (VR-12 physical health)[b]	49.40 (9.74)	49.76 (9.63)	−0.41	≤ .683
Alcohol/drug use				
Alcohol use (AUDIT-C)[c]	4.17 (3.07)	3.51 (2.21)	2.97	≤ .003
Substance abuse (BASIS-24) a	0.53 (0.74)	0.30 (0.53)	4.25	≤ .001
Drug Use (DAST)[d]	0.42 (0.88)	0.35 (0.63)	1.07	≤ .286

Note. AUDIT-C = Alcohol Use Disorders Identification Test; BASIS-24 = Behavior and Symptom Identification Scale; DAST = Drug Abuse Screening Test; MCS = Mental Component Score; OEF/OIF = Operation Enduring Freedom/Operation Iraqi Freedom; PCS = Physical Component Score; PTSD = posttraumatic stress disorder; PTSS = posttraumatic stress symptoms; VR-12 = Veterans Rand-12.
BASIS-24 scores range from 0–4; higher scores indicate greater symptom or problem severity or frequency.
MCS and PCS mean (SD) = 50 (10). Their ranges are unbounded. Higher scores indicate better mental health.
AUDIT-C scores range from 0–12; higher scores indicate greater risk of alcohol abuse.
DAST-10 scores range from 0–10; higher scores indicate greater risk of drug abuse.

$P < .001$); 7.4% of Marines and 3.4% of Army respondents screened positive for drug use compared with < 1% of Air Force or Navy respondents ($\chi^2_3 = 10.99$; $P < .001$).

DISCUSSION

This article extended previously published work in a number of ways. First, we obtained a broader sample than many previous studies, reporting results on a national stratified, random sample of Active and National Guard/Reserve military personnel from all branches of service who were not necessarily

Table 4. Service Branch Differences in Mental and Physical Health Status, Alcohol and Drug Use: United States, 2008-2009

	Army (n = 343), Mean (SD)	Air Force (n = 125), Mean (SD)	Marines (n = 27), Mean (SD)	Navy (n = 101), Mean (SD)	F	P
Mental/physical health						
PTSS (PTSD checklist)[a]	33.79 (14.76)	26.53 (12.67)	32.62 (14.48)	27.31 (10.01)	11.14	≤ .001
Depression/functioning (BASIS-24)[ab]	0.99 (0.80)	0.71 (0.63)	1.18 (0.97)	0.93 (0.78)	6.26	≤ .001
Interpersonal relations (BASIS-24)[ab]	1.22 (0.77)	0.90 (0.69)	1.41 (0.85)	1.16 (0.72)	8.47	≤ .001
Emotional lability (BASIS-24)[bc]	1.71 (1.05)	1.31 (0.91)	1.32 (0.67)	1.40 (0.95)	7.65	≤ .001
Psychotic symptoms (BASIS-24)[bc]	0.66 (0.87)	0.37 (0.67)	0.48 (0.62)	0.57 (0.86)	3.86	≤ .009
BASIS-24 overall score[ab]	1.10 (0.68)	0.80 (0.59)	1.16 (0.71)	0.98 (0.65)	7.45	≤ .001
MCS (VR-12 mental health)[ad]	40.44 (8.04)	42.60 (7.83)	39.53 (6.99)	39.35 (7.92)	4.03	≤ .007
PCS (VR-12 physical health)[de]	48.31 (9.89)	49.78 (10.07)	51.36 (9.33)	51.02 (7.98)	3.46	≤ .016
Alcohol/drug use						
Alcohol use (AUDIT-C)[af]	4.48 (3.13)	2.96 (2.02)	3.93 (2.63)	3.44 (2.59)	9.76	≤ .001
Substance abuse (BASIS-24)[ab]	0.59 (0.79)	0.21 (0.35)	0.54 (0.74)	0.27 (0.44)	12.50	≤ .001
Drug use (DAST)[ag]	0.44 (0.83)	0.18 (0.45)	0.78 (1.18)	0.28 (0.47)	10.80	≤ .001

Note. AUDIT-C = Alcohol Use Disorders Identification Test; BASIS-24 = Behavior and Symptom Identification Test; DAST = Drug Abuse Screening Test; MCS = Mental Component Score; PTSD = posttraumatic stress disorder; PTSS = posttraumatic stress symptoms; VR-12 = Veterans Rand-12.

Significant difference between Army and Marine and Air Force veterans.

BASIS-24 Scores range from 0-4; higher scores indicate greater symptom or problem severity or frequency.

Significant difference between Army and Air Force veterans.

MCS and PCS mean (SD) = 50 (10). Their ranges are unbounded. Higher scores indicate better mental health.

Significant difference between Marine and Navy and Army veterans.

AUDIT-C scores range from 0-12; higher scores indicate greater risk of alcohol abuse.

DAST-10 scores range from 0-10; higher scores indicate greater risk of drug abuse.

enrolled in Department of Veterans Affairs (VA) health care. Second, to allow for comparisons by gender we oversampled women to make up 50% of the sample. Third, rather than using brief screening tools, we included detailed, well-researched measures reflecting a wide range of mental health symptom and functioning domains, including PTSS, alcohol and drug use, and physical health functioning. Fourth, we applied 2 sets of weights to the data analysis, one to reflect the actual composition of the OEF/OIF force during the sampling interval, and another to account for nonresponse bias. Application of these weights provided more accurate estimates of mental health functioning and substance use problems, thus increasing generalizability of results.

We found that OEF/OIF veterans indicated significantly worse mental health functioning than did the general population based on multiple measures. Alcohol use was also potentially problematic, with 39% screening positive for "probable alcohol abuse," considerably higher than that reported by Hawkins et al.,[19] based on mandated screening of VA outpatients. This discrepancy might suggest that the context of the VA clinical setting could lead veterans to underreport their drinking in routine screening, resulting in underestimates of the severity of the problem. By contrast, physical health functioning assessed by the VR-12 was comparable to the US general population mean.[44] The relatively good physical health of our sample might be partly attributed to their youth and fitness compared with the general population.

Despite widespread publicity and concern about increasing rates of PTSD among OEF/OIF veterans, probable PTSD for this sample (13.9%) was within the range reported by other researchers and lower than rates reported in some studies.[2,4,28] A number of factors were identified as influencing reported rates of PTSD, including methodological factors (strictness of the definition, amount of time since return from deployment, sampling strategy, and response rates), as well as substantive factors (combat and other traumatic exposure).[21,47,48] Differences in PTSS or PTSD and other mental health problems as a function of postdeployment assessment time interval might be especially important to monitor as there was conflicting evidence regarding the impact of time on these conditions.[21] Kulka et al.[49] reported that depression, anxiety, and other mental health concerns subsided over time, whereas other researchers reported that PTSD sometimes had a delayed onset, resulting in higher rates over time.[21,50,51]

Tests of our hypotheses regarding subgroup differences on mental health, PTSS, alcohol, and drug use yielded mixed results. Higher rates of alcohol use in men, and worse mental health, PTSS, alcohol, and drug use among Army and Marine Corps veterans were observed, suggesting that these veteran subgroups were at higher risk for mental health problems. Although we were not aware of any significant differences in eligibility criteria for enlistment or commissioning in the different service branches that would lead to systematic predeployment differences among service personnel, demographic and cultural differences among the service branches as well as different stressors might contribute to their increased risk.

Contrary to our hypothesis, we found no gender differences in mental or physical health symptoms or functioning. It was important to note, however, that women experienced less intense combat than men.[52] Consequently, this finding did not preclude the possibility that women would be more vulnerable to combat stress when exposed at the same levels as men. To address this possibility more directly, another study based on this dataset examined whether associations between combat-related stressors and postdeployment mental health differed for women and men, and found no clinically significant differences.[52] The lack of significant gender differences might reflect improved training of female service members and the increased numbers of women currently in the military—15% now compared with less than 3% during World War II—as well as the fact that women's occupational roles in the military might be more similar to men's roles than in the past. The higher proportion of women in today's military might also provide social and emotional support that might increase their resilience.

Also contrary to our hypotheses, National Guard/Reserve Component veterans did not differ from Active component veterans with respect to mental or physical health functioning or substance use. The lack of differences between components might be because of changing expectations regarding deployment. As these wars continue, National Guard and other Reserve personnel are more likely to expect to be deployed. Consequently, they might be more psychologically and emotionally prepared and less vulnerable to deployment-related stresses. Similarly, the shift of combat operations from Iraq to Afghanistan might alter the balance between these 2 operations in terms of associated risks.

This study had a number of limitations. First, because of the retrospective design of the study, we could not infer that the physical and mental health status of respondents reflected the impact of deployment. It was possible that predeployment variations might account for the postdeployment differences. Second, we used only self-reported measures of mental health and substance use, which might be subject to bias. To minimize potential bias, we implemented the survey at least 3 months after participants had returned from deployment, and we conducted the survey independently of the Department of Defense or the participant's military unit. Thus, concerns about stigma regarding reporting mental health problems and potential evaluation regarding fitness for duty were minimized. Third, our response rate of 57% was based on the number of potential participants that we confirmed received the survey, but was 33% of the eligible participants, slightly lower than the 36% participation rate reported for the Millennium Cohort Study.[25] Although we weighted the data to address nonresponse, the weighting procedure assumed that the data were missing at random.[53] It was possible that nonresponse might have depended on unobserved information. For example, if military personnel with poor mental health were less likely to return the survey, then our results would only apply to a somewhat healthier segment of the population.

From clinical, public health and policy perspectives, the results of this study suggest a number of implications. First, continued multidimensional assessment of postdeployed veterans is valuable because previously identified findings may change as contextual factors, such as increasing numbers of women and the locus of combat, shift. Second, the context and timing of assessment (e.g., within one's unit, immediately after returning from deployment) have been shown to affect results. Consequently, we should strive to implement assessments in as neutral a context as possible to minimize (1) potential response bias because of concern about discrimination associated with admitting mental health or substance use problems, and (2) failure to report problems to avoid further mental health evaluation that would delay return to home. Third, continuing identification of those at highest risk for mental health and substance use problems, including examination of individual and deployment characteristics (e.g., race/ethnicity, education, income, combat exposure) is important for development and implementation of evidence-based interventions to increase resilience, as well as to enhance treatment when indicated.

ABOUT THE AUTHORS

Susan V. Eisen, Mark R. Schultz, Mark E. Glickman, A. Rani Elwy, Mari-Lynn Drainoni, and Princess E. Osei-Bonsu are with the Center for Health Quality, Outcomes and Economic Research (CHQOER), Edith Nourse Rogers Memorial Veterans Hospital, Bedford, MA. Susan V. Eisen, Mark E. Glickman, A. Rani Elwy, Mari-Lynn Drainoni, and Princess E. Osei-Bonsu are also with the Department of Health Policy and Management, Boston University School of Public Health, Boston, MA. Dawne Vogt is with the Women's Health Sciences Division, National Center for PTSD, VA Boston Healthcare System, Boston, and the Division of Psychiatry, Boston University School of Medicine, Boston. James Martin is with Bryn Mawr College, Bryn Mawr, PA.

CONTRIBUTORS

S. V. Eisen had overall responsibility and provided supervision for this study. S. V. Eisen, A. R. Elwy, M-L. Drainoni, J. Martin, and D. Vogt contributed to obtaining funding. S. V. Eisen, A. R. Elwy, D. Vogt, M. E. Glickman, M-L. Drainoni, and J. Martin contributed to the study concept, design, and acquisition of the data. S. V. Eisen, M. E. Glickman, and M. R. Schultz contributed to the statistical analysis. S. V. Eisen, M. R. Schultz, and P. E. Osei-Bonsu contributed to drafting the article. All authors contributed to the interpretation of data and to critical revision of the article for intellectual content.

ACKNOWLEDGMENTS

This research was funded by the Veterans Administration Health Services Research and Development (HSR&D; grant IAC 06-259-2; S. V. Eisen, PI), by the Center for Health Quality, Outcomes & Economic Research, a VA HSR&D Center of Excellence, and by Women's Health Sciences Division, National Center for PTSD, VA Boston Healthcare System.

We are most grateful to the veterans who participated in this study. We also thank Alexandra Howard, Patrick Furlong, and Nicole Del Vecchio for their assistance with data collection and management, with conference presentation materials, and with article preparation.

Some of the results reported in this article were presented at the Annual Academy Health Conference in June 2010 and at the Annual VA HSR&D conference in February 2011.

Note. The views expressed in this article are those of the authors and do not necessarily represent the views of the Department of Veterans Affairs or any of the institutional affiliations listed.

HUMAN PARTICIPANT PROTECTION

This study was approved by the institutional review board of the Edith Nourse Rogers Memorial Veterans Hospital.

REFERENCES

1. Smith TC, For the Millenium Cohort Study Team. The US Department of Defense Millennium Cohort Study: career span and beyond longitudinal follow-Up. *J Occup Environ Med.* 2009;51(10):1193–1201.

2. Hoge CW, Castro CA, Messer SC, McGurk D, Cotting DI, Koffman RL. Combat duty in Iraq and Afghanistan, mental health problems, and barriers to care. *N Engl J Med.* 2004;351:13–22.

3. Southwick SM, Morgan MD, Nagy LM, et al. Trauma-related symptoms in veterans of Operation Desert Storm: a preliminary report. *Am J Psychiatry.* 1993;150(10):1524–1528.

4. Hoge CW, Auchterlonie JL, Milliken CS. Mental health problems, use of mental health services, and attrition from military service after returning from deployment to Iraq or Afghanistan. *JAMA.* 2006;295(9):1023–1032.

5. Sutker PB, Davis JM, Uddo M, Ditta SR. War zone stress, personal resources, and PTSD in Persian Gulf War returnees. *J Abnorm Psychol.* 1995;104(3):444–452.

6. Vasterling JJ, Proctor SP, Amoroso P, Kane R, Heeren T, White RF. Neuropsychological outcomes of army personnel following deployment to the Iraq war. *JAMA.* 2006;296(5):519–529.

7. Vasterling JJ, Proctor SP, Friedman MJ, et al. PTSD symptom increases in Iraq-deployed soldiers: comparison with nondeployed soldiers and associations with baseline symptoms, deployment experiences, and postdeployment stress. *J Trauma Stress.* 2010;23(1):41–51.

8. Barrett DH, Doebbeling CC, Schwartz DA, et al. Posttraumatic stress disorder and self-reported physical health status among US military personnel serving during the Gulf War period. *Psychosomatics.* 2002;43:195–205.

9. Hoge CW, Terhakopian A, Castro CA, Messer SC, Engle CC. Association of posttraumatic stress disorder with somatic symptoms, health care visits, and absenteeism among Iraq War veterans. *Am J Psychiatry.* 2007;164(1):150–153.

10. Department of Defense. Operation Enduring Freedom/Operation Iraqi Freedom/Operation New Dawn US casualty status. 10/17/2011. Available at: http://www.defense.gov/news/casualty.pdf. Accessed October 18, 2011.

11. Kline A, Falca-Dodson M, Sussner B, et al. Effects of repeated deployment to Iraq and Afghanistan on the health of New Jersey Army National Guard Troops: implications for military readiness. *Am J Public Health.* 2010;100(2):276–283.

12. Hoge CW, McGurk D, Thomas JL, Cox AL, Engel CC, Castro CA. Mild traumatic brain injury in U.S. soldiers returning from Iraq. *N Engl J Med.* 2008;358(5):453–463.

13. Cohen BE, Marmar C, Ren L, Bertentahl D, Seal KH. Association of cardiovascular risk factors with mental health diagnoses in Iraq and Afghanistan war veterans using VA health care. *JAMA.* 2009;302(5):489–492.

14. Bernhardt A. Rising to the challenge of treating OEF/OIF veterans with co-occurring PTSD and substance abuse. *Smith Coll Stud Soc Work.* 2009;79:344–367.

15. Haskell SG, Gordon KS, Mattocks K, et al. Gender differences in rates of depression, PTSD, pain, obesity, and military sexual trauma among Connecticut war veterans of Iraq and Afghanistan. *J Womens Health (Larchmt).* 2010;19(2):267–271.

16. Maguen S, Lucenko BA, Reger MA, et al. The impact of reported direct and indirect killing on mental health symptoms in Iraq war veterans. *J Trauma Stress.* 2010;23(1):86–90.

17. Tolin DF, Foa EB. Sex differences in trauma and posttraumatic stress disorder: a quantitative review of 25 years of research. *Psychol Bull.* 2006;132(6):959–992.

18. Vogt DS, Pless AP, King LA, King DW. Deployment stressors, gender, and mental health outcomes among Gulf War I veterans. *J Trauma Stress*. 2005;18(2):115–127.

19. Hawkins EJ, Lapham GT, Kivlahan DR, Bradley KA. Recognition and management of alcohol misuse in OEF/OIF and other veterans in the VA: a cross-sectional study. *Drug Alcohol Depend*. 2010;109(1-3):147–153.

20. Jacobson IG, Ryan MAKK, Hooper TI, et al. Alcohol use and alcohol-related problems before and after military combat deployment. *JAMA*. 2008;300(6):663–675.

21. Milliken CS, Auchterlonie JL, Hoge CW. Longitudinal assessment of mental health problems among active and reserve component. *JAMA*. 2007;298(18):2141–2148.

22. Schell TL, Marshall GN. Survey of individuals previously deployed for OEF/OIF. In: Tanelian T, Jaycox LH, eds. *Invisible Wounds of War: Psychological and Cognitive Injuries, Their Consequences, and Services to Assist Recovery*. Santa Monica, CA: RAND Center for Military Health Policy Research; 2008:87–115.

23. Thomas JL, Wilk JE, Riviere LA, et al. Prevalence of mental health problems and functional impairment among active component and national guard soldiers 3 and 12 months following combat in Iraq. *Arch Gen Psychiatry*. 2010;67(6):614–623.

24. Bray RM, Olmsted KLRR, Williams J, Sanchez RP, Hartzell M. Progress toward healthy people 2000 objectives among U.S. military personnel. *Prev Med*. 2006;42(5):390–396.

25. Smith TC, Ryan MA, Wingard DL, et al. New onset and persistent symptoms of post-traumatic stress disorder self reported after deployment and combat exposures: prospective population based US military cohort study. *BMJ*. 2008;336:366–371.

26. Jakupcak M, Tull MT, McDermott MJ, Kaysen D, Hunt S, Simpson T. PTSD symptom clusters in relationship to alcohol misuse among Iraq and Afghanistan war veterans seeking post-deployment VA health care. *Addict Behav*. 2010;35(9):840–843.

27. Wells TS, LeardMann CA, Fortuna SO, et al. A prospective study of depression following combat deployment in support of the wars in Iraq and Afghanistan. *Am J Public Health*. 2010;100(1):90–99.

28. Lapierre CB, Schwegler AF, LaBauve BJ. Posttraumatic stress and depression symptoms in soldiers returning from combat operations in Iraq and Afghanistan. *J Trauma Stress*. 2007;20(6):933–943.

29. Welcome to DMDC. Available at: https://www.dmdc.osd.mil/appj/dwp/index.jsp. Accessed November 17, 2011.

30. Dillman DA. *Mail and Telephone Surveys*: The Total Design Method. New York: Wiley; 1978.

31. Fasoli DR, Glickman M, Eisen SV. Predisposing characteristics, enabling resources and need as predictors of utilization and clinical outcomes for veterans receiving mental health services. *Med Care*. 2010;48:288–295.

32. Eisen SV, Bottonari KA, Glickman ME, et al. The incremental value of self-reported mental health measures in predicting functional outcomes. *J Behav Health Serv Res*. 2011;38(2):170–190.

33. Ware J Jr, Kosinksi M, Keller SD. A 12-item short-form health survey (SF-12): construction of scales and preliminary tests of reliability and validity. *Med Care*. 1996;34:220–233.

34. Iqbal SU, Rogers W, Selim A, et al. The Veterans RAND 12-item health survey (VR-12): what it is and how it is used. Available at: http://www.chqoer.research.va.gov/docs/VR12.pdf. Accessed November 17, 2011

35. Eisen SV, Normand SLTT, Belanger A, Spiro A 3rd, Esch D. The Revised Behavior and Symptom Identification Scale (BASIS-24): reliability and validity. *Med Care*. 2004;42(12):1230–1241.

36. Weathers FW, Huska JA, Keane TM. *The PTSD Checklist (PCL)*. Boston, MA: National Center for PTSD; 1991.

37. Bush K, Kivlahan DR, McDonell MB, Fihn SD, Bradley KA. The AUDIT alcohol consumption questions (AUDIT-C): an effective brief screening test for problem drinking. Ambulatory Care Quality Improvement Project (ACQUIP). Alcohol Use Disorders Identification Test. *Arch Intern Med*. 1998;158(16):1789–1795.

38. Cocco KM, Carey KB. Psychometric properties of the Drug Abuse Screening Test in outpatients. *Psychol Assess*. 1998;10(4):408–414.

39. Kazis LE, Miller DR, Clark JA, et al. Improving the response choices on the veterans SF-36 health survey role functioning scales: results from the Veterans Health Study. *J Ambul Care Manage*. 2004;27(3):263–280.

40. Weathers F, Ford J. Psychometric properties of the PTSD checklist (PCL-C, PCL-S, PCL-M, PCL-PR). In: Stamm BH, ed. *Measurement of Stress, Trauma, and Adaptation.* Lutherville, MD: Sidran Press; 1996:250–251.

41. O'Keefe DJ. Colloquy: should familywise alpha be adjusted? Against familywise alpha adjustment. *Hum Commun Res.* 2003;29(3):431–447.

42. Rothman KJ. No adjustments are needed for multiple comparisons. *Epidemiology.* 1990;1(1):43–46.

43. Perneger TV. What's wrong with Bonferroni adjustments. *BMJ.* 1998;316(7139):1236–1238.

44. Selim AJ, Rogers W, Fleishman JA, et al. Updated U.S. population standard for the Veterans RAND 12-item Health Survey (VR-12). *Qual Life Res.* 2009;18(1):43–52.

45. Weathers FW, Litz BT, Herman DS, Huska JA, Keane TM. The PTSD Checklist (PCL): Reliability, Validity, and Diagnostic Utility. Paper presented at: Annual Meeting of International Society for Traumatic Stress Studies; October, 1993; San Antonio, TX.

46. Eisen SV, Gerena M, Ranganathan G, Esch D, Idiculla T. Reliability and validity of the BASIS-24 Mental Health Survey for Whites, African-Americans and Latinos. *J Behav Health Serv Res.* 2006;33:304–323.

47. Seal KH, Bertenthal D, Miner CR, Sen S, Marmar C. Bringing the war back home: mental health disorders among 103,788 US veterans returning from Iraq and Afghanistan seen at Department of Veterans Affairs facilities. *Arch Int Med.* 2007;167:476–482.

48. Ramchand R, Schell TL, Karney BR, Osilla KC, Burns RM, Caldarone LB. Disparate prevalence estimates of PTSD among service members who served in Iraq and Afghanistan: possible explanations. *J Trauma Stress.* 2010;23:59–68.

49. Kulka RA, Schlenger WE, Fairbank JA, Hough RL. *Trauma and the Vietnam War Generation: Report of Findings from the National Vietnam Veterans Readjustment Study.* New York: Brunner/Mazel; 1990.

50. Gabriel R, Neal LA. Lesson of the week: post-traumatic stress disorder following military combat or peace keeping. *BMJ.* 2002;324(7333):340–341.

51. Fear NT, Jones M, Murphy D, et al. What are the consequences of deployment to Iraq and Afghanistan on the mental health of the UK armed forces? A cohort study. *Lancet.* 2010;375(9728):1783–1797.

52. Vogt D, Vaughn R, Glickman ME, et al. Gender differences in combat-related stressors and their association with postdeployment mental health in a nationally representative sample of US OEF/OIF veterans. *J Abnorm Psychol.* 2011;120(4):797–806.

53. Rubin DB. Inference and missing data. *Biometrika.* 1976;63:581–592.

23

Reduced Mortality Among Department of Veterans Affairs Patients With Schizophrenia or Bipolar Disorder Lost to Follow-up and Engaged in Active Outreach to Return for Care

Chester L. Davis, ScD, MPH, Amy M. Kilbourne, PhD, Frederic C. Blow, PhD, John R. Pierce, MD, Bernard M. Winkel, EdD, Edward Huycke, MD, Robert Langberg, MA, David Lyle, Yancy Phillips, MD, and Stephanie Visnic, BA

Objectives. We determined whether contacting Department of Veterans Affairs (VA) patients with schizophrenia or bipolar disorders (serious mental illness [SMI]) who had dropped out of care for prolonged periods resulted in reengagement with VA services and decreased mortality.

Methods. We developed a list of patients with SMI who were last treated in fiscal years 2005 to 2006, and were lost to follow-up care for at least 1 year. VA medical centers used our list to contact patients and schedule appointments. Additional VA administrative data on patient utilization and mortality through May 2009 were analyzed.

Results. About 72% (2375 of 3306) of the patients who VA staff attempted to contact returned for VA care. The mortality rate of returning patients was significantly lower than that for patients not returning (0.5% vs 3.9%; adjusted odds ratio = 5.8; $P < .001$), after demographic and clinical factors were controlled.

Conclusions. The mortality rate for returning patients with SMI was almost 6 times less than for those who did not return for medical care. Proactive outreach might result in patients returning to care and should be implemented to reengage this vulnerable group.

Serious mental illness (SMI), including patients with schizophrenia and bipolar disorder, is associated with substantial functional impairment, morbidity, and premature mortality.[1,2] In a given year, Veterans Affairs (VA) treats more than 230 000 patients for SMI.[3] VA patients with SMI die on average 13 to 18 years younger than the US general population,[1] and this mortality gap exceeds 20 years in non-VA populations.[2] A key driver of premature mortality among VA and non-VA patients with mental disorders is medical comorbidity, and cardiovascular disease is the number 1 cause of death.[4] Persons with SMI have standard mortality ratios that are about 2.5 times greater than those of the general population.[2]

Improving access to medical care and the continuity of that care to reduce the risk of premature mortality among patients with SMI are important goals within VA and non-VA health care systems.[4,6,7] In a recent VA health services study, researchers reported that VA patients with schizophrenia with little care in the previous year were more likely to die than those without schizophrenia, suggesting that treatment dropouts in this group might be a significant risk factor in mortality and that efforts should be made to provide them treatment.[8] Similarly, patients with bipolar disorders as well as schizophrenia who were burdened by comorbid medical conditions might be prescribed medications that require regular monitoring (e.g., second-generation antipsychotics and mood stabilizers).[5]

Improving access to care for VA patients with schizophrenia or bipolar disorder has been a consistent priority goal, as stated in the Veteran Health Administration's (VHA) *Uniform Mental Health Services Handbook* and with Congress under the 1996 Public Law (104-262). Since the early 1990s, VA has modified its care-delivery system by moving from an inpatient to an outpatient model. Between 1993 and 2009, overall hospital admissions declined 33%, whereas the number of outpatient visits tripled.[9,10] Greater reliance has therefore been placed on community-based programs and ambulatory case management for veterans in general. Although veterans with SMI face substantial functional limitation and increased risk of hospitalization, there has been no national effort to date to facilitate reengagement among veterans with SMI who drop out of VA care.

In December 2010, the VHA's Office of the Medical Inspector (OMI) completed a landmark quality improvement project whose objectives were to identify and contact veterans with SMI who dropped out of care for a minimum of 1 year, and to offer them VA medical services. We described this project and presented the results on patient reengagement. We also compared mortality rates of patients returning to VA care after prolonged absences with mortality rates of patients who did not return.

METHODS

We identified patients with SMI, including schizophrenia (*International Classification of Disease-9th Revision-Clinical Modification*[11] [*ICD-9-CM*] codes 295.0–295.9) or bipolar disorders (*ICD-9-CM* codes 296.0–296.8), by using data from the VA National Psychosis Registry (NPR) in fiscal years (FYs) 2005 and 2006. The NPR is a continuous registry of all veterans diagnosed with psychosis who have received VHA services from FY 1988 to the present, based on inpatient and outpatient claims data from the VA's National Patient Care Database (NPCD). Patients were included in the NPR provided that they were treated for 1 of the qualifying diagnoses in inpatient or outpatient claims data files. Patients eligible to be included in this study had at least 1 SMI diagnosis and were lost to follow-up care for a minimum of 1 year and had no outpatient visits or inpatient stays of more than 2 days within the VA health care system. During FY 2005, there were 1913 patients diagnosed with SMI who were treated in VA facilities and dropped out of VA care for a minimum of 12 months. In FY 2006, there were 2958 patients diagnosed with SMI who were treated in VA facilities and dropped out of VA care for a minimum of 12 months. Overall, 4871 eligible patients diagnosed with SMI were included in this study and lost to follow-up VA care for a minimum of 1 year. For FY 2005, this was approximately 1% of the 173 637 patients with SMI who were treated in VA facilities. For FY 2006, this was approximately 2% of the 175 136 patients with SMI who were treated in VA facilities. A VA medical center (VAMC) institutional review board evaluated the protocol for this assessment and determined that it was a quality improvement effort, not research.

The list of patients was reduced further by identifying decedents. This was accomplished by matching patient identifiers—social security numbers and names—with those in the computerized death records, including date of death from the Social Security Administration (SSA) and the VA Beneficiary Identification Locator System (BIRLS) that were available in September 2007. For the remaining patients, their telephone numbers and addresses were added by matching patient identifiers with the VA National Enrollment Data file. Patients were then assigned to the VAMC where they had last received care. The lists of patients for each facility were then assembled and sent to the 138 VAMCs.

Each VAMC was asked to choose a point of contact (POC) to be responsible for following up on patients on their list who had dropped out of care. The majority of the VAMC points of contact were social workers (including VA local recovery or suicide prevention coordinators), nurses, and psychologists.

POCs were asked to review their patient lists before contacting patients and exclude those who met certain criteria. Each POC was asked to remove from their list those who had subsequently died according to their medical records (n = 80). Other veterans that POCs were requested to exclude from the study were those who were institutionalized (n = 806); were scheduled for clinic or emergency room visit (n = 449); had provided incorrect contact information (n = 81); were ineligible for VA care (n = 77); had to relocate to another state or region (n = 59); or other reasons (n = 43). Of the 80 patients reported to have died, we identified 40 who died before the start of the assessment from updated BIRLS and SSA death files and excluded them from the analysis. As a result, the assessment population for the analysis was reduced from 4871 to 3306 patients who staff attempted to contact and ask them to return for care.

The POCs used several methods to contact patients. About 96% (133 of 137) of the POCs telephoned the patients. About 90% of the POCs (124 of 137) sent a letter to each patient. Face-to-face contacts with patients were used at 106 VAMCs, and these included staff meeting patients on the street, in single room hotels, and meetings in shelters or group homes. Every POC completed a reporting form for each patient on their list. The reporting form consisted of structured questions about whether there was an attempt to contact the patient, whether contact was made, reasons for not contacting the patient, whether the patient was referred for care, and reasons the patient did not want care.

We used univariate statistics to describe the patients who dropped out of care, and bivariate analyses to compare the patient characteristics of those who POCs attempted to contact and returned for care versus those who did not return. We also queried VA administrative data files for the study period up to 20 months after initial contacts to determine use of VA services. Death rates and odds ratios were calculated to assess the difference in the probability of mortality up to May 1, 2009 (representing 21 months of follow-up time), by comparing patients who did and who did not return to VA for care. We employed Inquisite software (Allegiance, Austin, Texas) to conduct the surveys at VA facilities and SAS (version 9.1; SAS Institute, Cary, North Carolina) to process and analyze the data.

The study team conducted a multivariable analysis to determine whether not returning for VA care was associated with a greater probability of mortality, after adjusting for potential explanatory variables. Using logistic regression, we modeled the probability of death during the evaluation period, controlling for patient age, gender, marital status, Charlson Comorbidity Index,[12–14] mental health diagnoses, and whether the patient returned for VA care. We used the 20 comorbidities that compose the Charlson Comorbidity Index (based upon *ICD-9-CM* codes recorded in the NCPD files during the last 2 years of contact before the patient dropped out of treatment). The explanatory variables in the model were categorical and were converted into dummy-coded variables for patient age, gender (reference: male), marital status, mental health diagnosis, and Charlson Comorbidity Index. The coefficients (β) were the weights for the variables, and the SEs were the estimated errors for the weights. The Wald test statistic was calculated from the data and compared with the χ^2_1 distribution. The odds ratios and 95% confidence intervals were estimated for each variable in the model.

The Hosmer–Lemeshow goodness-of-fit test indicated that this model fit the data well ($P > .05$). Our model, with all of its independent variables, was a better predictive model compared with a model with just 1 variable, not returning to VA care: -2LogL, which decreased from 1459 to 1047. We conducted multicollinearity screening to test the assumption of independence among patients, and we did not find any multicollinearity concerns (variance inflation factor < 2.5). We tested the interaction between the variable mental health diagnosis and Charlson Comorbidity Index scores, and found that these terms were not statistically significant ($P > .05$). The C statistic was 0.89, which meant that the model predicted 89% of the data.

RESULTS

Using the NPR, 4871 patients diagnosed with SMI were lost to follow-up care for at least 1 year in FYs 2005 and 2006. Overall during the initial 7 months of the project, POCs tried to contact and report complete data for 3306 of the 4871 veterans who were last seen in VA facilities in FYs 2005 and 2006 and were lost to follow-up care for at least 1 year. The average length of time patients were lost to follow-up was 2.1 years for patients diagnosed with schizophrenia and 2.3 years for patients with bipolar disorder. In the year before dropping out of the VA system, many of the patients had been frequent users of VA health care services, averaging 18 VA outpatient visits and about 20 hospital discharges per 100 patients, with an average stay of 21 days.

Of the 3306 patients whom VA staff tried to contact, slightly more than 90% were men; 90% were not married; and about 88% were 64 years old or younger. Also, many patients had 1 or more medical comorbidities, including chronic pulmonary disease, diabetes, dementia, cerebrovascular disease, and cancer, which were diagnosed and treated in VA medical facilities (Table 1).

As of May 30, 2009, 2375 of 3306 patients (72%) had returned to VA facilities for mental health or medical treatment. At least 65% (1555 of 2375) of these patients who returned for care were contacted by the POCs during the first 7 months of this project. We did not require the POCs to report on their attempts to contact patients during the last 14 months of the study. From initial reengagement with VA facilities, these patients made a total of 44 171 clinic visits or about 28 visits per person during a 20-month follow-up period. The most frequent types of clinic visits were for mental health care (28%), followed by ancillary services (e.g., laboratory, pharmacy, radiology [18%]), specialist medical care (16%), substance abuse (10%), primary care (9%), or telephone consultations (6%).

In addition, 65% had at least 1 inpatient hospitalization since returning for care, with an average length of stay of 16 days. Moreover, 3% were admitted to VA Community Living Centers (formerly nursing homes), with an average stay of 90 days.

Of the 3306 patients who VA staff tried to contact during the first 7 months of the project, 643 (19%) did not accept a clinic appointment. Primary reasons that patients gave for not accepting a VA appointment included not having a perceived need for care, not satisfied with VA services, and distance or transportation barriers (Table 2).

About 2.2% (73 of 3306) of the target population died during the assessment period (Table 3). The mortality rate for the patients who did not return for VA care was 3.9%; the rate for patients who did return was 0.3%

Table 1. Demographics and Comorbidities of Target Patient Population: National Psychosis Registry, 2005–2006

	No. (%)
Gender	
Female	323 (9.8)
Male	2983 (90.2)
Marital status:	
Married	326 (9.9)
Not married	2980 (90.1)
Age	
< 65 y	2899 (87.7)
≥ 65 y	407 (12.3)
Comorbidities in Charlson Index (*ICD-9-CM* codes)	
Chronic pulmonary disease (490-496, 500-505, 506.4 508.1)	412 (12.5)
Diabetes (250.0, 250.1, 250.2, 250.3, 250.8, 250.9)	342 (10.3)
Dementia (290, 291.2, 292.82, 294.1, 294.10, 294.11, 294.8)	68 (2.1)
Cerebrovascular disease (430-438)	68 (2.1)
Chronic renal disease (403, 582, 583, 585, 586, 588, 404.2, 404.12, 404.92, 593.9)	56 (1.7)
Malignant neoplasm (140-165, 170-172, 174-195)	59 (1.8)
Congestive heart failure (398.91, 402.01-402.91, 404.3, 404.11, 404.13 494.91 404.93, 428)	46 (1.2)
Peripheral vascular disease (440.24, 443.81, 443.9 785.4)	46 (1.4)
Diabetes with complications (250.4, 250.5, 250.6 250.7)	39 (1.2)
Myocardial infarction (410.0-410.9, 414.8, 412)	92 (1.9)
Peptic ulcer disease (531, 532, 533, 534)	42 (1.3)
Cirrhosis (571)	46 (1.4)
Rheumatologic disease (710, 710.0, 710.1, 710.4, 714, 714.0-714.3, 714.30-714.33, 714.81, 720, 725)	21 (0.6)
Hemiplegia or paraplegia (342, 344)	11 (0.3)
AIDS (042, 043, 044)	16 (0.5)
HIV without AIDS (V08)	13 (0.4)
Hepatic failure (456.0, 456.1, 456.2, 456.20, 456.21)	7 (0.2)
Multiple myeloma or leukemia (203-208)	2 (0.1)
Metastatic solid tumor (196, 197, 198, 199)	2(0.1)
Lymphomas (200, 201, 202)	2 (0.1)

Note. ICD-9-CM = International Classification of Diseases-9th Revision-Clinical Modification.

Table 2. Primary Reasons Patients Gave for Not Accepting Department of Veterans Affairs (VA) Clinic Appointments: Office of Medical Inspector Survey, 2007

Reason	No. (%)
Did not perceive a need for care or clinic appointment	212 (33.0)
Were not satisfied with VA services	153 (23.8)
Did not have transportation to VA clinic	55 (8.6)
VA clinic was too far away	49 (7.6)
Wanted to solve problem by themselves	44 (6.8)
Did not have time for clinic appointment	17 (2.6)
Thought health problem would improve by itself	12 (1.9)
Could not get an appointment at the VA	7 (1.1)
All other reasons not listed above	94 (14.6)
Total	643 (100)

Table 3. Patient Mortality for Those Who Staff Attempted to Contact: National Psychosis Registry, 2005–2006, SSA and VA BIRLS Mortality Files, 2009

Variables	No. Died	Death Rate, %	χ^2	P	Patients, No. (%)
All patients	73	2.2	–	–	3306 (100.0)
Return to VA care	5	0.3			1555 (47.0)
Not returning to VA care	68	3.9	48.4	< .001	1751 (53.0)
Female	4	1.2			323 (9.8)
Male	69	2.3	1.6	.21	2983 (90.2)
Bipolar disorders	38	1.8			2119 (64.1)
Schizophrenia	35	3.0	4.7	0.03	1187 (35.9)
< 65 y	32	1.1			2899 (87.7)
≥ 65 y	41	10.1	133.0	< .001	407 (12.3)
Married	1	0.3			326 (9.9)
Not married or unknown	72	2.4	6.1	.013	2908 (90.1)
Charlson Comorbidity Score					
Level 0	30	1.3			2387 (72.2)
Level 1–2	32	3.9			826 (25.0)
Level 3–6	11	11.8			93 (2.8)
Elapsed time from last visit to death					
< 2 y	14	0.4			3218 (97.3)
≥ 2 y	59	67.1	1760	< .001	88 (2.7)

Note. BIRLS = Beneficiary Identification Locator System; SSA = Social Security Administration; VA = Veterans Affairs.

(Table 3). The difference between these rates was statistically significant ($\chi^2_1 = 122; P < .001$). We compared the mortality rate for patients who were lost to follow-up for less than 2 years with the rate for those lost to follow-up for 2 years or more. The difference between these rates was statistically significant ($\chi^2_1 = 1760; P < .001$).

For the multivariable analysis, we had complete data on 3306 persons. All of the explanatory variables were associated positively with patient mortality. After controlling for all variables, the odds of dying was about 6 times higher for those who did not return for VA care than for those who did return, after controlling for patient demographic and clinical variables (Table 4). Older patients were more likely to die than younger patients, and having a higher Charlson comorbidity score was associated with higher odds of death as well (Table 4).

DISCUSSION

In this quality improvement study, we identified VA patients with schizophrenia or bipolar disorders who did not return for care for at least 1 or 2 years or more after having been regularly seen in the VA health care system. We found that when contacted, 72% of these patients returned to VA for care. Also, we found that the mortality risk of patients who reengaged with

Table 4. Probability Model of Patient Mortality Showing Multivariable Results Adjusting for Patient Demographic and Clinical Factors: National Psychosis Registry, 2005–2006

Patient Variable	Coefficient, β (SE)	Wald	Odds Ratio (95% CI)
Intercept	−6.5 (0.9)	50.8	...
Did not return for care	1.8 (0.7)	5.7	5.8* (1.4, 24.4)
Age ⩾ 65 y (vs < 65 y)	1.8 (0.3)	45.1	5.9** (3.5, 10.0)
Male (vs female)	0.3 (0.5)	0.3	1.3 (0.4, 3.9)
Single (vs married)	0.2 (0.3)	0.6	1.3 (0.7, 2.3)
Schizophrenia (vs bipolar)	0.4 (0.3)	2.0	1.4 (0.8, 2.4)
Charlson score = 1 (vs 0)	0.7 (0.2)	8.2	2.0* (1.3, 3.8)
Charlson score = 2 (vs 0)	1.5 (0.4)	13.5	4.6* (2.0, 10.5)
Elapsed time from last visit to death: <2 y (vs ⩾ 2 y)	−0.9 (0.9)	1.0	0.4 (0.1, 2.4)

Note. CI = confidence interval.
*$P < .055$; **$P < .001$.

the VA health care system was almost 6 times lower than that for patients who did not return to care after adjusting for patient factors.

There is no operational definition of "lost to follow-up care" for either the VA health care system or for non-VA health care providers. Providing medical treatments on a continuous basis for patients with chronic mental and physical illnesses is considered to be a fundamental aspect of high-quality care. The absence of continuous care over time is considered by clinicians to be detrimental to the patient with schizophrenia or bipolar disorder. Patients who fail to see a physician or other health care provider, take prescribed medications, or complete the clinical course of treatment are at higher risk of not achieving desirable outcomes. Clinical guidelines recommend no fewer than 3 outpatient contacts per year for patients with schizophrenia or bipolar disorders.[15-17]

Although other studies on patient retention or disengagement used different definitions and measures, they corroborated our finding that irregular use of medical care was associated with suboptimal outcomes[18] or that consistent use of primary care was associated with increased survival.[19] Most of these studies of VA patients with schizophrenia or bipolar disorders who had long-term gaps in follow-up care were found to be at greater risk for experiencing poor health outcomes.[18-21]

This OMI study provided evidence that contacting patients who were lost to follow-up might play an important role in reengagement with the VA health care system. The rate of return (72%) observed in this study was almost 3 times greater than the 25% return rate observed in the study by Fischer et al, [18] in which disengaged mentally ill VA patients were not contacted. This high return rate might be due to 2 factors: (1) staff at VA facilities conducted outreach activities to reengage these patients, and (2) VA patients tended to be closely tied to the VA health care system.

Identifying and contacting patients who have dropped out of care is a key component of collaborative and medical home models.[22-24] Nonetheless, to our knowledge this was one of the first quality improvement studies that used a national administrative database to identify and follow up with disengaged patients who had chronic mental disorders. Although this form of panel management was used for chronic medical illnesses, it was applied to a lesser extent in those with a history of mental disorders. Recently, the VA Practice Guidelines for managing patients with bipolar disorder recommended the use of collaborative and chronic care model processes, along with standard pharmacotherapy and psychotherapy, including the systematic use of information technology (registries).[17]

Notwithstanding the use of national data and coordinated services across medical centers to identify and follow up with patients who had chronic mental disorders, there were limitations to this study that warrant consideration. First, the observational nature of this study and rapid need to identify all patients who dropped out of care precluded our ability to conduct a rigorous comparison of the outreach process to standard care. Second, we might have underestimated the rate at which patients returned to any health care provider because we did not query Medicare and other non-VA data sources to identify VA patients who returned to non-VA health care providers or facilities. Also, we did not know if these patients received treatment from non-VA health care providers during the time that they were lost to VA follow-up care. Consequently, those who returned to the VA for care might not have completely stopped using medical care services, regardless of auspices of the health care provider, and might have been in better health status than veterans who did not return to VA care. In addition, it is important to note that one should not infer from the results of our regression model that the VA's inability to provide follow-up care was the cause of mortality, because many patient and health care facility confounding variables were not included in this study. We did not have patient information on sociodemographic or clinical factors beyond what was available in VA administrative data that might have influenced the relationship between successful contact and mortality, including current homelessness, health behaviors, current psychiatric symptoms, dual use of VA and non-VA health care services, or social support. Finally, current limitations on the availability of comprehensive data necessary to mount a national quality improvement initiative made it difficult to generalize about how the results of this VA study might apply to other veterans who are not being treated for schizophrenia or bipolar disorder and other closed health care systems. We encourage the undertaking of further studies covering other SMI patient populations.

Despite these shortcomings, our study demonstrated that active follow-up of patients with SMI could result in patients returning to the VA health care system. Our findings also suggested that population-based panel management using large national databases could effectively identify and contact patients who have dropped out of care, even among a less stable population, such as the chronically mentally ill. Despite the proliferation of large-outcomes database research and measurement-based care (e.g., panel management, disease management registries), there has been little application of these processes at the population level for persons with SMI. VA's application of administrative data to clinical research and practice, as detailed in this study, demonstrated the clinical utility of these potentially rich data sources. To this end, VA should continue systematic data mining of its national databases to identify patients with chronic mental disorders who have had no contact or minimal contact with VA facilities. Most importantly, the VA staff should use directed and intensified outreach services to contact and schedule appointments for patients who have dropped out of care over prolonged periods of time.

Our study also pointed to suggestions for improving the efficiency of care for veterans with chronic mental disorders who dropped out of care. The VA health care system is an important part in the safety net for the nation's veterans.[25] At the time of this study, 138 VAMCs and their associated community-based outpatient clinics had a variety of service treatment options available and had outreach staff providing services. In addition, the *VA Uniform Mental Health Services Handbook* mandates that patients who call the VA to seek mental health care be contacted within 24 hours, and seen within 14 days. A similar mandate for patients with chronic mental disorders in need of medical care should be considered, because the majority of VA patients who were lost to follow-up for 1 year or more had at least 1 chronic condition, and there is growing awareness that the most common cause of mortality is medically related in this group.

Based on the results of this study, future VHA quality improvement efforts should consider using administrative database registries to identify and track patients with chronic mental disorders to coordinate and integrate appropriate care. In addition, the local recovery coordinator or other outreach staff at a medical center could receive a computerized alert when an elderly SMI patient who also has chronic pulmonary disease or diabetes misses a clinic appointment to enable effective reengagement in care. Also, when the patient returns for care, the ambulatory care clinic staff could be reminded to examine the patient for changes in physical as well as mental status. Further integration of these important outreach and reengagement processes into the VA's emerging medical home and primary care–mental health integration models[26,27] should also be considered to enhance continuity of care for this vulnerable group. By doing so, VA would be coordinating medical and mental health services in a way that enables persons with SMI to live more stable and meaningful lives within their communities.

ABOUT THE AUTHORS

Chester L. Davis, Edward Huycke, Robert Langberg, David Lyle, Yancy Phillips, John R. Pierce, and Bernard M. Winkel are with the Veterans Health Administration, Office of the Medical Inspector, Washington, DC. Frederic C. Blow, Amy M. Kilbourne, and Stephanie Visnic are with Veterans Health Administration, Serious Mental Illness Resource and Evaluation Center, Center for Clinical Management Research, Ann Arbor, MI.

CONTRIBUTORS

C. L. Davis, J. R. Pierce, F. C. Blow, A. M. Kilbourne, and B. M.Winkel conceptualized the study and study design. R. Langberg, D. Lyle, S. Visnic, and C. L. Davis acquired the data. C. L. Davis, J. R. Pierce, A. M. Kilbourne, F. C. Blow, E. Huycke, and Y. Phillips analyzed and interpreted the data. C. L. Davis and A. M. Kilbourne drafted the article. C. L. Davis, A. M. Kilbourne, R. Langberg, E. Huycke, Y. Phillips, F. C. Blow, J. R. Pierce, B. M. Winkel, D. Lyle, and S. Visnic wrote the critical revision of the article.

ACKNOWLEDGMENTS

This study would not have been possible without the critical review of the study proposal and results by Ira Katz, MD, former Chief Officer of Mental Health, Veterans Health Administration; Michael Kussman, MD, former Undersecretary for Health, Veterans Health Administration; Antonette Zeiss, PhD, Chief Officer Mental Health; Robert A. Petzel, MD, Undersecretary for Health, Veterans Health Administration; and Frank Cutler, former data analyst in Office of the Medical Inspector.

HUMAN PARTICIPANT PROTECTION

The Ann Arbor, Michigan VA Medical Center (VAMC) Institutional Review Board evaluated the protocol for this assessment and determined that it was a quality improvement effort, not research.

REFERENCES

1. Kilbourne AM, Ignacio RV, Kim HM, Blow FC. Datapoints: are VA patients with serious mental illness dying younger? *Psychiatr Serv.* 2009;60:589.

2. Colton CW, Manderscheid RW. Congruencies in increased mortality rates, years of potential life lost, and causes of death among public mental health clients in eight states. *Preventing Chronic Dis.* 2006;3(2):1–8.

3. Blow FC, McCarthy JF, Valenstein M, Visnic S, Mach J. *Care for Veterans with Psychosis in the Veterans Health Administration, FY07: 9th Annual National Psychosis Registry Report.* Ann Arbor, MI: Serious Mental Illness Treatment Research and Evaluation Center (SMITREC); 2008.

4. Kilbourne AM, Morden NE, Austin K, et al. Excess heart-disease-related mortality in a national study of patients with mental disorders: identifying modifiable risk factors. *Gen Hosp Psychiatry.* 2009;31(6):555–563.

5. Kilbourne AM, Cornelius JR, Han X, et al. General-medical conditions in older patients with serious mental illness. *Am J Geriatr Psychiatry.* 2005;13(3):250–254.

6. Druss BG, Bornemann TH. Improving health and health care for persons with serious mental illness: the window for US federal policy change. *JAMA.* 2010;303(19):1972–1973.

7. Horvitz-Lennon M, Kilbourne AM, Pincus HA. From silos to bridges: meeting the general health care needs of adults with severe mental illnesses. *Health Aff (Millwood).* 2006;25:659–669.

8. Copeland L, Zeber JE, Rosenheck RA, Miller AL. Unforeseen inpatient mortality among veterans with schizophrenia. *Med Care.* 2006;44(2):110.

9. Department of Veterans Affairs. Veterans Health Administration. *Journey of Change.* April, 1997: 1–57.

10. Office of Assistant Deputy Under Secretary for Health Policy and Planning. VHA at a Glance for selected workload statistics for FY 2009. Available at: http://vaww4.va.gov/VHAOPP/enroll01/VitalSignsPocketCards/FY09_4th_qtr.pdf. Accessed January 9, 2012.

11. *International Classification of Diseases, Ninth Revision, Clinical Modification.* Hyattsville, MD: National Center for Health Statistics; 1980.

12. Rush WA, O'Connor PJ, Goodman MJ. Validation of a Modified Charlson Score Using Health Plan Claims Data, Present at Academy of Health Services Health Policy Meeting, 2000.

13. McGregor JC, Kim P, Perencevich EN, et al. Utility of chronic disease score and the Charlson comorbidity index as comorbidity measures for use in epidemiologic studies of antibiotic-resistant organisms. *Am J Epidemiol.* 2005;161:483–493.

14. Hall WH, Ramanathan R, Narayan S, Jani AB, Vijayakumar S. An electronic application for rapidly calculating Charlson comorbidity score. *BMC Cancer.* 2004;4:94.

15. McEnvoy JP, Scheifler PL, Frances A. The Expert Consensus Guidelines Series: Treatment of schizophrenia. *J Clin Psychiatry.* 1999;60(suppl. 11):1–80.

16. Sachs GS, Printz DJ, Kahn A, Carpenter D, Docherty JP, The Expert Consensus Guidelines Series: treatment of bipolar disorder: 2000. *Postgrad Med.* 2000;(special no. 1):1–104.

17. Department of Veterans Affairs and Department of Defense. *VA/DoD Clinical Practice Guideline for Management of Bipolar Disorder in Adults,* Version 2.0. Washington, DC: Department of Veterans Affairs; 2009.

18. Fischer EP, McCarthy JF, Ignacio RV, et al. Longitudinal patterns in health system retention among veterans with schizophrenia or bipolar disorder. *Community Ment Health J.* 2008;44:321–330.

19. Copeland LA, Zeber JE, Wang CP, et al. Patterns of primary care among patients with schizophrenia or diabetes: a cluster analysis approach to the retrospective study of healthcare utilization. *BMC Health Serv Res.* 2009;9:127.

20. Kreyenbuhl J, Nossel I, Dixon LB. Disengagement from mental health treatment among individuals with schizophrenia and strategies for facilitating connections to care: a review of the literature. *Schizophrenia Bull.* 2009;35(4):696–703.

21. Felker B, Yazel J, Short D. Mortality and medical comorbidity among psychiatric patients: a review. *Psychiatric Serv.* 1996;47(12):1356–1363.

22. Bodenheimer T, Wagner EH, Grumbach K. Improving primary care for patients with chronic illness. *JAMA.* 2002;288(14):1775–1779.

23. Bodenheimer T, Wagner EH, Grumbach K. Improving primary care for patients with chronic illness: the chronic care model, part 2. *JAMA*. 2002;288(15):1909–1914.

24. Von Korff M, Gruman J, Schaefer J, Curry SJ, Wagner EH. Collaborative management of chronic illness. *Ann Intern Med*. 1997;127(12):1097–1102.

25. Wilson NJ, Kizer KW. The VA Health Care System: an unrecognized national safety net. *Health Aff*. 1997;16(4):200–204.

26. Kilbourne AM, Pirraglia PA, Lai Z, et al. Quality of general medical care among patients with serious mental illness: does colocation of services matter? *Psychiatr Serv*. 2011;63(8):922–928.

27. Post EP, Metzger M, Dumas P, Lehmann L. Integrating mental health into primary care within the Veterans Health Administration. *Fam Syst Health*. 2010;28(2):83–90.

24

Effects of Iraq/Afghanistan Deployments on Major Depression and Substance Use Disorder: Analysis of Active Duty Personnel in the US Military

Yu-Chu Shen, PhD, Jeremy Arkes, PhD, and Thomas V. Williams, PhD

Objectives. Our objective was to analyze the association between deployment characteristics and diagnostic rates for major depression and substance use disorder among active duty personnel.

Methods. Using active duty personnel serving between 2001 and 2006 (n = 678 382) and deployment information from the Contingent Tracking System, we identified individuals diagnosed with substance use disorders and major depression from TRICARE health records. We performed logistic regression analysis to assess the effect of deployment location and length on these diagnostic rates.

Results. Increased odds of diagnosis with both conditions were associated with deployment to Iraq or Afghanistan compared with nondeployed personnel and with Army and Marine Corps personnel compared with Navy and Air Force personnel. Increases in the likelihood of either diagnosis with deployment length were only observed among Army personnel.

Conclusions. There were increased substance use disorders and major depression across services associated with combat conditions. It would be important to assess whether the public health system has adequate resources to handle the increasing need of mental health services in this population.

The continuing presence of the US military in Iraq and Afghanistan has posed substantial mental health challenges to US military service members and mental health care systems.[1–7] Much media attention and research effort have focused on posttraumatic stress disorder (PTSD) among US servicemen returning from Iraq and Afghanistan (Operations Iraqi Freedom and Operations Enduring Freedom [OIF/OEF]) and less on other mental health outcomes. However, there are other mental health conditions that are more likely to be diagnosed among the active duty population, such as a substance use disorder, major depression, anxiety, and traumatic brain injury. Reports by the Mental Health Advisory Team (MHAT) have noted that the percentage of soldiers reporting symptoms of major depression and substance use disorders has been rising over the years,[6,7] and a recent Rand report pointed out the need to study these conditions as part of the broad spectrum of postdeployment mental health consequences.[3]

Most of the studies on this topic used convenience samples and focused on soldiers and Marines, with little attention paid to Navy and Air Force personnel. Two studies using convenience samples of soldiers or Marines returning from Iraq found that about 20% of these personnel required mental health treatment, 15% had depression, and 10% to 12% reported having substance use disorder problems.[8,9] Reports by MHAT, also focusing on soldiers and Marines, noted an increasing rate of depression and overall mental health problems over the years, and that the rate was positively associated with combat level.[6,7] A similar finding was echoed in a recent study using a convenience sample of 1200 soldiers—the authors found that witnessing atrocities (between rival Iraqi factions) and experiencing a personal threat were associated with significantly higher rates of alcohol misuse.[10] The most recent MHAT report also noted that Army-enlisted personnel had higher rates of mental health problems than did Marine-enlisted personnel.[6] These studies, although providing important information on the prevalence of mental health problems of deployed active duty populations, did not provide appropriate comparison groups among the nondeployed. The lack of proper comparison groups complicated efforts to attribute observed mental health problems to specific deployment-related experiences without the capacity to investigate corresponding background rates among the nondeployed active duty population. Although PTSD was typically triggered by witnessing a traumatic event—which was also part of the criteria for being diagnosed with the condition—major depression and substance use disorder could often be triggered by other events among the nondeployed population.[11]

A few studies included the nondeployed population and had mixed findings. Research based on the Millennium Cohort Study (MCS),[12,13] which used self-administered surveys and tracked both active duty personnel and those separated from the military, compared health outcomes for those deployed in support of the Iraq and Afghanistan wars with those not deployed. The MCS found that men and women deployed with combat exposure had, respectively, 1.32 and 2.13 times the odds of having depression compared with those not deployed[14] and found weak evidence of any impact of a combat deployment on drinking outcomes among active duty respondents.[15] Besides the MCS, 1 study, using a 2008 Department of Defense Health Related Behaviors Survey, found that service members with any combat deployment had significantly higher rates of heavy alcohol and cigarette use.[16] Finally, a study that examined the New Jersey Army National Guard members found previous deployment to be significantly linked to a higher rate of major depression and higher probability of binge drinking.[17]

In summary, many earlier investigations focused just on health needs among the Army and the Marines. When studies included all Armed Services, none distinguished between possible different effects across services.[12,14-16] Recent literature on other mental health conditions (in particular, PTSD) found that the mental health condition rates and the deployment effects differed across services.[6,18] Lastly, almost all studies relied on self-administered survey questions to identify mental health problems, where self-reported answers were subject to errors and misreporting and could lead to misdiagnoses of the conditions.

The objective of our study was to analyze, for each service branch, the association between deployment characteristics (location and duration) and the rates of diagnosis for major depression and substance use disorder among the active duty population. We examined a random sample of all active duty enlisted personnel serving between 2001 and 2006, focusing on the percentage of personnel diagnosed with major depression and substance use disorder and analyzing the 2 conditions separately for the 4 military services: Army, Marines, Navy, and Air Force.

METHODS

We combined several data sources from TRICARE and the Defense Manpower Data Center to form the basis of our analysis. First, we identified the active duty personnel population and obtained demographic and service information (such as age, gender, race, and rank) from the Defense Enrollment Eligibility Reporting System (DEERS). Second, we identified the date that each mental health condition was first diagnosed and related health information from the following sources: the Standard Inpatient Data Record, the Standard Ambulatory Data Record, and the TRICARE encounter data from services rendered in managed care support contracted facilities. The 4 data sources allowed us to capture the diagnoses from both the inpatient and outpatient settings and from all civilian and military health providers. Third, we did a random draw for each service from the entire DEERS database to obtain a 25% sample, and we linked OIF/OEF deployment characteristics and military occupational specialty (MOS) codes between 2001 and 2006 from the Contingency Tracking System for this sample.

Our data consisted of 678 382 unique enlisted personnel from all services. This represented roughly a 25% sample of the active duty population. Among the sample, 49% was Army, 14% Marine, 20% Navy, and 17% Air Force. Our sample was representative of the US Armed Forces active duty enlisted population—Appendix A (data available as a supplement to the online version of this article at http://www.ajph.org) shows the comparison of key demographic variables and the percentage diagnosed with major depression and substance use disorders between the active duty population from the 100% DEERS database and our analytic sample.

Outcome Measures

We analyzed 2 mental health conditions separately. The dependent variable in the depression analysis was whether an enlisted person was diagnosed with major depression (if the *International Classification of Diseases-9* [*ICD-9*][19] code was either 296.2 or 296.3) anytime between 2001 and 2006.[11] Likewise, the substance use disorder analysis identified persons who were diagnosed with substance use disorder (if the first 3 digits of the *ICD-9* code was 291 or 292, 303, 304, 305) during the study period. Because we could only identify conditions through *ICD-9* codes, we did not have information on which type of drugs were identified as the misused substance.

Statistical Models

Our goal was to provide comparison of incidences of major depression and substance use disorders between the nondeployed service members and those deployed to certain locations while controlling for underlying demographic and service characteristics. We used logistic regression models to assess the effect of deployment location and duration under OIF/OEF on the rate of major depression and substance use disorder within each service. Our key variables of interest were the deployment locations and deployment durations based on information of the last deployment. For those who were diagnosed with either mental health condition, "last deployment" referred to the last deployment before the service member was diagnosed with the condition. For example, if a person was diagnosed with major depression on March 2004 and their most recent deployment before this date was July 2003, we used deployment information from the July 2003 deployment. We provided details of the location and the duration categories in the following. Covariates included service affiliation and demographic characteristics as explained in the following. All models were estimated using Stata 11.[20]

Explanatory Variables

There were 3 categories of variables included in the models: deployment characteristics, service characteristics, and demographic information. We classified 4 categories of deployment locations: not deployed under OEF or OIF (the reference group), deployed to Iraq or Afghanistan, deployed at other known locations under OEF or OIF (such as Kuwait, Qatar, Saudi Arabia, Turkey), and deployed to classified or unknown locations. For duration, we classified the deployment length into 3 categories: short, if the length of the last deployment was less than 120 days (the reference group); medium, if the length was between 120 and 180 days; and long, if the length was greater than 180 days.

For service characteristics, we included rank and MOS categories. We categorized MOS codes into the following categories: combat arms (reference group), combat support, combat service support, aviation, medical, and other MOS. The occupational categories were proxies for potential differences in job stress that might have influenced a service member's probability of being diagnosed with the mental health conditions, independent of the deployment effect. We included the following demographic information in the models to control for potential differences in major depression and substance use disorder rates across the demographic dimensions: gender, race/ethnicity (White as the reference group, African American, Hispanic, Asian, and other races), marital status, and age. In a sensitivity analysis, we replaced age with length of service, and the results were similar between the two specifications. Lastly, we included year indicators to control for possible macro trends in major depression and substance use disorder rates over the study period in the overall active duty population.

RESULTS

Table 1 presents the descriptive statistics of the sample's deployment characteristics by service. The majority of the active duty personnel were not deployed under OIF/OEF: the percentages ranged from 62% in the Air Force to 77% in the Army. Not surprisingly, the Army and Marines had the highest share of enlisted members being sent to Iraq and Afghanistan (12% and 9%, respectively). The Navy only had 1% of its enlisted personnel deployed to

Table 1. Descriptive Statistics of Enlisted Personnel Deployment Characteristics, by Military Service Branch: 2001–2006

Deployment characteristics	Army, No. (%) or No.	Marines, No. (%) or No.	Navy, No. (%) or No.	Air Force, No. (%) or No.
Location of last OIF/OEF deployment				
Not deployed under OIF/OEF	257 873 (77%)	73 995 (75%)	86 754 (65%)	69 790 (62%)
Deployed to Afghanistan or Iraq	39 193 (12%)	8633 (9%)	1366 (1%)	5922 (5%)
Deployed to other nonclassified location	29 800 (9%)	11 586 (12%)	8556 (6%)	25 470 (23%)
Deployed to classified or unknown location	6682 (2%)	4310 (4%)	37 339 (28%)	11 113 (10%)
Duration of last OIF/OEF deployment among those that deployed				
Short (1–120 d)	91 885 (28%)	25 011 (25%)	42 106 (31%)	72 892 (65%)
Medium (120–180 d)	46 898 (14%)	25 644 (26%)	31 390 (23%)	27 590 (25%)
Long (more than 180 d)	194 796 (58%)	47 884 (49%)	60 499 (45%)	11 837 (11%)
Sample size	333 548	98 524	134 015	112 295

Note. OIF/OEF = Operations Iraqi Freedom and Operations Enduring Freedom.

Afghanistan or Iraq. The Navy had the highest share of its enlisted population being deployed to classified or unknown locations (28%), followed by the Air Force (10%). The Air Force appeared to serve a more supportive role, with 23% of their enlisted population being sent to known OIF/OEF missions other than Iraq andAfghanistan. Among those deployed, the Army and Marine Corps tended to have longer deployments: 58% and 49% of Army and Marine Corps personnel, respectively, had been deployed more than 180 days in their most recent deployment before being included in the sample, whereas 65% of deployed Air Force personnel had a tour length of less than 120 days.

Table 2 compares summary statistics of demographic and service characteristics by whether the service member was deployed to OIF/OEF. Although those deployed to OIF/OEF were similar on most dimensions to the control group, there were 2 notable differences: across all services, those deployed were more likely to be married and in the middle ranks (pay grade E4 and E5).

Table 3 presents the percentage of the active duty population who were diagnosed with each mental health condition by service. The top of Table 3 reports the rate of substance use disorder. The overall percentage of active duty population diagnosed with substance use disorder (regardless of deployment status) ranged from 6% in the Marine Corps to 9% in the Navy. Among the population diagnosed with a substance use disorder, 30% were because of alcohol use and 70% were because of drug use (see Appendix A; available online at http://www.ajph.org). In addition, 6% and 4% had major depression and PTSD as comorbid conditions, respectively (results not shown in Table 3). Deployment to Afghanistan and Iraq increased the incidence of substance use disorder substantially among Army and Marines Corps personnel: the rate of substance use disorder more than doubled in the Army (14.5% among those deployed to Afghanistan or Iraq vs 6% among the nondeployed; $P < .001$ in pairwise comparison) and almost doubled in the Marine Corps (9.3% vs 5%; $P < .001$). Among the small share of Navy personnel sent to Afghanistan or Iraq, their rate of substance use disorder diagnoses was comparable to the nondeployed Navy enlisted. A total of 7% of Air Force enlisted deployed to Iraq and Afghanistan were diagnosed with substance use disorder compared with 6% among the nondeployed population. Across all services, those deployed to other nonclassified OIF/OEF missions had similar substance use disorder rates as those deployed to Iraq or Afghanistan. Among Army and Air

246 | VETERAN SUICIDE

Table 2. Descriptive Statistics of Enlisted Personnel Demographic and Service Characteristics, by Military Service Branch and Deployment Status to OIF/OEF: 2001–2006

	Army		Marines		Navy		Air Force	
	Not Deployed, % or No.	Deployed, % or No.	Not Deployed, % or No.	Deployed, % or No.	Not Deployed, % or No.	Deployed, % or No.	Not Deployed, % or No.	Deployed, % or No.
Demographic Characteristics								
Gender								
Male	88%	89%	96%	97%	86%	87%	82%	85%
Female	12%	11%	4%	3%	14%	13%	18%	15%
Marital status								
Single	57%	42%	74%	54%	60%	47%	54%	39%
Married	43%	58%	26%	46%	40%	53%	46%	61%
Race								
White	65%	61%	72%	68%	59%	55%	75%	73%
Black	19%	22%	10%	11%	21%	23%	15%	16%
Hispanic	7%	6%	8%	10%	7%	8%	3%	4%
Asian	4%	3%	3%	3%	6%	6%	2%	2%
Other races	6%	7%	7%	8%	8%	8%	5%	5%
Age	27	29	23	25	26	28	27	31

(continued on next page)

Table 2. (*continued*)

	Army		Marines		Navy		Air Force	
	Not Deployed, % or No.	Deployed, % or No.	Not Deployed, % or No.	Deployed, % or No.	Not Deployed, % or No.	Deployed, % or No.	Not Deployed, % or No.	Deployed, % or No.
Service characteristics								
Military occupational specialty								
Combat arms	28%	28%	37%	38%	5%	5%	10%	10%
Combat support	11%	9%	16%	16%	9%	10%	0%	0%
Combat service support	26%	23%	27%	25%	5%	5%	75%	79%
Aviation			14%	15%	3%	3%		
Medical					3%	2%		
Other military occupational specialty	10%	10%						
	26%	30%	5%	5%	75%	74%	14%	10%
Rank								
E1-E3	41%	10%	70%	38%	48%	23%	45%	12%
E4	26%	37%	13%	30%	17%	25%	16%	24%
E5	15%	25%	9%	18%	17%	26%	19%	30%
E6	10%	16%	5%	7%	12%	17%	11%	19%
E7-E9	7%	11%	4%	7%	6%	10%	9%	16%
Sample size	294 814	88 614	80 373	27 275	97 378	52 821	84 285	51 149

Note. OIF/OEF = Operations Iraqi Freedom and Operations Enduring Freedom.

Table 3. Actual Percentage of Personnel Diagnosed With Substance Use Disorder and Major Depression, by Military Service Branch and Deployment Location and Length: 2001-2006

	Army, %, % (95% CI), or No.	Marines, %, % (95% CI), or No.	Navy, %, % (95% CI), or No.	Air Force, %, % (95% CI), or No.
Overall % diagnosed with substance use disorder	7.6%	6.0%	8.8%	6.1%
Based on location of last OIF/OEF deployment				
Not deployed under OIF/OEF	6.0 (6.0, 6.1)	5.0 (4.9, 5.2)	8.0 (7.8, 8.2)	5.9 (5.8, 6.1)
Deployed to Afghanistan or Iraq	14.8 (14.4,15.1)	9.3 (8.7, 9.9)	8.6 (7.2,10.2)	7.1 (6.5, 7.8)
Deployed to other nonclassified location	13.4 (13.0, 3.8)	8.6 (8.1, 9.2)	10.4 (9.8, 11.1)	7.1 (6.7, 7.4)
Deployed to classified or unknown location	4.9 (4.4,5.4)	8.7 (7.9, 9.6)	10.4 (10.1,10.8)	4.3 (3.9, 4.7)
Based on duration of Last OIF/OEF deployment				
Short (1-120 d)	11.2 (11.0, 11.9)	9.7 (9.0,10.5)	10.3 (9.8, 10.8)	6.1 (5.8, 6.3)
Medium (120-180 d)	12.6 (12.3, 13.5)	8.2 (7.6, 8.9)	10.9 (10.4, 11.5)	7.0 (6.5, 7.5)
Long (more than 180 d)	14.4 (14.1, 14.7)	8.8 (8.3, 9.3)	10.2 (9.8, 10.6)	6.5 (5.8,7.2)
Overall % diagnosed with major depression	2.5%	1.7%	2.4%	3.3%
Based on location of last OIF/OEF deployment				
Not deployed under OIF/OEF	1.7 (1.7, 1.8)	1.2 (1.1, 1.2)	2.2 (2.1, 2.3)	3.1 (3.0, 3.3)
Deployed to Afghanistan or Iraq	5.1 (4.9, 5.3)	3.8 (3.4, 4.2)	5.8 (4.6, 7.0)	3.5 (3.0, 4.0)
Deployed to other nonclassified location	5.7 (5.5, 6.0)	3.6 (3.2, 3.9)	3.5 (3.1, 3.9)	3.9 (3.6, 4.1)
Deployed to classified or unknown location	2.5 (2.2, 2.9)	2.3 (1.8, 2.7)	2.4 (2.3, 2.6)	2.3 (2.1, 2.6)
Based on duration of last OIF/OEF deployment				
Short (1-120 d)	4.6 (4.4, 5.0)	3.6 (3.1, 4.1)	2.7 (2.4, 3.0)	3.3 (3.1, 3.5)
Medium (120-180 d)	4.5 (4.2, 5.0)	3.5 (3.0, 3.9)	2.8 (2.5, 3.1)	3.8 (3.4, 4.2)
Long (more than 180 d)	5.4 (5.3, 5.7)	3.3 (3.0, 3.6)	2.7 (2.5, 2.9)	3.5 (3.0, 4.1)
Sample size	333 548	98 524	134 015	112 295

Note. OIF/OEF = Operations Iraqi Freedom and Operations Enduring Freedom.

Force personnel, those deployed to classified or unknown locations actually had lower substance use disorder rates than did the nondeployed group. Lastly, among Army soldiers deployed under OIF/OEF, the substance use disorder rate, which was higher than that in the other 3 services, increased as the tour length increased. We did not observe this trend in the other 3 services.

The bottom of Table 3 reports the rates of major depression by the service. The overall rate of major depression was much lower than that of substance use disorder: it ranged from 1.7% for the Marines Corps to 3.3% for the Air Force. However, major depression was more likely to be accompanied by other comorbid conditions; 25% had substance use disorder as a comorbid condition and 18% had PTSD (results not shown in Table 3). The rate of major depression was substantially higher in the population deployed to Iraq, Afghanistan, or other known nonclassified locations under OIF/OEF compared with the nondeployed population. The rate of major depression did not appear to substantially differ across different deployment durations.

Table 4 presents results from the logistic regressions in terms of odds ratios (ORs) and focuses only on the effect of deployment characteristics (the complete results for all variables are included in the Appendix, available online at http://www.ajph.org). The top of Table 4 shows that deployment under OIF/OEF significantly increased the odds of having a substance use disorder compared with those not deployed, although the magnitude varied somewhat across the services and locations. Among Army enlisted personnel, the odds of being diagnosed with substance use disorder was 4.05 times higher among those deployed to Iraq/Afghanistan than it was among those not deployed under OIF/OEF (95% confidence interval [CI] = 3.82, 4.30). Being deployed on other known OIF/OEF missions also increased the odds of having a substance use disorder by the same magnitude (OR = 3.72; 95% CI = 3.53, 3.93). Being deployed to a classified or unknown location (2% of the Army enlisted) increased the odds by a much smaller magnitude, although the effect was still highly significant (OR = 1.26; 95% CI = 1.12,1.41). The effects of being deployed to Iraq or Afghanistan and on other known OIF/OEF missions were comparable for the Marines; the odds of developing PTSD increased by 4.36 (95% CI =3.82, 4.97) and 3.12 (95% CI = 2.79, 3.48), respectively. Deployment to a classified or unknown location carried similar odds as the other locations for the enlisted Marines (OR = 3.03; 95% CI = 2.65, 3.47).

Table 4. Effect of Last Deployment's Location and Duration on the Rate of Substance Use Disorder and Major Depression, 2001-2006

	Army, OR (95% CI)	Marines, OR (95% CI)	Navy, OR (95% CI)	Air Force, OR (95% CI)
Substance use disorder				
Location of last deployment (reference group is not deployed under OIF/OEF)				
Deployed to Afghanistan or Iraq	4.05*** (3.82, 4.30)	4.36*** (3.82, 4.97)	1.77*** (1.45, 2.16)	1.76*** (1.56, 1.99)
Deployed to other nonclassified location	3.72*** (3.53, 3.93)	3.12*** (2.79, 3.48)	1.94*** (1.78, 2.12)	1.62*** (1.51, 1.75)
Deployed to classified or unknown location	1.26*** (1.12, 1.41)	3.03*** (2.65, 3.47)	1.82*** (1.71, 1.94)	1.05 (0.94, 1.16)
Duration of last deployment (reference group is short [< 120 d])				
Medium (120–180 d)	1.08** (1.00,1.16)	0.82*** (0.73, 0.93)	1.12*** (1.03, 1.21)	1.16*** (1.05, 1.27)
Long (longer than 180 d)	1.31*** (1.24, 1.39)	0.92 (0.82, 1.03)	1.06* (0.99, 1.14)	1.11 (0.97, 1.27)
Major depression				
Location of last deployment (reference group is not deployed under OIF/OEF)				
Deployed to Afghanistan or Iraq	3.52*** (3.21, 3.86)	4.51*** (3.66, 5.57)	3.25*** (2.50, 4.22)	1.45*** (1.22, 1.72)
Deployed to other nonclassified location	3.91*** (3.60, 4.24)	3.13*** (2.62, 3.74)	1.92*** (1.64, 2.24)	1.50*** (1.36, 1.66)
Deployed to classified or unknown location	1.56*** (1.32, 1.83)	2.00*** (1.57, 2.55)	1.39*** (1.22, 1.57)	0.97 (0.84, 1.11)
Duration of last deployment (reference group is short [< 120 d])				
Medium (120–180 d)	0.94 (0.84, 1.05)	1.01 (0.83, 1.23)	1.03 (0.88, 1.20)	1.20*** (1.06, 1.37)
Long (longer than 180 d)	1.20*** (1.10, 1.30)	0.89 (0.74, 1.07)	0.98 (0.86, 1.12)	1.16* (0.97, 1.38)
Sample size	333 548	98 524	134 015	112 295

Note. OIF/OEF = Operations Iraqi Freedom and Operations Enduring Freedom.

*P < .1; **P < .05; ***P < .01.

The effect of deployment location was much smaller for the Navy and the Air Force. For both, being deployed to Iraq or Afghanistan increased the odds of developing a substance use disorder by 1.8 times (95% CI = 1.56, 1.99) compared with those not deployed under OIF/OEF. For Navy personnel, being deployed to OIF/OEF locations other than Afghanistan or Iraq carried similar odds of having a substance use disorder (OR = 1.94; 95% CI = 1.78, 2.12 and OR = 1.82; 95% CI = 1.71, 1.94, for known and classified locations, respectively). For the Air Force, deployments to nonclassified locations increased the risk of having a substance use disorder by 1.62 times (95% CI = 1.51, 1.75), but deployments to a classified or unknown location did not affect the risk of having a substance use disorder.

Deployment duration appeared to be associated with substance use disorder diagnoses only among Army personnel. Compared with those who had a short tour length (< 120 days), Army soldiers whose last deployment was between 120 and 180 days were 1.08 times more likely to be diagnosed later with substance use disorder (95% CI = 1.00, 1.16), and those whose last deployment was more than 180 days had an OR of 1.31 (95% CI = 1.24, 1.39). A long deployment duration did not significantly increase the odds of having a substance use disorder for the other 3 services.

Although not the focus of this study, it was worth highlighting results of a few demographic and service variables. Appendix B (available as a supplement to the online article at http://www.ajph.org) shows that among the broad categories of MOS, enlisted personnel whose specialty was in the category combat arms had the highest odds of developing a substance use disorder. In general, being in a lower rank was associated with higher odds of having a substance use disorder, as was being White (compared with other racial/ethnic groups).

Table 4 shows the results from the major depression analysis (full results in Appendix C, available as a supplement to the online version of the article at http://www.ajph.org). Deployment to Iraq or Afghanistan was associated with higher odds of major depression. The highest OR was observed for the Marines (OR = 4.51; 95% CI = 3.66, 5.57), and the lowest OR was observed for the Air Force (OR = 1.45; 95% CI = 1.22, 1.72). Deployments to other nonclassified locations were also associated with higher odds of major depression, although the magnitude was lower for the Navy (OR = 3.25; 95% CI = 2.5, 4.22, for deployment to Afghanistan and Iraq; OR = 1.92; 95%

CI = 1.64, 2.24 for nonclassified locations). The ORs for classified or unknown locations were lower (OR ranged from 0.97 to 2 depending on the service), although these were still statistically significant for all services, except for the Air Force. Another result worth highlighting was that women had a much higher odds of developing major depression compared with men (see Appendix C, available online at http://www.ajph.org): the OR ranged from 4.04 for the Army to 7.71 for the Marines. Similarly, being married was also associated with a higher risk of major depression across all services. Lastly, in a sensitivity analysis, we analyzed alcohol and drug use disorders separately and found similarly strong associations between deployment location and either condition (Appendix D, available as a supplement to the online version of the article at http://www.ajph.org).

DISCUSSION

In this study, we found that in general, deployment under OIF/OEF increased the risks of being diagnosed with both substance use disorder and major depression substantially, although the magnitudes of the effects varied somewhat across services and across deployment locations. Deployment length, by contrast, was not strongly associated with these 2 mental health conditions, except among Army personnel. However, even in that case, the magnitude of the effect was much smaller than the magnitude of the effect because of deployment locations.

Our study provided valuable insight for the mental health readiness of the US Armed Services and implications for potential, continued support of ongoing operations and their post deployment health care needs. The Military Health System is currently a key focal point of military budget reviews; therefore, this study contributed important information to identify the need for sustained support of the services.

This study had a few limitations. First, our data did not allow for assessment of level of combat exposure. Therefore, we were unable to ascertain whether the adverse effect was because of deployment to a combat zone itself or because of direct combat exposure. We instead used the deployment location of Iraq and Afghanistan as a proxy for higher levels of combat stress, because troops deployed to OEF and OIF had increased likelihood of combat exposures compared with other deployed populations.[3]

Second, although we were able to include MOS, we did not have details on the specific assignments for any given deployment. Such details on assignment might provide additional insight on the underlying causes of adverse effects of deployments. Third, although our sample was representative of those who ever served in the US Armed Forces between 2001 and 2006, we most likely missed the more severe cases of the mental health conditions because those would show up in the VA system unless they were first diagnosed inside the TRICARE system. As a result, our overall percentages of major depression and substance use disorders understated the overall prevalence of the conditions, especially among the veteran population. Fourth, although we had the full deployment information of OIF/OEF missions, we were unable to capture other missions (e.g., those deployed to non-OIF/OEF missions, such as deployment to Haiti or Cuba, who would be in our control group). This likely made our estimated effects of deployment a conservative estimate, because the actual rate of major depression and substance use disorder was likely lower in the strictly nondeployed population.

Third, our sample was representative of all active duty personnel who served in the US Armed Forces between 2001 and 2006, including those who left the service but were eligible for TRICARE coverage for some part of the study period. TRICARE is the health care system of the Department of Defense that serves all uniformed services, activated National Guard and Reserve, retired military, and their families worldwide. Service members are automatically eligible for and enrolled in TRICARE when they remain on active duty. When veterans are separated from the military under other than dishonorable conditions, their health care is no longer provided by TRICARE but provided by the Department of Veterans Affairs (VA) health care system. Although we captured mental health status among recent veterans to include those who had diagnosed mental health problems while on active service, this was not a study of the general veteran population who were diagnosed in the VA health care system after separation from service. Although the military has implemented educational programs to reduce the amount of stigma associated with mental illness, such as the Army Campaign Plan for Health Promotion, Risk Reduction and Suicide Prevention, and the Suicide Prevention Council, our study could not address the extent to which mental health conditions remained undiagnosed among the active duty population who avoided seeking mental health treatment because of the stigma surrounding their illness.

Last, using clinical diagnoses likely underestimated the true rate of depression and substance use disorders among the active duty population because of underreporting as a result of the stigma associated with seeking mental health treatment—24% of enlisted members from OEF surveyed by MHAT in 2009 believed that seeking mental health care services would harm their careers (30% among those serving in OIF), and 30% among those in OEF (40% in OIF) believed that it would result in differential treatment by unit leadership and lost of confidence by unit members.[21,22] The degree of underreporting might be higher among those not deployed, because the deployed personnel were required to complete the Post-Deployment Health Assessment (PDHA), which screened for mental health problems and made referrals for treatment if needed. However, we did not expect the degree of underreporting to introduce any significant bias in our estimates for several reasons. For one, PDHA is administered to all deployed personnel, not just those deployed to OIF/OEF, so some of our control groups were also subject to the screening process. In addition, although PDHA was designed to screen for potential PTSD cases, it was not designed to explicitly screen for major depression and substance use disorder. Before the PDHA revision in April 2007, there was only 1 question related to depression as part of the PTSD screening, and 1 question related to whether a person was interested in receiving help for an alcohol problem.

With these caveats in mind, it was useful to compare our results to those from the MCS—the other major research effort that tracked population-based military cohort's health outcomes using self-administered surveys. It was not surprising that our overall rates of depression and substance use disorder because of alcohol were lower than those reported in MCS, because MCS identified conditions through surveys, whereas we identified conditions through TRICARE health records. The overall rate of new onset of depression in MCS was 4% (Wells et al[14]; Tables 2 and 3), whereas our overall rate of major depression was 2% (see the online appendixes, available at http://www.ajph.org). Note, however, MCS used screening questions that captured a broader spectrum of depression, whereas our clinical diagnoses were limited to just major depression. MCS did not have measures to capture drug use disorders, but reported percentages of respondents with drinking problems. By contrast, our analysis found a much higher OR associated with deployment to

Afghanistan or Iraq (i.e., deployed with combat exposures) for both conditions compared with the MCS findings.[14,15]

It was not surprising that deployment to Iraq and Afghanistan increased the odds of major depression and substance use disorders among service members, given that the combat exposure levels in those 2 locations were much higher in other locations. The magnitude of the adverse effect, however, was substantial, especially among those engaged in ground battle. The fact that we observed the largest adverse effect of deployment locations among Army and Marines likely reflected the different levels of direct combat exposure across services. Our calculations from the PDHA from the same time period showed that Army and Marine enlisted members had a much higher rate of seeing individuals killed during deployment or being inside destroyed vehicles compared with the Navy and Air Force. Other studies using the PDHA also documented that the majority of physical injuries from OIF occurred among Marine Corps personnel, followed by the Army.[23] The lower odds associated with classified location deployments might be caused by selection: those who were selected for covert operations might have been originally selected partly for having a stronger mental health readiness than the general deployed population; furthermore, they might have undergone better preparation and training. However, it was important to note that even among those deployed to the classified or unknown locations, the rate of both having a substance use disorder and major depression was still higher than that of the nondeployed population. The study also revealed a substantially higher risk of major depression among the female enlisted personnel, especially in the Marine Corps. This finding was consistent with previous literature that found that women had a higher likelihood of reporting symptoms of depression.[12,24,25] We could not ascertain, however, whether this might be because women more actively sought treatment of the depression symptoms, or that they were more likely to develop major depression in the military environment. However, evidence on gender and depression suggested that women were not more likely to seek treatment.[25]

Major depression and substance use disorders both require long-term treatment, and pose a substantial health care cost as well as psychological and social costs to the individual and society.[3,26,27] It is important for future research to link actual detailed combat experience and intensity to clinical data to better identify the types of combat experiences and environments that are triggers for these mental health conditions. Such insight would contribute to the design of training programs that can better mentally prepare the enlisted for their deployment assignments. Given the continuing US military presence in Afghanistan and other parts of the world, and the increasing trend in major mental health conditions reported in the US military, it would be important for the Department of Defense to assess whether the current system has adequate resources and manpower to handle the increasing number of active duty personnel who need mental health services.

ABOUT THE AUTHORS

Yu-Chu Shen is with the Graduate School of Business and Public Policy, Naval Postgraduate School, Monterey, CA, and the National Bureau of Economic Research, Cambridge, MA. Jeremy Arkes is with the Graduate School of Business and Public Policy, Naval Postgraduate School, Monterey, and the Rand Corporation, Santa Monica, CA. Thomas V. Williams is with Health Program Analysis and Evaluation, TRICARE Management Activity, Falls Church, VA.

CONTRIBUTORS

Y. Shen conceptualized the study concept and design, analyzed the data, performed the statistical analysis, drafted the article, and supervised the study. Y. Shen and T. V. Williams acquired the data and performed administration, technical, and material support. Y. Shen and J. Arkes obtained the funding. T. V. Williams and J. Arkes critically revised the article for important intellectual content. All three authors interpreted the data.

ACKNOWLEDGMENTS

Y. Shen and J. Arkes thank the Chief of Naval Personnel (N1) Manpower, Personnel, Training & Education Division for financial support. The authors thank Dennis Mar, Wendy Funk, and the staff at Defense Manpower Data Center and TRICARE Management Activity for assisting with data extraction, and Melissa Burke for data processing.

HUMAN PARTICIPANT PROTECTION

The study was approved by the Naval Postgraduate School's Institutional Review Board, TRICARE Management Activity privacy board, and the Office of Navy Medicine.

REFERENCES

1. Hoge CW, Auchterlonie JL, Milliken CS. Mental health problems, use of mental health services, and attrition from military service after returning from deployment to Iraq or Afghanistan. *JAMA*. 2006;295(9):1023–1032.

2. Hoge CW, Castro CA, Messer SC, McGurk D, Cotting DI, Koffman RL. Combat duty in Iraq and Afghanistan, mental health problems, and barriers to care. *N Engl J Med*. 2004;351(1):13–22.

3. Tanielian T, Jaycox LH. *Invisible Wounds of War: Psychological and Cognitive Injuries, Their Consequences, and Services to Assist Recovery*. Santa Monica, CA: Rand Corporation; 2008.

4. US Army. Operation Iraqi Freedom (OIF) Mental Health Advisory Team (MHAT) Report. 2003. Available at: http://www.armymedicine.army.mil/reports/mhat/mhat/mhat_report.pdf. Accessed May 11, 2009.

5. US Army. Operation Iraqi Freedom (OIF) Mental Health Advisory Team (MHAT-II) Report. 2005. Available at: http://www.armymedicine.army.mil/reports/mhat/mhat_ii/OIF-II_REPORT.pdf. Accessed May 11, 2009.

6. US Army. Operation Iraqi Freedom (OIF) Mental Health Advisory Team (MHAT-IV) Report. 2006. Available at: http://www.armymedicine.army.mil/reports/mhat/mhat_iv/MHAT_IV_Report_17NOV06.pdf. Accessed May 11, 2009.

7. US Army. Operation Iraqi Freedom (OIF) Mental Health Advisory Team (MHAT-III) Report. 2006. Available at: http://www.armymedicine.army.mil/reports/mhat/mhat_iii/MHATIII_Report_29May2006-Redacted.pdf. Accessed May 11, 2009.

8. Thomas JL, Wilk JE, Riviere LA, McGurk D, Castro CA, Hoge CW. Prevalence of mental health problems and functional impairment among active component and National Guard soldiers 3 and 12 months following combat in Iraq. *Arch Gen Psychiatry*. 2010;67(6):614–623.

9. Milliken CS, Auchterlonie JL, Hoge CW. Longitudinal assessment of mental health problems among active and reserve component soldiers returning from the Iraq war. *JAMA*. 2007;298(18):2141–2148.

10. Wilk JE, Bliese PD, Kim PY, Thomas JL, McGurk D, Hoge CW. Relationship of combat experiences to alcohol misuse among U.S. soldiers returning from the Iraq war. *Drug Alcohol Depend*. 2010;108(1-2):115–121.

11. *Diagnostic and Statistical Manual of Mental Disorders, Fourth Edition*. Washington, DC; American Psychiatric Association; 1994.

12. Smith TC, Jacobson IG, Hooper TI, et al. Health impact of US military service in a large population-based military cohort: findings of the Millennium Cohort Study, 2001-2008. *BMC Public Health*. 2011;11(1):69.

13. Smith TC, Zamorski M, Smith B, et al. The physical and mental health of a large military cohort: baseline functional health status of the Millennium Cohort. *BMC Public Health*. 2007;7:340.

14. Wells TS, Leardmann CA, Fortuna SO, et al. A prospective study of depression following combat deployment in support of the wars in Iraq and Afghanistan. *Am J Public Health*. 2010;100(1):90–99.

15. Jacobson IG, Ryan MAKK, Hooper TI, et al. Alcohol use and alcohol-related problems before and after military combat deployment. *JAMA*. 2008;300(6): 663–675.

16. Bray RM, Pemberton MR, Lane ME, Hourani LL, Mattiko MJ, Babeu LA. Substance use and mental health trends among U.S. military active duty personnel: key findings from the 2008 DoD Health Behavior Survey. *Mil Med*. 2010;175(6): 390–399.

17. Kline A, Falca-Dodson M, Sussner B, et al. Effects of repeated deployment to Iraq and Afghanistan on the health of New Jersey Army National Guard troops: implications for military readiness. *Am J Public Health*. 2010;100(2):276–283.

18. Shen YC, Arkes J, Kwan BW, Tan LY, Williams TV. Effects of Iraq/Afghanistan deployments on PTSD diagnoses for still active personnel in all four services. *Mil Med*. 2010;175(10):763–769.

19. *International Classification of Diseases. Ninth Revision*. Geneva, Switzerland: World Health Organization; 1994.

20. StataCorp. *Stata Statistical Software: Release 11*. College Station, TX: StataCorp LP; 2009.

21. US Army. Mental Health Advisory Team (MHAT) 6: Operation Enduring Freedom 2009 Afghanistan. 2009. Available at: http://www.armymedicine.army.mil/reports/ mhat/mhat_vi/MHAT_VI-OEF_Redacted.pdf. Accessed August 11, 2011.

22. US Army. Mental Health Advisory Team (MHAT) VI: Operation Iraqi Freedom 07-09. 2009. Available at: http://www.armymedicine.army.mil/reports/mhat/mhat_vi/ MHAT_VI-OIF_Redacted.pdf. Accessed August 11, 2011.

23. MacGregor AJ, Shaffer RA, Dougherty AL, et al. Psychological correlates of battle and nonbattle injury among Operation Iraqi Freedom veterans. *Mil Med.* 2009;174(3):224–231.

24. Ebmeier KP, Donaghey C, Steele JD. Recent developments and current controversies in depression. *Lancet.* 2006;367(9505):153–167.

25. Angst J, Gamma A, Gastpar M, et al. Gender differences in depression. Epidemiological findings from the European DEPRES I and II studies. *Eur Arch Psychiatry Clin Neurosci.* 2002;252(5):201–209.

26. Stoudemire A, Frank R, Hedemark N, Kamlet M, Blazer D. The economic burden of depression. *Gen Hosp Psychiatry.* 1986;8(6):387–394.

27. Greenberg PE, Kessler RC, Birnbaum HG, et al. The economic burden of depression in the United States: how did it change between 1990 and 2000? *J Clin Psychiatry.* 2003;64(12):1465–1475.

25

Patterns of Treatment Utilization Before Suicide Among Male Veterans With Substance Use Disorders

Mark A. Ilgen, PhD, Kenneth R. Conner, PsyD, Kathryn M. Roeder, BA, Frederic C. Blow, PhD, Karen Austin, MPH, and Marcia Valenstein, MD

Objectives. We sought to describe the extent and nature of contact with the health care system before suicide among veterans with substance use disorders (SUDs).

Methods. We examined all male Veterans Health Administration patients who died by suicide between October 1, 1999, and September 30, 2007, and who had a documented SUD diagnosis during the 2 years before death (n = 3132).

Results. Over half (55.5%; n = 1740) of the male patients were seen during the month before suicide, and 25.4% (n = 796) were seen during the week before suicide. In examining those with a medical visit in the year before suicide (n = 2964), most of the last visits before suicide (56.6%; n = 1679) were in a general medical setting, 32.8% (n = 973) were in a specialty mental health setting, and 10.5% (n = 312) were in SUD treatment.

Conclusions. Men with SUDs who died from suicide were frequently seen in the month before their death. Most were last seen in general medical settings, although a substantial minority of those with SUDs was seen in specialty mental health settings.

Suicide represents a major public health concern.[1] Over 30 000 suicides occur in the United States each year, and suicide is a leading cause of death and years of potential life lost among Americans aged 18 to 65 years.[2] Individuals with substance use disorders (SUDs) are at high risk for suicidal behaviors, including suicide attempts and fatal suicides.[3–5] For example, survey data indicate that the risk of lifetime suicide attempt is nearly 6 times greater among individuals with SUDs than among the general population.[4] Data from SUD treatment settings also indicate that individuals treated for cocaine dependence,[6] opiate dependence,[7] and various other SUDs[8-10] have high lifetime prevalence rates of suicide attempts. Data on suicide mortality show similar results, including cohort studies showing that individuals treated for alcohol, opiate, intravenous drug, and stimulant use disorders are at high risk for eventual suicide[5] and controlled postmortem studies showing that alcohol and other SUDs confer risk for suicide.[11] Moreover, alcohol use disorders are the second most prevalent disorders among suicide decedents, following only mood disorders.[12]

Existing evidence indicates that between 24% and 69% of suicide decedents contact a health care professional during the month before suicide, with 23% to 47% having a health care contact in the week before suicide.[13-19] However, relatively little is known about how individuals with SUDs interact with the health care system before suicide. Understanding which SUD patients may be at heightened risk for suicide, as well as treatment patterns before suicide, is essential to develop effective interventions to prevent suicide among this large at-risk population.

The goals of this study were 2-fold. First, we aimed to describe the demographic and clinical characteristics of male patients with SUDs who died by suicide, as well as the nature of their contacts with the health care system during the year before suicide. The decision was made to focus on male patients because of concerns about low numbers of female patients utilizing Veterans Health Administration (VHA) services. Second, we examined the factors associated with the setting of care on the last visit before suicide. Such information was needed to aid in the development of more precise risk models for suicide among male patients with SUDs and to identify promising service contact points for suicide prevention interventions.

METHODS

Study data were obtained from the Veterans Affairs (VA) National Patient Care Database (NPCD) and the National Death Index (NDI). Study methods were approved by the Ann Arbor VA's institutional review board.

Sample

As outlined previously,[20] we comprehensively identified all VHA patients who died by suicide from October 1, 1999, to September 30, 2007 (fiscal years [FYs]

2000–2007; N = 16 892). To identify VA patients who died by suicide from FY 2000–FY 2007, we first identified all individuals who used VA services based on treatment records in the NPCD during this period. We then examined whether these individuals had any record of contact with a VHA treatment provider in FY 2008 or FY 2009 and, thus, were known to be alive through the end of the observation period (end of FY 2007). For these individuals, no NDI searches were conducted. NDI searches conducted for the remaining individuals with no VA utilization in FY 2008 or FY 2009 revealed 16 892 suicides from FY 2000 to FY 2007. Among this sample, we identified individuals who had at least 1 SUD diagnosis documented in electronic medical records by a VA clinician during the 2 years before death. A total of 3227 patients with previous SUDs (according to the previously described criteria) were alive at the beginning of FY 2000 (October 1, 1999) and died by suicide by the end of FY 2007 (September 30, 2007). This sample of 3227 patients represents 18.5% of all VHA suicides. Over 97% (n = 3132) of these suicides occurred among men, and the remaining analyses focused on these 3132 male suicide decedents with a SUD diagnosis in the 2 years before death.

Measures

Cause of death.
The NDI is considered the "gold standard" for mortality assessment information.[21] The NDI includes national data regarding dates and causes of death for all US residents, derived from death certificates filed in state vital statistics offices. The NDI data request included Social Security Number, last name, first name, middle initial, date of birth, race/ethnicity, gender, and state of residence. Frequently, NDI searches yield multiple records that are potential matches. Established procedures described by Sohn et al.[22] were used to identify "true matches" from the set of available matches. Using NDI data, we identified dates and causes of death. Suicide deaths were identified using the *International Classification of Diseases-10* (*ICD-10*) codes X60–X84 and Y87.0.[23]

Demographic information.
Demographic information available for each patient included age in years (categorized into 18–44 years old, 45–64 years old, and ≥ 65 years old), and race (categorized into White, Black, unknown or other, and missing). Reliable

data on other demographic characteristics (e.g., employment, salary) were not available in the present sample.

Substance use disorder and other psychiatric diagnoses.

SUD and mental disorder diagnoses were based on *International Classification of Diseases, Ninth Revision, Clinical Modification* (*ICD-9-CM*) diagnostic codes,[24] reflecting clinical diagnoses made by VA treatment providers during their clinical encounters. The current VA clinical records system uses *ICD-9-CM*.

Specific SUDs examined were any diagnoses of intoxication, withdrawal, abuse, or dependence involving alcohol, cocaine, cannabis, opiates, amphetamines, barbiturates, or multiple substances, or other. The multiple substances or other category included individuals with an *ICD-9* clinical diagnosis of "polysubstance abuse" or "polysubstance dependence" as well as individuals with a rarer SUD diagnosis (e.g., inhalant abuse). Participants could be diagnosed with multiple SUDs. Presence or absence of the following psychiatric diagnoses during the 2 years before suicide was also examined: major depression, schizophrenia, bipolar disorder I or II, posttraumatic stress disorder (PTSD), other anxiety disorder, and any personality disorder. An indicator was also created for each patient to reflect the presence of 2 or more nonsubstance use related mental health conditions.

Treatment utilization.

Information in the NPCD was examined to generate indicators of care within the 12 months before suicide. The following indicators were utilized to reflect care received within 7, 30, and 90 days, and within the year before death: any SUD treatment, any mental health treatment, and any other medical treatment. Most of the visits in the "other medical treatment" category were outpatient medical care visits in the following settings: primary care (21.8%), admission or screening (13.6%), and telephone triage (4.4%). Overall, 20.3% of visits occurred with a prescribing provider, 14.2% occurred in an emergency room, 13.3% were telephone visits, and 1.1% were psychotherapy visits. Additionally, the specific setting of care of the last visit was examined and categorized into the following 3 mutually exclusive categories: SUD, mental health, or other medical. If a participant received more than 1 type of care on the last visit, the setting of care of the last visit was coded using the following hierarchy: (1) inpatient or outpatient SUD; (2) inpatient or outpatient mental health; and (3) inpatient or outpatient general medical treatment. Additionally, we developed a measure of number of days between last treatment contact and suicide.

Analyses

Descriptive statistics of the sample were completed using frequencies or means, as appropriate. Bivariate analyses were completed examining the patient characteristics associated with receiving care on the last visit in different settings (i.e., SUD, mental health, or other medical treatment). Finally, a multivariate multinomial logistic regression analysis[25] was completed, which examined the adjusted association between patient characteristics and likelihood of completing their last visit before suicide death in SUD or mental health treatment relative to other medical treatment on the last visit before suicide.

RESULTS

The previously mentioned methods identified 3132 suicides among male VA patients from FY 2000–FY 2007 who had at least 1 SUD diagnosis during the 2 years before death. As described in Table 1, this sample was 6.2% Black (n = 193) and 75.8% White (n = 2394). Alcohol use disorders were the most common type of SUD, affecting 83.4% of the sample (n = 2611), with other or polysubstance abuse being the second most common SUD (31.9%; n = 999). Psychiatric comorbidity was prevalent, and the most common psychiatric condition in suicide decedents with SUDs was depression (31.9%; n = 1000). Moreover, almost half (48.1%; n = 1507) of suicide decedents with SUDs were diagnosed with 2 or more psychiatric problems in the 2 years before death.

Timing and Type of Treatment Before Suicide

Data on treatment contacts before suicide are presented in Table 2. The majority of the total sample (94.6%; n = 2964) had some contact with the VHA during the year preceding suicide. Over half (55.5%; n = 1740) were seen at a VA facility during the month before death, and 25.4% (n = 796) were seen during the week before suicide. In the year before suicide, 32.8% (n = 1026) of the sample was seen in SUD treatment, 69% (n = 2163) in mental health treatment, and 89.4% (n = 2800) in other medical treatment settings.

Table 1. Sample Characteristics of Male Veterans With Substance Use Disorders Who Died by Suicide: Fiscal Years 2000–2007

Characteristic	Total (n = 3132), No. (%)
Race	
White	2374 (75.8)
Black	193 (6.2)
Other	35 (1.1)
Missing	530 (16.9)
Age, y	
18–44	1108 (35.4)
45–64	1723 (55.0)
≥ 65	247 (7.9)
Missing	54 (1.7)
Psychiatric conditions	
Major depression	1000 (31.9)
Other anxiety disorder	858 (27.4)
PTSD	721 (23.0)
Bipolar disorder	582 (18.6)
Personality disorder	472 (15.1)
Schizophrenia	403 (12.9)
≥ 2 Psychiatric conditions	1507 (48.1)
Substance abuse	
Alcohol	2611 (83.4)
Cocaine	512 (16.4)
Cannabis	478 (15.3)
Opiate	426 (13.6)
Barbiturate	191 (6.1)
Amphetamine	150 (4.8)
Other or polysubstance	999 (31.9)

Note. PTSD = posttraumatic stress disorder.
Suicides occurred from fiscal years 2000 to fiscal year 2007 among men with at least 1 substance use disorder diagnosis 2 years before date of death.

Data from male patients who had some contact with the VHA during the year before suicide (n = 2964) were used in subsequent analyses of treatment patterns. For these analyses, treatment received on the last visit before suicide was classified into 3 groups: (1) SUD treatment (10.5%; n = 312); (2) mental health treatment (32.8%; n = 973); or (3) any other medical contact (56.6%; n = 1679). Bivariate analyses revealed significant differences among these 3 groups (Table 3). Fewer Black patients received mental health treatment, and

Table 2. Recent Treatment Before Suicide Among Male Veterans: Fiscal Year 2000-2007

	Total (n = 3132), No.(%)
Overall: any treatment or contact	
7 d prior	796 (25.4)
30 d prior	1740 (55.6)
90 d prior	2378 (75.9)
1 y prior	2964 (94.6)
Categories of treatment: any substance abuse treatment	
7 d prior	125 (4.0)
30 d prior	318 (10.2)
90 d prior	533 (17.0)
1 y prior	1026 (32.8)
Any mental health treatment	
7 d prior	382 (12.2)
30 d prior	930 (29.7)
90 d prior	1461 (46.7)
1 y prior	2163 (69.1)
Any other medical contact	
7 d prior	480 (15.3)
30 d prior	1337 (42.7)
90 d prior	2057 (65.7)
1 y prior	2800 (89.4)

older patients were significantly more likely to receive other medical treatment on their last VA visit before suicide. As expected, patients with psychiatric diagnoses were significantly more likely to receive mental health treatment at their last visit. Major depression diagnosis (43.4%) and having 2 or more psychiatric diagnoses (68.1%) were most highly related to treatment in a mental health setting. Last visits among patients with alcohol, cocaine, opiate, amphetamines, or other or polysubstance use disorders were significantly more likely to be in a SUD setting, although patients with alcohol use disorders were also seen quite frequently in mental health and other medical settings.

Adjusted Models of Factors Associated With Treatment Setting Before Suicide

A series of multivariable analyses were conducted to examine the relative impact of predictors of setting for a patient's last visit before suicide (Table 4).

Table 3. Patient Characteristics and Treatment Received on Last Visit Before Suicide Among Male Veterans: Fiscal Year 2000–2007

Characteristic or Treatment Received	Total Sample[a] (n = 2964; 100%), %	SUD (n = 312; 10.5%), %	Mental Health (n = 973; 32.8%), %	Other Medical Contact (n = 1679; 56.6%), %	χ^2	P
Race						
White	76.5	74.0	79.5	75.2	7.4	.025
Black	6.1	3.9	6.2	6.5	3.2	.199
Other	1.2	1.0	1.1	1.3	0.2	.896
Missing	16.3	21.2	13.3	17.1	12.8	.017
Age, y						
18–44	35.3	43.5	42.2	29.7	51.8	< .001
45–64	56.5	53.5	54.7	58.2	4.3	.114
≥ 65	8.2	3.0	3.1	12.1	77.7	< .001
Psychiatric conditions						
Major depression	32.8	33.7	43.4	26.6	79.0	< .001
Other anxiety disorder	28.3	23.1	34.6	25.6	29.4	< .001
PTSD	23.9	21.5	30.9	20.3	39.8	< .001
Bipolar disorder	19.2	15.4	29.6	13.9	101.4	< .001
Personality disorder	15.4	11.9	23.5	11.3	77.4	< .001
Schizophrenia	13.1	5.8	24.5	7.9	165.6	< .001
≥ 2 Psychiatric conditions	49.5	42.3	68.1	40.0	202.8	< .001
Substance abuse						
Alcohol	83.4	89.1	79.1	84.8	22.3	< .001
Cocaine	16.3	27.2	18.9	12.8	47.2	< .001
Cannabis	15.4	19.2	19.7	12.2	31.2	< .001
Opiate	13.9	21.2	12.7	13.3	15.3	.005
Barbiturate	6.3	5.1	8.7	5.1	14.9	.006
Amphetamine	4.8	7.7	6.4	3.3	19.7	< .001
Other or polysubstance	32.3	43.3	33.4	29.5	23.6	< .001

Note: PTSD = posttraumatic stress disorder; SUD = substance use disorder.
Patients receiving treatment in year before suicide.

Table 4. Predictors of Type of Treatment Received at Last Visit Before Suicide, Adjusting for Race, Age, and Psychiatric and Substance Use Disorders Among Male Veterans: Fiscal Year 2000-2007

	SUD (n = 301), OR (95% CI)	Mental Health (n = 966), OR (95% CI)
Race		
Black (vs White)	0.42* (0.22, 0.79)	0.71 (0.49, 1.03)
Other (vs White)	0.80 (0.23, 2.73)	0.91 (0.41, 2.01)
Missing (vs White)	1.39 (0.99, 1.95)	1.11 (0.86, 1.43)
Age, y		
18-44 (vs ≥ 65)	4.40** (2.16, 8.94)	3.88** (2.54, 5.94)
45-64 (vs ≥ 65)	3.19 (1.59, 6.39)	2.81** (1.86, 4.25)
Psychiatric conditions		
Major depression	1.32 (0.99, 1.76)	1.48** (1.22, 1.79)
Other anxiety disorder	0.77 (0.54, 1.11)	0.97 (0.78, 1.21)
PTSD	0.98 (0.67, 1.41)	1.22 (0.98, 1.53)
Bipolar disorder***	0.95 (0.64, 1.40)	1.48* (1.18, 1.86)
Schizophrenia[†]	0.64 (0.37, 1.09)	2.57** (1.99, 3.32)
Personality disorder***	0.74 (0.48, 1.13)	1.24 (0.97, 1.58)
≥ 2 Psychiatric conditions***	1.04 (0.68, 1.59)	1.80** (1.38, 2.35)
Substance abuse		
Alcohol[†]	1.79* (1.19, 2.70)	0.69* (0.55, 0.86)
Cocaine***	2.05** (1.45, 2.88)	1.22 (0.94, 1.57)
Cannabis	1.10 (0.77, 1.58)	1.04 (0.82, 1.33)
Opiate***	1.35 (0.95, 1.92)	0.68* (0.52, 0.89)
Barbiturate***	0.76 (0.42, 1.38)	1.39 (0.98, 1.98)
Amphetamine	1.45 (0.85, 2.49)	1.26 (0.84, 1.89)
Other or polysubstance[†]	1.52* (1.14, 2.03)	0.70* (0.57, 0.85)

Note. CI = confidence interval; OR = odds ratio; PTSD = posttramautic stress disorder; SUD = substance use disorder. Observations used: n = 2910. Reference category is patients with "other medical contact" on last visit before suicide (n = 1643).
*P < .05 and **P < .001, for association with either SUD or mental health treatment; ***P < .05 and [†]P < .001, for significant difference between SUD and mental health treatment.

In these analyses, Black male veterans with SUDs who died from suicide were less likely to be seen in SUD treatment settings than mental health or general medical settings. Older veterans were far less likely to be seen in SUD treatment than in mental health or general medical settings. Most of the psychiatric conditions (i.e., depression, bipolar disorder, schizophrenia, personality disorder, and multiple psychiatric conditions) were associated with an increased likelihood of being treated in specialty mental health treatment before suicide, relative to other medical settings. Alcohol, cocaine, and other or polysubstance use disorders were associated with a greater likelihood of receiving care in SUD treatment as the last setting of care before suicide. Additionally, alcohol, opiate, and other or polysubstance use disorders were associated with lower likelihood of receiving care in mental health treatment as the last setting of care before suicide compared with other medical settings.

DISCUSSION

Our findings on service utilization before suicide confirmed as well as extended previous work on health service use before suicide.[13-18] We confirmed that male patients with SUDs who died from suicide often had contact with VHA providers before their deaths. Approximately 26% of male VHA patients with SUDs who died by suicide made contact with a VHA treatment provider within 1 week and 56% within 1 month of suicide. We extended previous work by examining the types of treatment settings in which patients with SUD diagnoses were last seen. We found that the majority of these contacts were within medical settings, although both specialty mental health and SUD treatment programs had contact with a sizable portion of SUD patients on the last visit before suicide. Consistent with the symptom profile of patients, those men with more severe psychopathology were more likely to be seen last in specialty mental health care settings, whereas those diagnosed with alcohol, cocaine, and polysubstance use disorders were more likely to be seen last in SUD treatment settings.

The large number of suicides in male veterans with SUDs was consistent with previous research.[26] This previous research found that the risk of suicide associated with a SUD was lower than that for bipolar disorder or depression, but higher than that for schizophrenia, PTSD, and other anxiety disorders. The present data showed that SUD patients at risk for suicide received care in a variety of treatment settings and not solely specialty SUD treatment. A lower percentage of male VHA patients with a SUD diagnosis were seen in specialty SUD treatment than either mental health or general medical treatment. The results of the adjusted and unadjusted analyses indicated that specific patient factors were associated with the setting of last care before suicide. Thus, future research on suicide prevention is needed in both specialty SUD treatment as well as other VHA treatment settings, for example, research on the impact of suicide screening and targeted intervention efforts on rates of suicidal behavior in SUD patients in different treatment venues.

These results must be viewed in light of the study's limitations. Classification of cause of death was based on data from the NDI. Although the NDI is widely regarded as the best national-level source of mortality data,[21] misclassification of cause of death could have influenced the present results. In addition, the sample consisted solely of patients receiving treatment services from the VHA, and the results of this study might not be generalizable to other patient populations. Moreover, all diagnoses were made during visits with VHA treatment providers (some of whom did not have a mental health background) and could be expected to differ from results that would be obtained with structured diagnostic research interviews. Further, the way that the sample was constructed might have increased the estimated rates of treatment utilization in those with SUDs before suicide; specifically, because a diagnosis of a SUD from a VHA treatment provider in the 2 years before suicide was required for inclusion in the sample, individuals within the sample were, by definition, in some form of contact with the VHA system in the 2 years before death. Our sample was also large and represented approximately 19% of all VA suicides during the observation period. Findings based on this large sample are likely to be important for understanding the role of the treatment system in suicides of VHA patients with SUDs. It is also important to note that the analyses did not allow for the examination of the extent to which specific treatment settings might have reduced or increased suicide risk. Instead, the analyses were intended to help identify settings in which veterans received care before suicide to inform future research efforts.

To our knowledge, ours is the first study to describe the nature and setting of care provided to men with SUDs before suicide within an integrated health care setting. Most of these patients were in general contact with the health care system in the period before death, which could provide the potential for future evaluations of suicide risk detection and intervention strategies based in specialty SUD treatment as well as other mental health treatment and medical care settings. A high proportion of male VA SUD patients were seen within a month before suicide in a wide range of treatment settings, suggesting the value of conducting risk reduction research and evaluation across a broad spectrum of care.

ABOUT THE AUTHORS

Mark A. Ilgen, Frederic C. Blow, and Marcia Valenstein are with the Serious Mental Illness Treatment Research and Evaluation Center (SMITREC), Department of Veterans Affairs, Ann Arbor, MI, and the Department of Psychiatry, University of Michigan, Ann Arbor. Kenneth R. Conner is with the Canandaigua VA Center of Excellence, Canandaigua, NY, and the Department of Psychiatry, University of Rochester School of Medicine, Rochester, NY. Kathryn M. Roeder is with the Department of Psychiatry, University of Michigan, Ann Arbor. Karen Austin is with SMITREC, Department of Veterans Affairs, Ann Arbor.

CONTRIBUTORS

M.A. Ilgen, K.M., Roeder, F.C. Blow, M. Valenstein, and K.R. Conner designed the study and wrote the article. K. Austin conducted all of the study analyses. All of the authors take responsibility for the final article.

ACKNOWLEDGMENTS

This work was supported with pilot project funding from the Canandaigua VA Center of Excellence (XVA 41-043).

Note. The views expressed in this report are those of the authors, and do not necessarily represent those of the Canandaigua VA Center of Excellence.

HUMAN PARTICIPANT PROTECTION

Study methods were approved by the Ann Arbor VA's institutional review board.

REFERENCES

1. Office of the Surgeon General. *The Surgeon General's Call to Action to Prevent Suicide.* Washington, DC: Department of Health and Human Services, US Public Health Service; 1999.

2. Centers for Disease Control and Prevention. Web-based Injury Statistics Query and Reporting System: Leading Causes of Death Reports. Available at: http://www.cdc.gov/injury/wisqars/index.html. Accessed March 1, 2010.

3. Borges G, Walters EE, Kessler RC. Associations of substance use, abuse and dependence with subsequent suicidal behavior. *Am J Epidemiol.* 2000;151(8):781–789.

4. Kessler RC, Borges G, Walters EE. Prevalence of and risk factors for lifetime suicide attempts in the national comorbidity survey. *Arch Gen Psychiatry.* 1999;56(7):617–626.

5. Wilcox HC, Conner KR, Caine ED. Association of alcohol and drug use disorders and completed suicide: an empirical review of cohort studies. *Drug Alcohol Depend.* 2004;76(Suppl):S11–S19.

6. Roy A. Childhood trauma and suicidal behavior in male cocaine dependent patients. *Suicide Life Threat Behav.* 2001;31(2):194–196.

7. Darke S, Ross J, Lynskey M, Teesson M. Attempted suicide among entrants to three treatment modalities for heroin dependence in the Australian Treatment Outcome Study (ATOS): prevalence and risk factors. *Drug Alcohol Depend.* 2004;73(1):1–10.

8. Ilgen MA, Jain A, Lucas E, Moos R. Substance use-disorder treatment and a decline in attempted suicide during and after treatment. *J Stud Alcohol Drugs.* 2007;68(4):503–509.

9. Conner KR, Swogger MT, Houston RJ. A test of the reactive aggression-suicidal behavior hypothesis: is there a case for proactive aggression? *J Abnorm Psychol.* 2009;118(1):235–240.

10. Wines JD Jr, Saitz R, Horton NJ, Lloyd-Travaglini C, Samet JH. Suicidal behavior, drug use and depressive symptoms after detoxification: a 2-year prospective study. *Drug Alcohol Depend.* 2004;76(Suppl):S21–29.

11. Yoshimasu K, Kiyohara C, Miyashita K. Suicidal risk factors and completed suicide: meta-analyses based on psychological autopsy studies. *Environ Health Prev Med.* 2008;13(5):243–256.

12. Cavanagh JT, Carson AJ, Sharpe M, Lawrie SM. Psychological autopsy studies of suicide: a systematic review. *Psychol Med.* 2003;33(3):395–405.

13. Barraclough B, Bunch J, Nelson B, Sainsbury P. A hundred cases of suicide: clinical aspects. *Br J Psychiatry.* 1974;125(0):355–373.

14. Cheng AT. Mental illness and suicide. A case-control study in east Taiwan. *Arch Gen Psychiatry.* 1995;52(7):594–603.

15. Robins E, Murphy G, Wilkinson RH Jr, Gassner S, Kayes J. Some clinical considerations in the prevention of suicide based on a study of 134 successful suicides. *Am J Public Health Nations Health.* 1959;49(7):888–899.

16. Seager CP, Flood RA. Suicide in Bristol. *Br J Psychiatry.* 1965;111(479):919–932.

17. Squires TJ, Busuttil A. Elderly suicides in the Lothian and borders region of Scotland, 1983–1988. *Med Sci Law.* 1991;31(2):137–146.

18. Andersen UA, Andersen M, Rosholm JU, Gram LF. Contacts to the health care system prior to suicide: a comprehensive analysis using registers for general and psychiatric hospital admissions, contacts to general practitioners and practising specialists and drug prescriptions. *Acta Psychiatr Scand.* 2000;102(2):126–134.

19. Smith EG, Craig TJ, Ganoczy D, Walters H, Valenstein M. Treatment of veterans with depression who die from suicide: timing and quality of care at last VHA visit. *J Clin Psychiatry.* 2011;72(5)622–629.

20. McCarthy JF, Valenstein M, Kim HM, Ilgen M, Zivin K, Blow FC. Suicide mortality among patients receiving care in the Veterans Health Administration health system. *Am J Epidemiol.* 2009;169(8):1033–1038.

21. Cowper DC, Kubal JD, Maynard C, Hynes DM. A primer and comparative review of major US mortality databases. *Ann Epidemiol.* 2002;12(7):462–468.

22. Sohn MW, Arnold N, Maynard C, Hynes DM. Accuracy and completeness of mortality data in the Department of Veterans Affairs. *Popul Health Metr.* 2006;4:2.

23. World Health Organization. *International Statistical Classification of Diseases and Related Health Problems, 10th Revision (ICD-10).* 2nd ed. Geneva, Switzerland: World Health Organization; 2004.

24. US Department of Health and Human Services. *ICD-9-CM. The International Classification of Diseases, 9th Revision, Clinical Modification.* Washington, DC: US Government Printing Office; 1980.

25. Böhning D. Multinomial logistic regression algorithm. *Ann Inst Stat Math.* 1992;44(1):197–200.

26. Ilgen MA, Bohnert ASBB, Ignacio RV, McCarthy JF, Valenstein MM, Kim HM, et al. Psychiatric diagnoses and risk of suicide in patients treated by the Department of Veterans Affairs. *Arch Gen Psychiatry.* 2010;67(11):1152–1158.

Sleep Disturbance Preceding Suicide Among Veterans

Wilfred R. Pigeon, PhD, Peter C. Britton, PhD, Mark A. Ilgen, PhD, Ben Chapman, PhD, and Kenneth R. Conner, PsyD, MPH

Objectives. We examined the role of sleep disturbance in time to suicide since the last treatment visit among veterans receiving Veterans Health Administration (VHA) services.

Methods. Among 423 veteran suicide decedents from 2 geographic areas, systematic chart reviews were conducted on the 381 (90.1%) who had a VHA visit in the last year of life. Veteran suicides with a documented sleep disturbance (45.4%) were compared with those without sleep disturbance (54.6%) on time to death since their last VHA visit using an accelerated failure time model.

Results. Veterans with sleep disturbance died sooner after their last visit than did those without sleep disturbance, after we adjusted for the presence of mental health or substance use symptoms, age, and region.

Conclusions. Findings indicated that sleep disturbance was associated with time to suicide in this sample of veterans who died by suicide. The findings had implications for using the presence of sleep disturbance to detect near-term risk for suicide and suggested that sleep disturbance might provide an important intervention target for a subgroup of at-risk veterans.

Sleep disturbance is prevalent in and strongly associated with a variety of psychiatric and medical conditions.[1,2] Several reviews[3–5] and commentaries[6–8] have highlighted associations of sleep disturbance and suicidal thoughts and behaviors. Insomnia (difficulty initiating or maintaining sleep) and nightmares are the sleep disturbances most commonly associated with suicidal thoughts and behaviors, although some work suggests that sleep disordered breathing and periodic limb movement disorder may also pose risks.[9]

Until recent years, empirical data were almost entirely based on studies of suicidal ideation and nonlethal suicide attempts, with unclear generalization to suicide deaths (hereafter referred to as "suicide"). There is, however, small but growing empirical literature linking sleep disturbance and suicide from cohort studies and investigations using postmortem case–control designs. A Finnish national cohort study of 21 to 64 year-old adults was linked with Finland's National Death Registry to analyze the association of nightmares and suicide over a mean follow-up of approximately 14 years.[10] In adjusted models, the relative risk (RR) for suicide was 1.57 (95% confidence interval [CI] = 1.12, 2.19) for occasional nightmares and 2.05 (95% CI = 1.06, 3.97) for frequent nightmares compared with the no nightmares referent group. Adjusted analyses were not conducted. In Japan, a community cohort of adults aged 30 to 79 years were surveyed, with a mean follow-up of approximately 7 years.[11] Difficulty maintaining sleep was associated with suicide with an age-adjusted RR of 2.4 (95% CI = 1.3, 4.3) and a fully adjusted RR of 2.1 (95% CI = 1.1, 3.9). A 10-year, multisite, observational cohort of older adults (age ⩾ 65 years) in the United States was used to compare suicides to control participants drawn from the larger sample.[12] Higher sleep quality scores were found to be protective from suicide with an odds ratio (OR) of 0.72 (95% CI = 0.58, 0.87). A Canadian postmortem case–control investigation compared adults who killed themselves during an episode of major depressive disorder to living patients of comparable age and gender with major depressive disorders.[13] In unadjusted models, insomnia symptoms were associated with suicide (OR 2.37; 95% CI = 1.21, 4.66), and this remained a significant finding after adjusting for the presence of other psychopathologies (OR 1.78; 95% CI = 1.22, 2.58). In a US case–control study of adolescent suicide,[14] hypersomnia and insomnia distinguished suicides from control participants in unadjusted analyses. In adjusted analyses, insomnia in the past week was associated with suicide at a statistically significant level (OR 5.3; 95% CI = 1.4, 20.4). Although samples, methods, and types of sleep disturbance varied across these studies, the findings consistently indicated an association of sleep disturbances to suicide.

We are aware of no other published empirical studies of sleep disturbance and suicide in a veteran population. VHA is the largest integrated health care system in the United States. Veterans who receive VHA care are at increased risk for suicide compared with the US general population.[15] More than 1800 VHA users die by suicide each year, representing at least 5% of suicides in the United States annually. Accordingly, suicide prevention among veterans is both a national and VHA priority.[16] Sleep disturbances are prevalent in military returnees from Iraq and Afghanistan with posttraumatic stress disorder[17] or with mild traumatic brain injury.[18] Moreover, VHA users have high rates of sleep disturbance overall,[19] compelling the study of sleep disturbance and suicide in this population.

The purpose of our study was to examine sleep disturbance and suicide in a sample of veterans who used Veterans Health Administration (VHA) services and died by suicide. More specifically, we focused on the impact of sleep disturbance on time to death among veteran suicide decedents by comparing a subgroup of suicide decedents with sleep disturbance to a subgroup without sleep problems. Another analysis of this sample showed that mental disorders predicted time to suicide,[20] informing our approach to examine sleep disturbance in time to death in the present study.

METHODS

We collected data from all 423 veterans who died by suicide between fiscal years 2000 and 2006 and who received VHA services in Veterans Integrated Service Network 2 (VISN 2), which is located in upstate New York and north central Pennsylvania (n = 130), or from VISN 11 (n = 293), which is located in central Illinois, Indiana, Michigan, and northwest Ohio. Of these 423 veteran suicide decedents, 381 (90.8%) received VHA services during their last year of life. All had complete data on the variables included in the final analysis, although 2 participants were missing data for race/ethnicity.

Procedure

Data for the study were obtained in a 2-step process. First, identification of veterans was carried out by the VISN 11 Serious Mental Illness Training, Research, and Education Center, which created a National Suicide Registry by linking data from the VHA National Patient Care Database and the National Center for Health Statistic's (NCHS) National Death Index (NDI). The NDI is considered the "gold standard" for mortality assessment information because data are derived from death certificates filed in state vital statistics offices and checked for accuracy by NCHS.[21] The registry contains information on all patients identified from the NPCD who used VHA services in fiscal years 2000 to 2007, did not have any record of VHA service use in fiscal year 2008 or 2009, and were subsequently identified to have died by suicide by cross-matching to the NDI using social security number, last name, first name, middle initial, date of birth, race/ethnicity, gender, and state of residence. Previously established procedures were used to identify "true" matches.[22] Data for the present study were drawn from this registry for veterans receiving care from VHA in VISN 2 or VSIN 11 from 2000 to 2006.

The second step in obtaining data used the VHA Computerized Patient Record System (CPRS), which contains demographic information and all clinical notes about care provided within the VHA system. Notes can be written in free form or using templates and typically include information about the patient's presenting problem and the type of care provided. CPRS data provide information about symptoms, stressors, and disorders that may or may not be tied to specific visit encounters or treatment plans.

Chart reviews of CPRS records of each of the identified suicide decedents were conducted at the Center of Excellence for Suicide Prevention located at the VA Medical Center in Canandaigua, New York. When demographic data were not available in the expected CPRS data fields (e.g., race/ethnicity), the record was searched for references to such data. A chart review tool developed for a previous study of veterans treated for depression[23] was used to systematically assess and extract data on documented symptoms of depression, anxiety, alcohol use disorders, illicit drug use, prescription drug misuse, mania, schizophrenia, and sleep disturbance symptoms in the year before suicide. Symptoms were recorded whether they reached a diagnostic threshold or not, necessitating the use of chart reviews (as opposed to relying merely on aggregate electronic data). Inter-rater agreement on reported variables ranged from substantial to outstanding and are provided in the following; readers may reference Britton et al.[20] on this issue for agreement on additional variables not reported here.

For each patient record, we used 2 or more independent coders who, after initial coding, met to compare results and resolve discrepancies to create a consensus record for use in analyses. When a clear consensus could not be reached, the coding decisions were staffed at a weekly consensus conference. Percentage agreement was calculated to assess the inter-rater reliability between independent raters.

Measures

Number of days between last visit and death.
The primary outcome for the study was date of the last visit in CPRS, and date of death from the NDI was used to calculate days between last visit and death, which served as the primary outcome variable.

Sleep disturbance.
Chart reviews identified information on documented sleep complaints. The sleep item assessed the presence of sleep problems in patients' charts. Coders were instructed to code sleep symptoms if any of a wide variety of sleep problems was noted, including trouble falling asleep, staying asleep, sleeping too much, as well as waking up too early. Patients were also identified as having sleep problems if sleep aids were prescribed or if a sleep diagnosis was documented. In assessments based on sleep medications alone, an inclusive approach was used for the "last year," whereby sleep symptoms were documented if sleep aids were prescribed at any time during the year. For the last visit codes, a more conservative approach was taken. Namely, when use of prescription sleep medications was accompanied by a notation that the patient was sleeping well or sleep was improved, these were coded as having no sleep symptoms at the last visit. Average percentage agreement between raters for sleep disturbance was 89.3% for last year codes and 86.2% for last visit codes.

Psychiatric symptoms.
Chart reviews assessed documented symptoms whether they reached a diagnostic threshold (e.g., depressive symptoms) as well as diagnoses (e.g., depressive disorder), referred to from here forward simply as symptoms. Average percentage agreement between pairs of raters on symptoms was as follows: depression (95.0% last year, 84.7% last visit), mania (93.7% last year, 96.4% last visit), anxiety (90.5% last year, 89.9% last visit), psychotic symptoms (94.3% last year, 93.4% last visit), alcohol use disorder (87.2% last year, 85.3% last visit), illicit drug use (91.0% last year, 91.6% last visit), and misuse of prescription drugs (85.8% last year, 92.4% last visit). Results of the chart review were dichotomized to create 2 categories, individuals with and without symptoms of mental disorders, which included substance use.

Data Analysis

The comparison of interest was between suicide decedents with sleep disturbance in the year preceding death and those without sleep disturbance. Unadjusted comparisons between these groups were made using the χ^2 test. For comparisons with sample sizes less than 5, we used the Fisher exact 2-sided test.

To identify variables that would be entered into the multivariate analysis, we conducted univariate Cox proportional hazard regression models. Variables that were statistically associated with time to death ($P < .05$) were entered into the multivariate model. Backward elimination was used to trim the model because it avoided the potential biases of forward selection procedures.[24,25]

Variables that were statistically associated with time to death ($P < .05$) were kept in the model. Diagnostics revealed that sleep problems violated the proportional hazards assumption of the Cox model. Although treating sleep as a time-varying covariate was an option, we decided to use an accelerated failure time (AFT) model because such models make no proportionality assumption and they model the survival time rather than hazard rate, allowing estimation of the actual time after contact to suicide rather than the chance of instantaneous failure over the follow-up.[26] In a cohort where all persons died and the probability of death was 1, the time to event might provide a more informative outcome than would the instantaneous probability of death. To fit the AFT data with a survival distribution most appropriate to the data, we compared several different distributions with the Akaike Information Criterion statistic,[27] which identified the log-normal AFT model to be a better fit than the log-logistic, Weibull, and Gompertz models.[28] We reran all univariate and multivariate analyses using the log-normal AFT model and only reported these results. As is the practice in reporting results from AFT models, we reported survival time as time ratios with 95% CIs, where values less than 1 represented a decrease in survival time (and values greater than 1 represented a prolonged survival time).[26] Median time to event for the referent group (those without sleep disturbance) was calculated from the reverse log of the model intercept coefficient (i.e., exp[coefficient]); median time to event for the sleep disturbance group was exp(intercept coefficient minus absolute value of sleep coefficient). All analyses were conducted with STATA 10 (Stata Corporation: College Station, Texas).

RESULTS

Of the 381 suicide decedents analyzed, 173 (45.4%) had clinician-documented sleep disturbance, and 208 (54.6%) had no recorded sleep problems. Age, gender, minority status, and the presence of psychiatric or substance abuse symptoms were associated with sleep problems (Table 1), whereas no such associations were present for VISN or region.

In univariate log-normal AFT analyses, sleep problems, psychiatric or substance abuse symptoms, gender, and VISN or region had significant associations with time to death. Accordingly, these 5 variables were entered into the multivariate analysis (Table 2). Following backward elimination, gender and age did not contribute to the model and were removed. The final

Table 1. Demographics of Veterans Health Administration Suicide Decedents With and Without Sleep Disturbance: VISN 2 and VISN 11, Fiscal Year 2000–2006

Variables	With Sleep Disturbance, No. (%)	Without Sleep Disturbance, No. (%)	χ^2	P
Gender			6.06	.03[a]
Male	164 (94.8)	206 (99.0)		
Female	9 (5.2)	2 (1.0)		
Race/ethnicity			5.66	.02
White	150 (86.7)	159 (76.4)		
Minority	23 (13.3)	47 (22.6)		
Age, y			25.87	< .001[a]
18–34	3 (1.7)	8 (3.8)		
35–54	45 (26.0)	26 (12.5)		
55–74	88 (50.9)	85 (40.9)		
≥ 75	37 (21.4)	89 (42.8)		
Region			0.45	.5
VISN 2	51 (29.5)	68 (32.7)		
VISN 11	122 (70.5)	140 (67.3)		
Diagnosis[b]			72.69	< .001
Yes	157 (90.8)	104 (50.0)		
No	16 (9.2)	104 (50.0)		

Note. VISN = Veterans Integrated Service Network. For veterans with a sleep disturbance, the sample size was n = 173 (45.4%); for veterans without sleep disturbance, the sample size was n = 208 (54.6%).
[a]Calculated via the Fisher exact test.
[b]Diagnosis was the presence of psychiatric or substance abuse symptoms or diagnosis.

Table 2. Survival Time Ratios for the Log-normal Accelerate Failure Time (AFT) Model for Veteran Suicides With and Without Sleep Disturbance: VISN 2 and VISN 11, Fiscal Year 2000–2006

Variable	Univariate Analyses		Multivariate Analysis	
	Coefficient	Survival Time Ratio (95% CI)	Coefficient	Survival Time Ratio (95% CI)
Sleep	−1.01	0.36 (0.28, 0.47)	−0.84	0.43 (0.33, 0.56)
Diagnosis	−0.92	0.40 (0.30, 0.52)	−0.62	0.54 (0.40, 0.71)
Age Group	−0.05	0.95 (0.80, 1.13)	...	...
Gender	0.89	2.45 (1.10, 5.42)	...	...
White	−0.30	0.74 (0.52, 1.04)	...	...
VISN 2	−0.44	0.64 (0.48, 0.86)	−0.45	0.64 (0.49, 0.82)
Constant	...[a]	...	5.16	...

Note. CI = confidence interval; VISN = Veterans Integrated Service Network.
[a]The intercept varied depending on the univariate model.

model for time to death included sleep disturbance, psychiatric or substance abuse symptoms, and VISN or region. Sleep disturbance predicted a 57% loss in survival time after control for the presence of psychiatric or substance abuse symptoms and region (Table 2). Specifically, the average veteran without sleep problems died 174 days after their last contact with VHA (exp[5.16]), whereas the average veteran with sleep problems died 75 days after their last contact (exp[5.16–0.84]). A survival curve was plotted to illustrate the survival rates for both groups over the follow-up period (Figure 1).

DISCUSSION

In this article, we examined the contribution of sleep disturbance to time to death after the last visit in a sample of veterans in VHA care that died by suicide. The group with recorded sleep disturbance died more quickly after their last visit, after control for the presence of age, region, and symptoms of several mental disorders that conferred risk for suicide, including substance use disorders. The central finding that sleep disturbance predicted shorter time to suicide among suicide decedents provided important information on clinician-observed risk factors for imminent suicide risk and had implications for suicide prevention and treatment efforts.

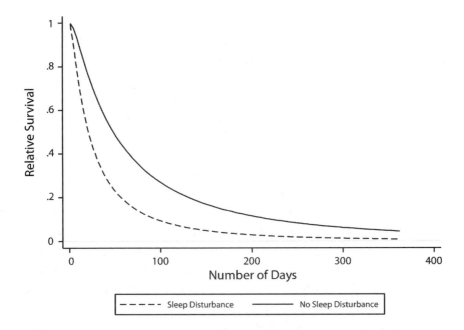

Figure 1. Survival time preceding suicide among veterans with and without sleep disturbance: VISN 2 and VISN 11, Fiscal Year 2000–2006.

Note. VISN = Veterans Integrated Service Network. The dashed line is sleep disturbance in the year preceding death; the solid line represents no sleep disturbance in the year preceding death.

Although numerous studies examined the heterogeneity among suicide decedents by comparing subgroups of suicides,[29–31] this might be the first such undertaking to compare suicide decedents on the basis of sleep disturbance. Given the considerable heterogeneity among individuals who died by suicide,[29,30] including among veterans,[31] it was suggested that prevention and treatment efforts be tailored to distinct subgroups of vulnerable patients who might require different prevention and intervention strategies.[32] Veterans receiving VHA services who present with sleep disturbance, particularly in the face of other suicide risk factors, might represent one such subgroup.

Limitations of the study included data derived from chart reviews, and although coding between raters was done reliably, information about the reliability, validity, or completeness of the information contained in the charts was not available, and it was not possible in this study to control for charting practices of providers. Although a strength of the study was the ability to control for a number of factors, some conditions such as traumatic brain injury and a number of specific mental disorders were not available for analyses. In addition, generalizability to VHA patients in other regions of the country who were not sampled was unclear, as was generalizability to non-VHA samples. The study also did not distinguish among types of sleep disturbance. Finally, unlike studies that assessed sleep disturbance as a risk factor for suicide using a nonsuicide comparison group, in our study, all veterans died by suicide, ruling out inferences about sleep disturbance as a causal risk factor for suicide.

To our knowledge, the present analysis was the first to examine the heterogeneity among suicide decedents using sleep disturbance as the probe and adds to the small but growing literature on sleep disturbance and suicide. Looking forward, there are several reasons to accelerate research on sleep disturbance and suicide. First, because sleep disturbances may also precede depression,[33] such disturbances provide an opportunity to begin monitoring early in the development of a recognized risk for suicide. Second, we believe that veterans generally may be more ready to acknowledge sleep disturbances before reporting psychiatric symptoms such as depression or anxiety, although this idea requires empirical study. Third, the strong association between sleep disturbance and time to suicide also indicates a potential entrée for novel preventive interventions. Efficacious and evidence-based approaches for major sleep disorders are available[34] and appear to have an impact on reducing psychiatric symptoms that are associated with suicide (e.g., depression and anxiety)[35-38]; therefore, the mechanisms of action may work through multiple pathways. Research is therefore needed to test the potential of sleep interventions as viable standalone or adjuvant suicide prevention interventions.

ABOUT THE AUTHORS

Wilfred R. Pigeon is with VISN 2 Center of Excellence for Suicide Prevention, Canandaigua Veteran Affairs Medical Center, Canandaigua, NY, Center for Integrated Healthcare, Syracuse Veteran Affairs Medical Center, Syracuse, NY, and the Department of PsychiatrySleep and Neurophysiology Research Laboratory, University of Rochester School of Medicine and Dentistry, Rochester, NY. Peter C. Britton and Kenneth R. Conner are with the VISN 2

Center of Excellence for Suicide Prevention, Canandaigua Veteran Affairs Medical Center, Canandaigua, and the Department of Psychiatry, University of Rochester School of Medicine and Dentistry, NY. Ben Chapman is with at the Department of Psychiatry, University of Rochester School of Medicine and Dentistry, Rochester, NY. Mark A. Ilgen with the VISN 11 Serious Mental Illness Treatment Resource and Evaluation Center (SMITREC), Department of Veteran Affairs Medical Center, Ann Arbor, MI, and the Department of Psychiatry, University of Michigan Medical School, Ann Arbor.

CONTRIBUTORS

P. C. Britton, M. A.Ilgen, and K. R. Conner designed the original study from which the present study was derived. W. R. Pigeon, P. C. Britton, and K. R. Conner designed the present study. P. C. Britton conducted the analysis in consultation with B. Chapman. W. R. Pigeon took the lead in writing. All of the authors contributed to the writing and review of the article.

ACKNOWLEDGMENTS

This study was funded by the Department of Veterans Affairs (VA), VISN 2 Center of Excellence for Suicide Prevention.

The authors would like to thank Heather Walters for training the coders, Liam Cerveny, Suzanne Dougherty, Sharon Fell, Elizabeth Schifano, and Patrick Walsh for conducting the chart reviews, and Brady Stephens for creating and managing the database.

Note. VA had no role in study design; in the collection, analysis and interpretation of data; in the writing of the article; or in the decision to submit the article for publication.

HUMAN PARTICIPANT PROTECTION

The study protocol was approved by the Syracuse VA Medical Center Institutional Review Board.

REFERENCES

1. Pigeon WR. Insomnia as a risk factor for disease. In: Buysee DJ, Sateia MJ, eds. *Insomnia: Diagnosis and Treatment.* New York: Informa Healthcare; 2010: 31–41.

2. Taylor DJ, Mallory LJ, Lichstein KL, Durrence HH, Riedel BW, Bush AJ. Comorbidity of chronic insomnia with medical problems. *Sleep*. 2007;30:213–218.

3. Liu X, Buysse DJ. Sleep and youth suicidal behavior: a neglected field. *Curr Opin Psychiatry*. 2006;19:288–293.

4. Singareddy RK, Balon R. Sleep and suicide in psychiatric patients. *Ann Clin Psychiatry*. 2001;13:93–101.

5. Bernert RA, Joiner TE. Sleep disturbances and suicide risk: a review of the literature. *Neuropsychiatr Dis Treat*. 2007;3:735–743.

6. Agargun MY, Besiroglu L. Sleep and suicidality: do sleep disturbances predict suicide risk? *Sleep*. 2005;28:1039–1040.

7. Kohyama J. More sleep will bring more serotonin and less suicide in Japan. *Med Hypotheses*. 2010;75(3):340.

8. Pigeon WR, Caine ED. Insomnia and the risk for suicide: does sleep medicine have interventions that can make a difference? *Sleep Med*. 2010;11:816–817.

9. Krakow B, Artar A, Warner TD, et al. Sleep disorder, depression, and suicidality in female sexual assault survivors. *Crisis*. 2000;21:163–170.

10. Tanskanen A, Tuomilehto J, Viinamaki H, Vartiainen E, Lehtonen J, Puska P. Nightmares as predictors of suicide. *Sleep*. 2001;24:844–847.

11. Fujino Y, Mizoue T, Tokui N, Yoshimura T. Prospective cohort study of stress, life satisfaction, self-rated health, insomnia, and suicide death in Japan. *Suicide Life Threat Behav*. 2005;35:227–237.

12. Turvey CL, Conwell Y, Jones MP, et al. Risk factors for late-life suicide: a prospective, community-based study. *Am J Geriatr Psychiatry*. 2002;10:398–406.

13. McGirr A, Renaud J, Seguin M, et al. An examination of DSM-IV depressive symptoms and risk for suicide completion in major depressive disorder: a psychological autopsy study. *J Affect Disord*. 2007;97:203–209.

14. Goldstein TR, Bridge JA, Brent DA. Sleep disturbance preceding completed suicide in adolescents. *J Consult Clin Psychol*. 2008;76:84–91.

15. McCarthy JF, Valenstein M, Kim HM, Ilgen M, Zivin K, Blow FC. Suicide mortality among patients receiving care in the Veterans Health Administration Health System. *Am J Epidemiol.* 2009;169:1033–1038.

16. Blue Ribbon Report Group. *Report of the blue ribbon work group on suicide prevention in the Veteran population.* 2008. Available at: http://www.mentalhealth.va.gov/suicide_prevention/Blue_Ribbon_Report-FINAL_June-30-08.pdf. Accessed May 6, 2011

17. Friedman MJ. Posttraumatic stress disorder among military returnees from Afghanistan and Iraq. *Am J Psychiatry.* 2006;163:586–593.

18. Hoge CW, McGurk D, Thomas JL, Cox AL, Engel CC, Castro CA. Mild traumatic brain injury in US soldiers returning from Iraq. *N Engl J Med.* 2008;358:453–463.

19. Mustafa M, Erokwu N, Ebose I, Strohl K. Sleep problems and the risk for sleep disorders in an outpatient veteran population. *Sleep Breath.* 2005;9:57–63.

20. Britton PC, Ilgen MA, Valenstein M, Knox K, Claassen CA, Conner KR. Differences between veteran suicides with and without psychiatric symptoms. *Am J Public Health.* 2012;102(Suppl 1):S125–S130.

21. Cowper DC, Kubal JD, Maynard C, Hynes DM. A primer and comparative review of major US mortality databases. *Ann Epidemiol.* 2002;12:462–468.

22. Sohn MW, Arnold N, Maynard C, Hynes DM. Accuracy and completeness of mortality data in the Department of Veterans Affairs. *Popul Health Metr.* 2006;4:2.

23. Valenstein M, Kim HM, Ganoczy D, et al. Higher-risk periods for suicide among VA patients receiving depression treatment: prioritizing suicide prevention efforts. *J Affect Disord.* 2009;112:50–58.

24. Hosmer DW, Lemeshow S. *Applied Logistic Regression.* New York: Wiley; 1989.

25. Sauerbrei W, Royston P, Binder H. Selection of important variables and determination of functional from for continuous predictors in multivariate model building. *Stat Med.* 2007;26:5512–5528.

26. Wei LJ. The accelerated failure time model: a useful alternative to the Cox regression model in survival anlysis. *Stat Med.* 1992;11:1871–1879.

27. Burnham KP, Anderson DR. *Model Selection and Inference: A Practical Information-Theoretical Approach.* New York: Springer-Verlag; 2002.

28. Cleves MA, Gould WW. *An Introduction to Survival Analysis Using Stata.* 2nd ed. College Station, TX: Stata Press; 2008.

29. Conwell Y, Duberstein PR, Cox C, Herrmann JH, Forbes NT, Caine ED. Relationships of age and axis I diagnoses in victims of completed suicide: a psychological autopsy study. *Am J Psychiatry.* 1996;153:1001–1008.

30. Rich CL, Fowler RC, Fogarty LA, Young D. San Diego suicide study. 3. Relationships between diagnoses and stressors. *Arch Gen Psychiatry.* 1988;45:589–592.

31. Ilgen MA, Conner KR, Valenstein M, Austin K, Blow FC. Violent and nonviolent suicide in veterans with substance-use disorders. *J Stud Alcohol Drugs.* 2010;71:473–479.

32. Kaplan KJ, Harrow M. Psychosis and functioning as risk factors for later suicidal activity among schizophrenia and schizoaffective patients: a disease-based interactive model. *Suicide Life Threat Behav.* 1999;29:10–24.

33. Baglioni C, Battagliese G, Feige B, et al. Insomnia as a predictor of depression: a meta-analytic evaluation of longitudinal epidemiological studies. *J Affect Disord.* 2011;135:10–19.

34. Pigeon WR, Crabtree VM, Scherer MR. The future of behavioral sleep medicine. *J Clin Sleep Med.* 2007;3:73–79.

35. Fava M, McCall WV, Krystal A, et al. Eszopiclone co-administered with fluoxetine in patients with insomnia coexisting with major depressive disorder. *Biol Psychiatry.* 2006;59:1052–1060.

36. Manber R, Edinger JD, Gress JL, Pedro-Salcedo MGSS, Kuo TF, Kalista T. Cognitive behavioral therapy for insomnia enhances depression outcome in patients with comorbid major depressive disorder and insomnia. *Sleep.* 2008;31:489–495.

37. Raskind MA, Peskind ER, Hoff DJ, et al. A parallel group placebo controlled study of prazosin for trauma nightmares and sleep disturbance in combat veterans with post-traumatic stress disorder. *Biol Psychiatry.* 2007;61:928–934.

38. Ulmer C, Bosworth H, Edinger J, Calhoun P, Almirall D. A brief intervention for sleep disturbance in PTSD: pilot study findings. *J Gen Intern Med.* 2010;25:206.

27

Suicide Mortality Among Patients Treated by the Veterans Health Administration From 2000 to 2007

Frederic C. Blow, PhD, Amy S. B. Bohnert, PhD, Mark A. Ilgen, PhD, Rosalinda Ignacio, MS, John F. McCarthy, PhD, Marcia M. Valenstein, MD, and Kerry L. Knox, PhD

Objectives. We sought to examine rates of suicide among individuals receiving health care services in Veterans Health Administration (VHA) facilities over an 8-year period.

Methods. We included annual cohorts of all individuals who received VHA health care services from fiscal year (FY) 2000 through FY 2007 (October 1, 1999–September 30, 2007; N = 8 855 655). Vital status and cause of death were obtained from the National Death Index.

Results. Suicide was more common among VHA patients than members of the general US population. The overall rates of suicide among VHA patients decreased slightly but significantly from 2000 to 2007 ($P < .001$). Male veterans between the ages of 30 and 64 years were at the highest risk of suicide.

Conclusions. VHA health care system patients are at elevated risk for suicide and are appropriate for suicide reduction services, although the rate of suicide has decreased in recent years for this group. Comprehensive approaches to suicide prevention in the VHA focus not only on recent returnees from Iraq and Afghanistan but also on middle-aged and older Veterans.

Reducing suicide within the United States is a national priority.[1,2] Over 30 000 individuals in the US die by suicide every year, with an annual age-adjusted rate of approximately 11 suicides per 100 000 persons.[3] Recent public and policy attention has focused on suicide among veterans generally and among individuals receiving services from the Veterans Health Administration

(VHA). VHA patients are more likely to have characteristics related to higher risk of suicide, including older age, male gender, and substantial medical and psychiatric morbidities.[4,5] Recent studies provide inconsistent information regarding the relative risk of suicide in veterans. Kaplan et al.[6] found that male veterans who responded to the US National Health Interview Survey were twice as likely to report a suicide attempt as nonveteran males. Additionally, McCarthy et al.[7] found that, compared with rates for the general US population, suicide rates of VHA users in 2000 to 2001 were 1.66 times higher in men and 1.87 times higher in women. By contrast, other studies of specific cohorts of Veterans have failed to find that the risk of suicide is substantially higher than that found in the general population, except within specific high-risk subgroups (e.g. veterans with a mental disorder).[8-14] Similarly, a recent large-scale study of older men found that Veteran status did not significantly increase suicide risk.[15]

Research regarding changes over time in suicidal behaviors is also limited. Kessler et al.[16] found that rates of nonfatal suicide attempts did not change over nearly 2 decades. In the general US population, suicide rates increased 2%–3% from 1999 through 2005.[17] However, changes in suicidal behaviors observed in the general population may not apply to Veterans generally and to high-risk individuals receiving VHA services in particular, who may be more accessible for suicide prevention efforts.

Monitoring suicide rates among Veterans is also important because of concerns regarding the impact of the conflicts in Iraq (Operation Iraqi Freedom [OIF]) and Afghanistan (Operation Enduring Freedom [OEF]). OEF/OIF Veterans have elevated rates of psychiatric and substance use disorders,[18-21] and Congress has mandated implementation of a comprehensive VHA suicide prevention program, which began in 2007.[22] However, a 2008 report observed that suicide rates among OEF/OIF Veterans were not greater than those among the general population.[13] Better data are needed to examine whether suicide rates among VHA patients have changed since the start of the wars in Iraq and Afghanistan, as well as to assess the general stability of rates among patients receiving health care in the VHA, which is the largest integrated health system in the United States. Data on trends in suicide rates among VHA patients also would provide a baseline for assessing the potential impact of initiatives designed to reduce suicide risk.

Our study documents potential changes in the rates of suicide among all male and female users of VHA services between fiscal years (FYs) 2000 and 2007. Yearly rates of suicide in Veterans seeking treatment at the VHA were also compared with rates of suicide within the general US population over this time period, both overall and within demographic subgroups defined by age and gender. Based on prior research of Veterans receiving VHA services,[7] we hypothesized that the rate of suicide would be elevated among VHA patients compared with the general population.

METHODS

For our study, we included all patients who utilized VHA services between Fiscal Years 2000 and 2007 (FY00 and FY07). Fiscal years begin on October 1st of the prior calendar year and continue through September 30th of the calendar year (e.g., FY00 includes October 1, 1999 to September 30, 2000). A total of 8 855 655 individuals received inpatient or outpatient VHA services between FY00 and FY07. Of those, 101 959 individuals (1.2%) were excluded because of invalid or missing data or non-US residences. The Veterans Affairs (VA) Ann Arbor institutional review board approved this project. Annual demographic information on the VHA user population is available in Appendix 1 (available as a supplement to the online version of this article at http:www.ajph.org).

Data Sources

Data came from the VA's National Patient Care Database (NPCD) and the Centers for Disease Control and Prevention's (CDC's) National Death Index (NDI). NPCD records all VHA inpatient or outpatient visits. NDI data identified vital status and cause of death and were acquired for VA program planning. NDI searches were conducted for all individuals with VHA use between FY00 and FY07 and who did not receive VHA services during FY08, thereby obviating costly searches for individuals whose VHA use post-FY07 indicated survival through the end of FY07. The NDI compiles death records from state vital statistics offices, and it has the greatest sensitivity in determining vital status among population-level sources.[23] Established procedures identified "true" matches when the search resulted in multiple potential matches.[24]

The CDC's Web-based Injury Statistics Query and Reporting System (WISQARS)[25] was used to compare VHA suicide rates to those of the general population. WISQARS provides suicide rates by age and gender in the US population.

Measures

Age categories included those aged 18 to 29 years, 30 to 64 years, and 65 years and older; these were chosen to represent young, middle, and older adulthood, respectively, and because suicide rates are relatively stable within each of these groups. Because information regarding race/ethnicity was not consistently available in the NPCD, race/ethnicity was not included in analyses. Suicide deaths were identified using *International Classification of Diseases, Tenth Revision,* codes X60–X84, Y87.0, and U03.[26]

For each annual cohort, patients were included if they received VHA services in either that year or the prior fiscal year and were alive at the start of that year. For example, an individual who used VHA services in FY00 and survived all of FY01 contributed one year of risk time for suicide in FY01. If an individual did not use VHA services in FY00 but did in FY01 and was alive at the end of FY01, the individual was considered to have entered the cohort of VHA patients half way through the year (on average) and contributed half of a person-year toward the suicide rate for FY01. If an individual met criteria to be defined as part of the cohort of VHA patients for a given fiscal year as already defined died in that fiscal year from any cause, their contribution toward the person-years calculation for that fiscal year was also half a year.

Analyses

We calculated annual rates of suicide by dividing the number of suicides observed in each fiscal year by the person-years accrued during that period, multiplied by 100 000. We calculated confidence intervals with the Poisson method for all rates.[27]

To compare VHA rates to those of the general population, we calculated Standardized Mortality Ratios (SMRs) for age and gender subgroups for each year, using the WISQARS data as the reference group.[28] Data from WISQARS were categorized by calendar year and rates of suicide for the VHA are organized by fiscal year. Although this was not an exact temporal match, SMRs were calculated for time periods with a 9-month overlap for each 12-month period. We used indirect standardization[29] which uses age-specific mortality rates from the standard US population to derive expected deaths in the VA user population. We calculated 95% confidence intervals for the SMRs using an exact method based on the Poisson distribution,[27] and the rate among the VHA population was considered significantly higher than that among the general population when the confidence interval did not include zero. We further tested changes over time in the rate of suicide between FY00 and FY07 by creating Poisson regression models. Poisson regression is a generalized linear modeling technique based on the Poisson distribution and provides standardized parameter estimates (B) that represent the estimated difference in the log of expected counts, holding other variables constant. The procedure models the count of suicides given the total population at risk, with a separate observation for each year.

RESULTS

From FY00 to FY07, annual VHA rates of suicide mortality ranged from 34.3 to 39.8 suicides per 100 000 person-years (Figure 1a). Figure 1b and 1c displays the age-stratified rates of suicide for male and female VHA users. Among male VHA users, the annual rates of suicide ranged from 36.4 to 43.1 suicides per 100 000 person-years, while among female VHA users, the annual rates of suicide ranged from 9.8 to 13.7. The rate of suicide was lower among male VHA users aged 65 years and older than among male VHA users age 30–64; in all years, the lower limit of the confidence interval around the rate of suicide for male VHA users aged 30–64 years was greater than the upper limit of the confidence interval around the rate of suicide for male VHA users aged 65 years and older (Table 1).

Table 2 reports the SMRs for comparisons of suicide mortality among VHA users compared with the general US population, by age and gender subgroups. Over 8 years, SMRs for suicide for all VHA users ranged from 1.42 to 1.66 (Figure 2a). Each year, the lower limit of the 95% confidence interval exceeded 1.0, indicating excess suicide mortality. This was also observed for the SMRs for each age group (18–29 years, 30–64 years, and 65 years and older) when male and female VHA users were combined, except in FY01 among VHA users between the ages of 18 and 29. From FY00 to FY07, the SMRs for the

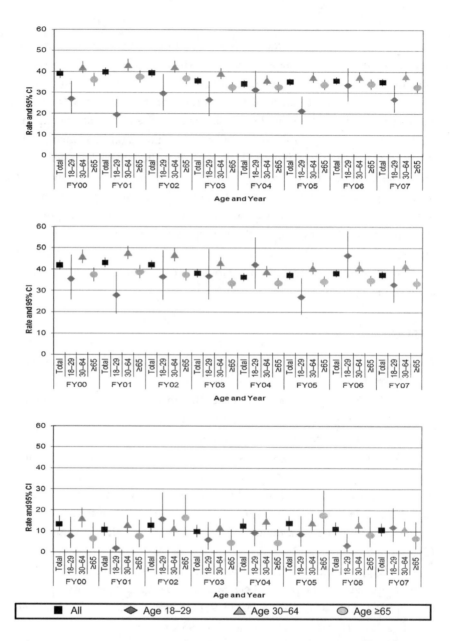

Figure 1. Rate per 100 000 person-years and 95% confidence intervals (CIs) of suicide by age and fiscal year (FY), among (a) all Veterans Health Administration (VHA) users, (b) male VHA users, and (c) female VHA users: FY2000–FY2007.

middle age group (30–64 years) were consistently higher than that for the oldest age group (65 years and older), and confidence intervals did not overlap. There was insufficient statistical power to compare the excess suicide mortality in the youngest age group with that in the other age groups.

Figures 2b and 2c present the total and age-group specific SMRs for men and women. Among male VHA users in the age groups of 30–64 years and 65 years and older, the SMR of suicide mortality was stable and significantly elevated over all years (ranges of 1.69–2.14 and 1.12–1.24, respectively). For male patients, excess suicide mortality was higher for middle age than for older groups, with nonoverlapping confidence intervals. For male VHA users aged 18–29 years, the range of SMRs from FY00 to FY07 was 1.38–2.35. The SMR for men aged 65 years and older was below that of men aged 18–29 years (with nonoverlapping 95% confidence intervals) for FY02, FY03, FY04, and FY06.

The suicide rate for VHA users decreased between FY00 and FY07, with a parameter estimate for each FY of -0.022 ($P < .001$, after control for age and gender). Examining confidence intervals for the annual rates in Table 1 indicates the rate of suicide decreased most notably around FY03. Gender- and age-stratified Poisson regression modeling indicated that the rate of suicide decreased for men aged 30–64 years (B $= -0.025$; $P < .001$) and men aged 65 years and older (B $= -0.020$,; $P = .007$).

Inspection of the annual rates and their confidence intervals in Figure 1b suggests the drop in the suicide rate was most pronounced around FY03 for men aged 30–64 years because the lower limit of the confidence intervals for FY01 and FY02 are greater than the upper limit of the confidence intervals for the rates of FY04 through FY07 in this age–gender group. The confidence intervals around the estimates of the rate of suicide for the smaller group of those aged 18–29 years were wide and overlapped for all years; no significant changes were found in rates of suicide in this group (B $= 0.015$; $P = .49$).

As demonstrated in Figure 1c, the rate of suicide for female VHA users was less stable over time than for male VHA users; confidence intervals were wide, particularly for women aged 18–29 years and aged 65 years and older. No significant time trends in the suicide rate were found among female VHA users; age–group stratified models resulted in standardized parameter estimates between -0.021 and 0.029 (all $P > .05$). Consequently, it cannot be concluded that the overall trends represent true changes in the rate of suicide for these groups.

Table 1. Number of Suicides and Suicide Rates per 100 000 Person-Years Among VHA Users, by Gender and Age: Fiscal Year (FY) 2000–FY2007

	FY2000		FY2001		FY2002		FY2003		FY2004		FY2005		FY2006		FY2007	
	Suicides, No.	Rate (95% CI)	Suicides, No	Rate (95% CI)	Suicides, No	Rate (95% CI)	Suicides, No	Rate (95% CI)	Suicides, No	Rate (95% CI)	Suicides, No	Rate (95% CI)	Suicides, No	Rate (95% CI)	Suicides, No	Rate (95% CI)
All VHA users																
Total	1453	39.0 (37.0, 41.0)	1609	39.8 (37.9, 41.8)	1741	39.4 (37.5, 41.2)	1694	35.7 (34.1, 37.5)	1692	34.3 (32.7, 36.0)	1785	35.2 (33.6, 36.9)	1855	35.8 (34.2, 37.5)	1841	35.1 (33.5, 36.8)
Age 18–29 y	47	27.0 (19.8, 35.3)	32	19.5 (13.4, 26.8)	46	29.7 (21.7, 38.9)	41	26.6 (19.1, 35.4)	52	31.4 (23.4, 40.4)	40	21.3 (15.2, 28.3)	71	33.6 (26.2, 41.8)	64	26.9 (20.7, 33.8)
Age 30–64 y	863	42.0 (39.2, 44.8)	925	43.2 (40.5, 46.0)	960	42.3 (39.7, 45.1)	943	39.2 (36.7, 41.7)	904	36.0 (33.7, 38.4)	969	37.4 (35.0, 39.7)	995	37.5 (35.2, 39.9)	1024	37.9 (35.6, 40.3)
Age ≥ 65 y	543	36.2 (33.2, 39.3)	652	37.6 (34.8, 40.6)	735	36.8 (34.2, 39.5)	710	32.6 (30.2, 35.0)	736	32.7 (30.4, 35.1)	776	33.9 (31.6, 36.4)	789	34.1 (31.7, 36.5)	753	32.7 (30.4, 35.1)
Male VHA users																
Total	1401	41.9 (39.8, 44.2)	1566	43.1 (41.0, 45.3)	1689	42.1 (40.1, 44.1)	1653	38.2 (36.4, 40.1)	1638	36.4 (34.7, 38.2)	1724	37.3 (35.5, 39.1)	1805	38.2 (36.5, 40.0)	1791	37.5 (35.8, 39.3)
Age 18–29 y	43	35.5 (25.7, 46.8)	31	27.9 (19.0, 38.6)	38	36.5 (25.9, 49.0)	38	36.8 (26.1, 49.5)	47	42.2 (31.0, 55.1)	35	27.1 (18.9, 36.0)	69	46.5 (36.2, 58.1)	56	32.9 (24.8, 42.0)
Age 30–64 y	819	46.0 (42.9, 49.2)	888	47.8 (44.7, 51.0)	927	46.9 (43.9, 50.0)	908	43.1 (40.3, 45.9)	858	39.0 (36.5, 41.7)	924	40.7 (38.1, 43.3)	952	41.0 (38.4, 43.6)	986	41.8 (39.2, 44.5)
Age ≥ 65 y	539	37.5 (34.4, 40.7)	647	38.8 (35.9, 41.9)	724	37.5 (34.8, 40.3)	707	33.5 (31.1, 36.0)	733	33.6 (31.2, 36.0)	765	34.4 (32.0, 36.9)	784	34.8 (32.4, 37.2)	749	33.4 (31.1, 35.9)
Female VHA users																
Total	52	13.3 (10.0, 17.2)	43	10.6 (7.7, 14.0)	52	12.7 (9.5, 16.4)	41	9.8 (7.1, 13.1)	54	12.5 (9.4, 16.0)	61	13.7 (10.5, 17.4)	50	11.0 (8.2, 14.3)	50	10.6 (7.9, 13.8)
Age 18–29 y	4	7.6 (2.1, 16.6)	1	1.9 (0.1, 7.0)	8	15.7 (6.8, 29.3)	3	5.9 (1.2, 14.3)	5	9.2 (3.0, 18.8)	5	8.5 (2.8, 17.4)	2	3.2 (0.4, 8.8)	8	11.8 (5.1, 21.2)
Age 30–64 y	44	16.1 (11.7, 21.1)	37	13.0 (9.2, 17.5)	33	11.3 (7.8, 15.5)	35	11.7 (8.2, 15.9)	46	14.8 (10.8, 19.3)	45	14.0 (10.2, 18.3)	43	13.0 (9.4, 17.2)	38	11.1 (7.9, 14.9)
Age ≥ 65 y	4	6.4 (1.7, 14.0)	5	7.5 (2.4, 15.3)	11	16.3 (8.1, 27.3)	3	4.5 (0.9, 10.8)	3	4.5 (0.9, 10.9)	11	17.6 (8.8, 29.5)	5	8.2 (2.7, 16.8)	4	6.6 (1.8, 14.5)

Note. VHA = Veterans Health Administration; CI = confidence interval.

Table 2. Standardized Mortality Ratio of Suicide Fatality (With 95% Confidence Intervals [CIs]), by Gender and Age Group: VHA Users, FY2000–FY2007

	FY2000, SMR (95% CI)	FY2001, SMR (95% CI)	FY2002, SMR (95% CI)	FY2003, SMR (95% CI)	FY2004, SMR (95% CI)	FY2005, SMR (95% CI)	FY2006, SMR (95% CI)	FY2007, SMR (95% CI)
All VHA users								
Total	1.66 (1.58, 1.75)	1.63 (1.55, 1.71)	1.56 (1.49, 1.63)	1.46 (1.39, 1.53)	1.42 (1.36, 1.49)	1.44 (1.38, 1.51)	1.49 (1.42, 1.55)	1.43 (1.37, 1.50)
Age 18–29 y	1.79 (1.32, 2.34)	1.32 (0.90, 1.82)	2.02 (1.48, 2.64)	1.87 (1.35, 2.49)	2.10 (1.57, 2.71)	1.46 (1.04, 1.94)	2.23 (1.74, 2.78)	1.74 (1.34, 2.19)
Age 30–64 y	2.16 (2.02, 2.31)	2.13 (1.99, 2.27)	2.02 (1.89, 2.15)	1.86 (1.74, 1.98)	1.71 (1.60, 1.82)	1.76 (1.65, 1.88)	1.74 (1.64, 1.85)	1.69 (1.59, 1.80)
Age ≥ 65 y	1.21 (1.11, 1.31)	1.24 (1.15, 1.34)	1.19 (1.11, 1.28)	1.12 (1.04, 1.21)	1.16 (1.07, 1.24)	1.18 (1.09, 1.26)	1.22 (1.14, 1.31)	1.17 (1.09, 1.26)
Male VHA users								
Total	1.64 (1.56, 1.73)	1.63 (1.55, 1.71)	1.55 (1.47, 1.62)	1.45 (1.38, 1.52)	1.41 (1.34, 1.48)	1.42 (1.36, 1.49)	1.48 (1.41, 1.55)	1.43 (1.36, 1.50)
Age 18–29 y	1.76 (1.28, 2.33)	1.38 (0.94, 1.91)	1.81 (1.28, 2.44)	1.89 (1.34, 2.54)	2.08 (1.53, 2.71)	1.39 (0.97, 1.89)	2.35 (1.83, 2.94)	1.65 (1.25, 2.11)
Age 30–64 y	2.14 (2.00, 2.29)	2.13 (1.99, 2.27)	2.03 (1.90, 2.16)	1.86 (1.74, 1.98)	1.69 (1.58, 1.81)	1.75 (1.64, 1.87)	1.74 (1.63, 1.85)	1.70 (1.60, 1.81)
Age ≥ 65 y	1.21 (1.11, 1.31)	1.24 (1.14, 1.33)	1.18 (1.09, 1.27)	1.12 (1.04, 1.21)	1.16 (1.07, 1.24)	1.16 (1.08, 1.25)	1.22 (1.14, 1.31)	1.17 (1.09, 1.26)
Female VHA users								
Total	2.50 (1.87, 3.22)	1.93 (1.40, 2.55)	2.22 (1.66, 2.86)	1.71 (1.23, 2.27)	2.02 (1.52, 2.59)	2.29 (1.75, 2.89)	1.76 (1.31, 2.28)	1.62 (1.20, 2.10)
Age 18–29 y	2.18 (0.59, 4.78)	0.55 (0.01, 2.05)	4.27 (1.84, 7.69)	1.66 (0.34, 3.99)	2.34 (0.76, 4.79)	2.16 (0.70, 4.43)	0.80 (0.10, 2.23)	2.87 (1.24, 5.17)
Age 30–64 y	2.67 (1.94, 3.52)	2.07 (1.46, 2.79)	1.75 (1.21, 2.40)	1.78 (1.24, 2.42)	2.08 (1.52, 2.72)	2.06 (1.50, 2.70)	1.83 (1.32, 2.42)	1.48 (1.05, 1.99)
Age ≥ 65 y	1.58 (0.43, 3.47)	1.93 (0.63, 3.95)	3.98 (1.99, 6.65)	1.18 (0.24, 2.85)	1.19 (0.25, 2.87)	4.41 (2.20, 7.37)	2.11 (0.69, 4.33)	1.71 (0.46, 3.74)

Note. VHA = Veterans Health Administration; CI = confidence interval; FY = fiscal year.

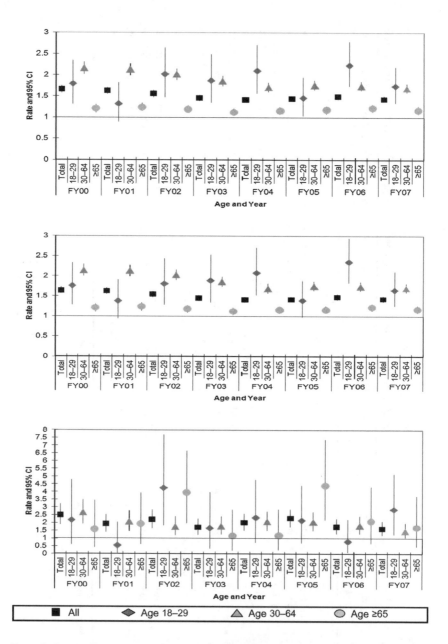

Figure 2. Standardized mortality ratios and 95% confidence intervals (CIs) of suicide, by age and fiscal year (FY), as compared with the general population among (a) all Veterans Health Administration (VHA) users, (b) male VHA users, and (c) female VHA users: FY2000–FY2007.

The estimated SMRs for males aged 30–64 years were consistently lower between FY04 to FY07 than for FY00 to FY02, with nonoverlapping confidence intervals. This shift suggests that suicide risk for male VHA users aged 30–64 years decreased relative to men of the same age in the general population around FY03. Age-stratified SMRs for suicide mortality among female VHA users had wide confidence intervals and did not indicate a consistent trend in suicide rates for female VHA users relative to females in the United States.

DISCUSSION

In each of the 8 years from 2000 to 2007, suicide was consistently more common among those who used VHA services than in the general US age- and gender-matched population. However, Poisson regression tests indicate that rates among VHA users decreased over time (B $= -0.022$; $P < .001$). Rates of suicide in the most recent years were significantly lower than those found in the earlier portion of the observation period, with the middle year of 2003 serving as a transition year. This shift in 2003 may signify an increased awareness and sensitivity to mental health issues in the VHA following the initiation of OIF, which began the same year; Seal et al.[30] found that rates of mental health diagnoses increased significantly after the start of OIF among first-time users of VHA services returning from Iraq and Afghanistan over a 2-year period. The reductions in suicide rates found in the present study appear to be largely driven by lower rates of suicide after 2004 among men aged 30–64 years, and, to a lesser degree, by men in the 65 years and older age group. Although suicide rates decreased over time among male veterans in the middle age group, their rates remained consistently higher than either older or younger veterans. These results differ from the typical pattern observed in the United States, in which rates of suicide are highest in older males.[3]

Examining suicide in veterans over the past several years is of particular importance because of the potential impact of the conflicts in Iraq and Afghanistan on suicide risk. These concerns are largely driven by recent findings documenting an elevated prevalence of suicide risk factors among individuals who served in Iraq or Afghanistan.[4,5] However, suicide has multiple causal pathways that are influenced by a variety of components, such as biological (e.g., gender), socioeconomic (e.g., employment status), and other factors (e.g., access to firearms) and confer increased risk of suicidal behaviors and suicide among specific cohorts.[2,15,16,31] Mental health problems associated with these recent conflicts may not directly lead to increased rates of suicide among VHA users. No increase in rates of suicide was observed since the start of the conflict in Afghanistan; in fact, we observed a statistically significant ($P < .001$) decrease in the suicide rate among VHA health system users between FY00 and FY07. These results are broadly consistent with a prior report noting no significant difference between rates of suicide in a smaller cohort of recent returnees from Iraq and Afghanistan and the general population.[13]

Our study evaluated rates in the entire population of VHA patients, which provided a greater precision to detect smaller differences than prior research on Veteran suicides. This is consistent with the fact that the SMRs calculated in the present study often fell within the 95% confidence intervals reported in many of the studies with null results.[8–15] Additionally, many prior reports on suicide rates among Veteran populations were limited by determining vital status from data from the Beneficiary Identification Records Locator Subsystem (BIRLS) and Social Security Administration (SSA) files[10,32] which have poorer sensitivity to detect vital status than does the NDI.[23]

These data are particularly important for any nationwide suicide prevention efforts. For example, between 2000 and 2007, the 13 626 suicides found among adults seen in the VHA represented 5.5% of the total 248 179 US adult suicides during this time period; while the VHA provides care for approximately 5 000 000 patients per year, representing approximately 2% of the US population. Our findings establish a baseline for examining the potential impact of comprehensive suicide-reduction strategies. Prior research in smaller European countries has examined changes in regional or even national suicide rates as a method for determining the impact of broad-based suicide-reduction programs.[33–35] By establishing clear data on the baseline rates of suicide among users of VHA system, more specific data are available on the potential impact of VHA suicide prevention efforts.

In our study, middle-aged men were at the highest risk for suicide. It is not known why these individuals were at elevated risk, but several potential explanations exist. Within the VHA system, these individuals represent Vietnam-era veterans who may be a cohort at higher risk for suicide caused by overall morbidity, or to ongoing social, economic or psychiatric difficulties.

Also, recent data indicates that suicide rates among middle-aged adults in the US have increased over the past 7 years.[17] It is possible that the factors leading to this broad increase in this age group are particularly difficult for Veterans. Additionally, our results support the focus of VHA's ongoing efforts at suicide prevention. Although it is clearly important to target recent returnees, VA's approach to suicide prevention among veterans also includes an emphasis on targeting veterans from past conflicts.[15]

An important limitation of our study is that we did not have reliable data on race across all years. Data on military duty characteristics and prior research indicates that National Guard veterans may have a particularly high rate of suicide.[36,37] Because there is a several year lag in the dissemination of US mortality data, the analyses we present do not include data from more recent years. The population is predominantly male and of middle age, thus estimates in other subgroups of individuals are less precise. Our study focused on examining SMRs in specific age and gender subgroups; however, we did not control for other differences in case mix. The methods for calculating risk in the present study are novel and it is possible that differing methods for calculating risk would have yielded other results. However, the results were consistent to ± 0.2 when compared with an a prior publication[7] that used an exact method to calculate rates for FY01. Additionally, the precision of the estimation of SMRs was diminished by the fact that the last 3 months of every calendar year were included in the subsequent fiscal year. However, the general lack of change in the rates of suicide in the United States increases the likelihood that this had minimal impact on the calculation of SMRs. The comparison group for calculating SMRs includes some veterans, likely diminishing the differences between groups used in our primary analyses. Finally, our sample was restricted to veterans utilizing VHA services, which represents approximately 20% of all veterans in the United States (≥ 5.5 million out of ≥ 24 million).[38]

Despite these limitations, to our knowledge this is the first comprehensive study of suicide mortality among patients receiving health care in a large national health care system. These findings indicate that there has been no increase in suicide rates among the VHA population of patients since the start of the conflicts in Iraq and Afghanistan; in fact, suicide rates among the VHA patient population have decreased since FY2000. However, VHA users are at increased risk for suicide compared with individuals the same age and gender in the general population. Comprehensive approaches to suicide prevention in the VHA should focus not only on recent returnees but also on middle-aged and older Veterans.

ABOUT THE AUTHORS

Frederic C. Blow, Amy S. B. Bohnert, Mark A. Ilgen, Rosalinda Ignacio, John F. McCarthy, and Marcia M. Valenstein are with the Department of Veterans Affairs, Serious Mental Illness Treatment Resource and Evaluation Center (SMITREC) and Health Services Research and Development Center of Excellence, Ann Arbor, MI, and the Department of Psychiatry, University of Michigan Medical School, Ann Arbor. Kerry L. Knox is with Department of Veterans Affairs, Center of Excellence for Suicide Prevention, Canandaigua, NY, and the Department of Psychiatry, University of Rochester Medical School, Rochester, NY.

CONTRIBUTORS

F. C. Blow led the project design and led the writing. F. C. Blow and J. F. McCarthy designed and oversaw data collection. R. Ignacio conducted data analysis with help from A. S. B. Bohnert. M. A. Ilgen, A. S. B. Bohnert, J. F. McCarthy, M. M. Valenstein, and K. L. Knox assisted in projected design. M. A. Ilgen and A. S. B. Bohnert aided in writing sections of the article, and all authors provided substantive feedback on drafts.

ACKNOWLEDGMENTS

This work was supported by the Department of Veterans Affairs, Veterans Health Administration, Office of Mental Health Services. Input from VA's Office of Mental Health Services shaped the design and conduct of the study, the collection, management, analysis, and interpretation of the data, and the preparation, review, and approval of the manuscript.

HUMAN PARTICIPATION STATEMENT

Approval was granted to this study by the Ann Arbor VA Human Subjects Committee.

REFERENCES

1. Office of the Surgeon General. *The Surgeon General's Call to Action to Prevent Suicide.* Washington, DC: Department of Health and Human Services, US Public Health Service, 1999.

2. Institute of Medicine. *Reducing Suicide: A National Imperative.* Washington, DC: National Academies Press; 2002.

3. Centers for Disease Control and Prevention. *Web-based Injury Statistics Query and Reporting System: Leading Causes of Death Reports.* Atlanta, GA: Centers for Disease Control and Prevention; 2008.

4. Agha Z, Lofgren RP, VanRuiswyk JV, Layde PM. Are patients at Veterans Affairs Medical Centers sicker? *Arch Intern Med.* 2000;160:3252–3257.

5. Lambert MT, Fowler DR. Suicide risk factors among veterans: risk management in the changing culture of the Department of Veterans Affairs. *J Ment Health Admin.* 1997;24:350–358.

6. Kaplan MS, Huguet N, McFarland BH, Newsom JT. Suicide among male veterans: a prospective population-based study. *J Epidemiol Community Health.* 2007;61:619–624.

7. McCarthy JF, Valenstein M, Kim HM, Ilgen M, Zivin K, Blow FC. Suicide mortality among patients receiving care in the Veterans Health Administration health system. *Am J Epidemiol.* 2009;169:1033–1038.

8. Boyle CA, Decoufle P. Postdischarge mortality from suicide and motor-vehicle injuries among Vietnam-era veterans. *N Engl J Med.* 1987;317:506–507.

9. Watanabe KK, Kang HK. Military service in Vietnam and the risk of death from trauma and selected cancers. *Ann Epidemiol.* 1995;5:407–412.

10. Bullman TA, Kang HK. The risk of suicide among wounded Vietnam veterans. *Am J Public Health.* 1996;86:662–667.

11. Cypel Y, Kang H. Mortality patterns among women Vietnam-era veterans: results of a retrospective cohort study. *Ann Epidemiol.* 2008;18:244–252.

12. Kang HK, Bullman TA. Mortality among US veterans of the Persian Gulf War. *N Engl J Med.* 1996;335:1498–1504.

13. Kang HK, Bullman TA. Risk of suicide among US veterans after returning from the Iraq or Afghanistan war zones. *JAMA*. 2008;300:652–653.

14. Thomas TL, Kang HK, Dalager NA. Mortality among women Vietnam veterans, 1973–1987. *Am J Epidemiol*. 1991;134:973–980.

15. Miller M, Barber C, Azrael D, Calle E, Lawler E, Mukamal K. Suicide among US veterans: a prospective study of 500,000 middle-aged and elderly men. *Am J Epidemiol*. 2009;170:494–500.

16. Kessler RC, Berglund P, Borges G, Nock M, Wang PS. Trends in suicide ideation, plans, gestures, and attempts in the United States, 1990–1992 to 2001–2003. *JAMA*. 2005;293:2487–2495.

17. Hu G, Wilcox HC, Wissow L, Baker SP. Mid-life suicide: an increasing problem in US Whites, 1999–2005. *Am J Prev Med*. 2008;35:589–593.

18. Hoge CW, Auchterlonie JL, Milliken CS. Mental health problems, use of mental health services, and attrition from military service after returning from deployment to Iraq or Afghanistan. *JAMA*. 2006;295:1023–1032.

19. Milliken CS, Auchterloni JL, Hoge CW. Longitudinal assessment of mental health problems among active and reserve component solidiers returning from the Iraq War. *JAMA*. 2007;298:2141–2148.

20. Seal KH, Bertenthal D, Miner CR, Sen S, Marmar C. Bringing the war back home: mental health disorders among 103 788 US veterans returning from Iraq and Afghanistan seen at Department of Veterans Affairs facilities. *Arch Intern Med*. 2007;167:476–482.

21. West AN, Weeks WB. Mental distress among younger veterans before, during, and after the invasion of Iraq. *Psychiatr Serv*. 2006;57:244–248.

22. *Joshua Omvig Veterans Suicide Prevention Act of 2007*, Pub. L. No. 110-110, 121 Stat. 1031.

23. Cowper DC, Kubal JD, Maynard C, Hynes DM. A primer and comparative review of major US mortality databases. *Ann Epidemiol*. 2002;12:462–468.

24. Sohn MW, Arnold N, Maynard C, Hynes DM. Accuracy and completeness of mortality data in the Department of Veterans Affairs. *Popul Health Metr*. 2006;4:2.

25. National Center for Injury Prevention and Control. Office of Statistics and Programming. WISQARS Fatal Injuries: Mortality Reports. Available at: http://www.cdc.gov/injury/wisqars/fatal.html. Accessed September 3, 2010.

26. World Health Organization. *International Statistical Classification of Diseases and Related Health Problems, 10th Revision.* Geneva, Switzerland: World Health Organization; 2004.

27. Ulm K. A simple method to calculate the confidence interval of a standardized mortality ratio (SMR). *Am J Epidemiol.* 1990;131:373–375.

28. Hennekens C. *Buring J. Epidemiology in Medicine.* Boston, MA: Little, Brown and Company; 1987.

29. Pagano M, Gauvreau K. *Principles of Biostatistics.* 2nd edition. Belmont, CA: Wadsworth Inc., 2000.

30. Seal KH, Metzler TJ, Gima KS, Bertenthal D, Maguen S, Marmar CR. Trends and risk factors for mental health diagnoses among Iraq and Afghanistan veterans using Department of Veterans Affairs health care, 2002–2008. *Am J Public Health.* 2009;99(9):1651–1658.

31. Kaplan MS, McFarland BH, Huguet N. Firearm suicide among veterans in the general population: findings from the national violent death reporting system. *J Trauma.* 2009;67:503–507.

32. Bullman TA, Kang HK. Posttraumatic stress disorder and the risk of traumatic deaths among Vietnam veterans. *J Nerv Ment Dis.* 1994;182:604–610.

33. Rihmer Z, Rutz W, Pihlgren H. Depression and suicide on Gotland. An intensive study of all suicides before and after a depression-training programme for general practitioners. *J Affect Disord.* 1995;35:147–152.

34. Rutz W, von Knorring L, Walinder J. Long-term effects of an educational program for general practitioners given by the Swedish Committee for the Prevention and Treatment of Depression. *Acta Psychiatr Scand.* 1992;85:83–88.

35. Szanto K, Kalmar S, Hendin H, Rihmer Z, Mann JJ. A suicide prevention program in a region with a very high suicide rate. *Arch Gen Psychiatry.* 2007;64:914–920.

36. Zoroya G. More Army Guard, Reserve soldiers committing suicide. USA Today. Published January 20, 2011. Available at: http://www.usatoday.com/news/military/ 2011-01-20-suicides20_ST_N.htm. Accessed February 26, 2011.

37. Department of Defense (DOD). Army releases December and 2010 suicide data. Published January 19, 2011. Available at: http://www.defense.gov/utility/ printitem.aspx?print=http://www.defense.gov/Releases/ Release.aspx?ReleaseID=14213. Accessed February 26, 2011.

38. Department of Veterans Affairs. National Center for Veterans Analysis and Statistics data. Available at: http://www.va.gov/vetdata/index.asp. Accessed July 5, 2011.

28

Suicide Among Veterans in 16 States, 2005 to 2008: Comparisons Between Utilizers and Nonutilizers of Veterans Health Administration (VHA) Services Based on Data From the National Death Index, the National Violent Death Reporting System, and VHA Administrative Records

Ira R. Katz, MD, PhD, John F. McCarthy, PhD, Rosalinda V. Ignacio, MS, and Janet Kemp, RN, PhD

Objectives. We sought to compare suicide rates among veterans utilizing Veterans Health Administration (VHA) services versus those who did not.

Methods. Suicide rates from 2005 to 2008 were estimated for veterans in the 16 states that fully participated in the National Violent Death Reporting System (NVDRS), using data from the National Death Index, NVDRS, and VHA records.

Results. Between 2005 and 2008, veteran suicide rates differed by age and VHA utilization status. Among men aged 30 years and older, suicide rates were consistently higher among VHA utilizers. However, among men younger than 30 years, rates declined significantly among VHA utilizers while increasing among nonutilizers. Over these years, an increasing proportion of male veterans younger than 30 years received VHA services, and these individuals had a rising prevalence of diagnosed mental health conditions.

*Conclusions.*The higher rates of suicide for utilizers of VHA among veteran men aged 30 and older were consistent with previous reports about which veterans utilize VHA services. The increasing rates of mental health conditions in utilizers younger than 30 years suggested that the decreasing relative rates in this group were related to the care provided, rather than to selective enrollment of those at lower risk for suicide.

Since the start of the wars in Afghanistan and Iraq, there has been increasing interest in suicide among American military veterans. This reflects a number of important issues. First, veterans constitute a sizeable population that has been identified as being at increased risk for suicide by some[1,2] but not all,[3] research studies. Second, there is increasing evidence that suicide may be a consequence of the stresses related to the experience of deployment and combat.[4] Third, there have been concerns about the extent to which the Veterans Health Administration (VHA), the Department of Veterans Affairs (VA) health care system, has addressed the needs of veterans, especially those who have returned from service in Operation Enduring Freedom (OEF) and Operation Iraqi Freedom (OIF), the wars in Afghanistan and Iraq.

Since the start of OEF and OIF, there have been a number of reports on rates and risk factors for death from suicide among all American veterans, independent of whether they have received VHA health care services,[1-3,5-9] as well as a greater number of reports on those who utilize VHA services,[10-22] and on mixed samples.[23] Currently, the literature is not clear as to whether rates in veterans as a whole are higher than those for other Americans after controlling for demographic variables. However, there is evidence for increased rates in veterans utilizing VHA health care services. To date, there have been no reports of comparisons between veterans who utilize VHA services (utilizers) and those who do not (nonutilizers). This information is critical to advance a population-based approach to suicide prevention in veterans; to evaluate how the burden of suicide is distributed in the total veteran population; and to assess how completely VHA, the nation's largest integrated health care system, addresses the needs of the population it was established to serve.

Comparisons between suicide rates among veterans who are VHA utilizers versus nonutilizers can also provide information on the impact of recent changes in the VHA and the patients it serves. Toward the end of 2005, VHA began to implement a mental health strategic plan based on recommendations from the President's New Freedom Commission on Mental Health[24] as well as recognition of the mental health needs of returning veterans. At the same time, VHA began to increase the budget for mental health services to support this strategy. As a result of these enhancements, systemwide VA mental health staffing increased 26.1%, from 13 667 at the start of 2005 to 17 234 at the end of 2008. Over this same period, the total number of veterans seen per year in VHA increased 3.6%, from 5.02 million in 2005 to 5.20 million in 2008; the number with diagnosed mental health conditions increased 15.0%, from 1.45 to 1.69 million; and the percentage of veteran patients with mental health conditions increased by 11.1%, from 28.9% to 32.1%.[25]

Veterans returning from OEF and OIF are all eligible for VHA services during the first 5 years after they return from deployment without additional requirements. For veterans who served in previous eras, VHA eligibility is determined by factors such as service-connected health conditions, disability, age, and income.[26] The differences in eligibility requirements, as well as differences in the recency of deployment and the acuity of deployment-related conditions, suggest the importance of testing for differences between age groups both when comparing suicide rates in veterans who are VHA utilizers versus nonutilizers and when evaluating changes in rates over time.

For our study, we compared rates of suicide and assessed changes over time among veterans who utilized VHA health care services and those who did not, by gender, age group, and year. Given greater morbidity among those veterans who received VHA services, we hypothesized that suicide rates were higher among veterans who were VHA utilizers than those who were nonutilizers. Given the magnitude of VHA mental health enhancements, we hypothesized that rates among VHA utilizers would decrease over time. Finally, given greater acuity of mental health problems in OEF and OIF veterans, we hypothesized that among VHA utilizers decreases in rates would be greater among younger than older veterans.

METHODS

Suicide rates for veterans using VHA health services and for other veterans were estimated using VHA administrative data, vital status, and cause of death records from the National Center for Health Statistics' National Death Index (NDI),[27] and state-level information on suicides among veterans, by gender and age, from the Center for Disease Control and Prevention's National Violent Death Reporting System (NVDRS).[28] Clinical information from the VHA's electronic health records was not utilized because it was not available for those who did not utilize VHA services.

Suicide rates, expressed as suicide deaths per 100 000 person-years, were estimated for veterans in the 16 states that fully participated in NVDRS from 2005 to 2008 (Alaska, Colorado, Georgia, Kentucky, Maryland, Massachusetts, New Jersey, New Mexico, North Carolina, Oklahoma, Oregon, Rhode Island, South Carolina, Utah, Virginia, and Wisconsin).

Suicide mortality among individuals receiving VHA services was estimated using VHA administrative data included in the National Patient Care Database and NDI data using previously described methods.[19,21] Briefly, we identified all patients with VHA inpatient or outpatient encounters from 2005 to 2008 who had no VHA encounters in subsequent years, and we queried the NDI to determine these individuals' vital status, and, for those who died, their cause of death. To estimate state-level suicide rates, VHA users who died from suicide were assigned to specific states based on the location of the VHA medical center where they last received services. Rates among VHA users were estimated for each year, sex, and age group (18–29, 30–64, and 65 years and older), using the total number of suicides among those who received VHA services in the 16 NVDRS states, divided by the total number of veterans receiving care from VHA medical centers in those states.

The NVDRS provided information on the total number of suicide deaths among veterans, independent of whether they received VHA services, by year, sex, and age category for each of the 16 states from 2005 to 2008 based on the methods detailed in their coding manual.[29] NVDRS data included information on each decedent's veteran status, which was used in previous studies.[2,8,9] This was assessed from an indicator of whether the decedent ever served in the US Armed Forces, which was derived from the standardized death certificates in the NVDRS states and is included in a section that is usually completed by funeral directors on the basis of all of the information and reports available to them.[30,31] For each year, gender, and age group, suicide rates among all veterans in the NVDRS states were estimated from the total number of veteran suicides identified by NVDRS divided by the total number of veterans in those states. Data on the size of the total veteran population, and for veterans who were VHA utilizers versus nonutilizers, were derived from the Veteran Population (VetPop) 2007 file[32] maintained by the VA.

The nature of the data use agreements between NVDRS and the states precluded disclosure of identifying information on decedents. Consequently, suicide rates for nonutilizers were estimated indirectly, using the relevant numerators and denominators for the 16 states. The numerators were estimated from the total number of veterans identified as having died from suicide in NVDRS data for the 16 states minus the number of suicide deaths among VHA utilizers in these states. Denominators were estimated by subtracting the number of individuals served by VA facilities in the NVDRS states from the total number of veterans in those states as indicated from the VetPop 2007 data.

Statistical analyses were conducted using Predictive Analytics SoftWare Statistics 18 (SPSS Statistics, Hong Kong). Comparisons of suicide rates were conducted using the generalized linear modeling command, with Poisson log linear modeling for counts.

RESULTS

Suicide counts, populations, and rates in the 16 states for 2005–2008, overall and by VHA user status, are presented in Table 1 for veteran women and in Table 2 for veteran men. These provided information by year for veterans in the 16 states, overall and by age category.

Among all veteran women in the 16 states, approximately 21.8% utilized VHA services: 28.1% of veteran women younger than 30 years, 22.2% of those aged 30 to 64 years, and 15.5% of those 65 years and older. There were no significant changes in suicide rates between 2005 and 2008. Suicide rates for veteran women were lower than those observed for men, overall, for each of the age categories and among both VHA utilizers and nonutilizers. The relatively low numbers of suicides among women in these states precluded meaningful comparisons between rates in utilizers and nonutilizers across the years.

For veteran men in the 16 states, approximately 17.9% utilized VHA services: 15.5% of those younger than 30 years, 16.2% of those aged 30–64 years, and 20.8% of those 65 years and older. The proportion of veterans younger than 30 years who utilized VHA health care increased significantly

Table 1. Suicide Counts, At Risk Populations, and Suicide Rates Among Veteran Women, Overall and by Veterans Health Administration User Status: 16 National Violent Death Reporting System States, 2005–2008

Ages, y	All Veteran Women			VA Utilizer Women			VA Nonutilizer Women		
	Suicides, No.	Population, No.	Suicide Rate	Suicides, No.	Population, No.	Suicide Rate	Suicides, No.	Population, No.	Suicide Rate
2005									
All	50	527 208	9.48	9	110 904	8.12[a]	41	416 304	9.85
18-29	10	59 507	16.81[a]	0	16 102	0.00[a]	10	43 405	23.04[a]
30-64	36	387 007	9.30	8	82 765	9.67[a]	28	304 242	9.20
≥ 65	4	80 694	4.96[a]	1	12 036	8.31[a]	3	68 658	4.37[a]
2006									
All	65	536 668	12.11	16	114 654	13.96[a]	49	422 014	11.61
18-29	9	59 280	15.18[a]	2	16 931	11.81[a]	7	42 349	16.53[a]
30-64	53	396 950	13.35	13	85 751	15.16[a]	40	311 199	12.85
≥ 65	3	80 438	3.73[a]	1	11 972	8.35[a]	2	68 466	2.92[a]
2007									
All	72	545 600	13.20	21	119 327	17.60	51	426 521	11.96
18-29	9	58 791	15.31[a]	2	17 269	11.58[a]	7	41 769	16.76[a]
30-64	60	407 003	14.74	19	90 338	21.03[a]	41	316 665	12.95
≥ 65	3	79 806	3.76[a]	0	11 720	0.00[a]	3	68 086	4.41[a]
2008									
All	55	517 566	10.63	18	118 812	15.15[a]	37	398 754	9.28[a]
18-29	9	58 614	15.35[a]	4	15 988	25.02[a]	5	42 626	11.73[a]
30-64	43	376875	11.41	14	88 531	15.81[a]	29	288 344	10.06
≥ 65	3	82 077	3.66[a]	0	14 293	0.00[a]	3	67 784	4.43[a]

[a]Rates based on small sample sizes must be interpreted with caution, as they are sensitive to small differences in counts.

Table 2. Suicide Counts, at Risk Populations, and Suicide Rates Among Veteran Men, Overall and by Veteran Health Administration User Status: 16 National Violent Death Reporting System States, 2005-2008

Ages, y	All Veteran Men			VA Utilizer Men			VA non-Utilizer Men		
	Suicides, No.	Population, No.	Suicide Rate	Suicides, No.	Population, No.	Suicide Rate	Suicides, No.	Population, No.	Suicide Rate
2005									
All	1767	6 193 444	28.53	423	1151 260	36.74	1344	5 042 184	26.66
18-29	100	222 255	44.99	17	31 966	53.18[a]	83	190 289	43.62
30-64	931	3 636 370	25.60	217	594 346	36.51	714	3 042 024	23.47
≥ 65	736	2 334 819	31.52	189	524 948	36.00	547	1 809 871	30.22
2006									
All	1600	6 118 208	26.15	396	1 049 666	37.73	1204	5 068 542	23.75
18-29	104	229 848	45.25	15	33 827	44.34[a]	89	196 021	45.40
30-64	900	3 575 049	25.17	219	548 316	39.94	681	3 026 733	22.50
≥ 65	596	2 313 311	25.76	162	467 523	34.65	434	1 845 788	23.51
2007									
All	1787	6 052 918	29.52	391	1 072 818	36.45	1396	4 980 100	28.03
18-29	137	241 339	56.77	18	38 544	46.70[a]	119	202 795	58.68
30-64	965	3 490 677	27.65	216	563 769	38.31	749	2 926 908	25.59
≥ 65	685	2 320 902	29.51	157	470 504	33.37	528	1 850 398	28.53
2008									
All	1843	5 982 534	30.81	435	1 085 111	40.09	1408	4 897 423	28.75
18-29	144	250 070	57.58	14	42 113	33.24[a]	130	207 957	62.51
30-64	992	3 406 930	29.12	248	575 991	43.06	744	2 830 939	26.28
≥ 65	707	2 325 534	30.40	173	467 007	37.04	534	185 8527	28.73

[a]Rates based on small sample sizes must be interpreted with caution, as they are sensitive to small differences in counts.

from 14.3% in 2005 to 16.8% in 2008 (average of 0.87% per year). There were no significant changes over time for those aged 30–64 years or for those aged 65 years and older.

Further, among all veteran men, for those aged 30–64 years and those aged 65 years and older, there were no significant changes in suicide rates over time (Figure 1). For each of these groups, suicide rates for utilizers were consistently higher than for nonutilizers (Figure 2).

However, for all men younger than 30 years, suicide rates increased from 2005 to 2008 (Poisson log linear model; Wald χ^2_1 = 5.559; P = .018), with significant increases among nonutilizers (Wald χ^2_1 = 9.204; P = .002) but no significant increases among utilizers (Table 2; Figure 1). When models considered both differences between years and between VHA utilizers versus nonutilizers, the interaction term was significant (Wald χ^2_1 = 4.949; P = .026), reflecting decreasing suicide rates in utilizers compared with nonutilizers over time (Figure 2). In 2005, rates were 21.9% higher in young male utilizers than in nonutilizers; by 2008, rates among young male utilizers were 46.8% lower (Figure 2).

A number of the findings reported here identified veteran men younger than age 30 as an important subgroup. Men younger than age 30 as a proportion of the total number of men in the 16 states receiving VA health care services increased from 2.8% in 2005 to 3.2% in 2006, to 3.6% in 2007, and

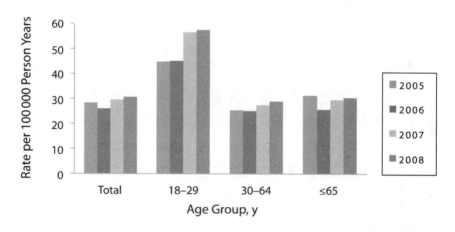

Figure 1. Suicide rates among veteran men, by year and age group: 16 National Violent Death Reporting System states, 2005-2008

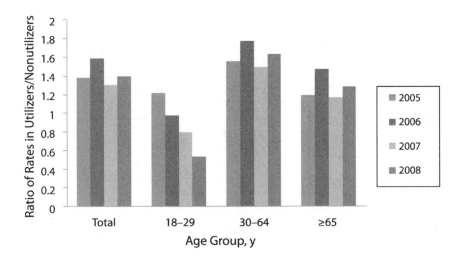

Figure 2. Ratio of suicide rates among veteran men utilizing Veterans Affairs health care services and among nonutilizers, by year and age group: 16 National Violent Death Reporting System states, 2005-2008

to 3.9% in 2008 (Table 2). During this period, there were also substantial increases (> 50%) in the proportion of these young men who served in Afghanistan or Iraq, and in those diagnosed with a substance use disorder, depression, posttraumatic stress disorder (PTSD), another anxiety disorder, or any mental health condition. There were marginal increases in the proportion with diagnoses of bipolar disorder and decreases in the proportion with diagnoses of schizophrenia (Table 3).

DISCUSSION

The findings reported here are important for 2 reasons. First, they demonstrated the feasibility and utility of linking information from NVDRS, NDI, and VHA sources to compare outcomes in veterans who utilized VHA healthcare services and those who did not. Second, they constituted the first reported comparison of suicide rates between veteran utilizers and nonutilizers.

The findings presented here demonstrated that for veteran men overall, for those aged 30–64 years, and for those 65 years and older, suicide rates among VHA utilizers were persistently higher than for nonutilizers. Other findings

Table 3. OEF/OIF Status and Clinical Characteristics of Veteran Men Younger Than 30 Years Utilizing the Veterans Health Administration: 16 National Violent Death Reporting System States, 2005–2008

	2005, %	2006, %	2007, %	2008, %
OEF/OIF	3.60	47.61	57.57	63.75
SUD	5.28	6.33	8.18	10.36
Depression	11.28	12.70	15.30	18.23
PTSD	7.93	11.50	16.65	21.68
Other anxiety	5.17	6.08	7.93	9.71
Bipolar	1.95	2.00	2.19	2.37
Schizophrenia	1.27	1.23	1.16	1.08
Any MH condition	23.16	27.04	33.53	39.42

Note. MH = mental health; OEF/OIF = Operation Enduring Freedom/Operation Iraqi Freedom; PTSD = posttraumatic stress disorder; SUD = substance use disorder.

demonstrated important trends among veteran men younger than 30 years. The number of these veterans and the proportion of them using VHA services increased from 2005–2008. Suicide rates increased in the overall population of young veteran men in parallel with the rates in VHA service nonutilizers, as opposed to nonsignificant changes in VHA service utilizers. Most significantly, from 2005–2008, there were dramatic decreases in suicide rates in young male VHA utilizers relative to nonutilizers. We noted that in the general US population in the 16 states, the Web-based Injury Statistics Query and Reporting System/NVDRS web site indicated that suicide rates in 2008 were 19.4 per 100 000 among men age 18 to 29 years, and 25.1 and 28.3 among men age 30–64 and 65 years and older, respectively. Finally, findings were consistent with previous reports that suicide rates were higher for men than for women, both in veteran and nonveteran populations.[19,33] Given the lower prevalence of suicide in women and the relatively low proportion of veterans who were women, it was not feasible to compare rates among veteran women by VHA utilization status in the 16 NVDRS states. Consequently, this discussion focused on findings among veteran men.

The results for all veteran men, for those aged 30–64 years and for those aged 65 years and older, were consistent with reported comparisons of suicide rates between VHA utilizers and age- and gender-matched individuals in the general population.[19] As discussed previously,[19] these findings might be related to selection of those who were more likely to be mentally ill, chronically ill, disabled, and economically disadvantaged by the eligibility criteria for enrollment in VHA.[26] Several lines of investigation supported selective use of VHA services by those with risk factors for suicide. Research conducted before the first Gulf War demonstrated that high illness levels and service connected disability were associated with use of VA health care services.[34] Research between the first Gulf War and OEF/OIF demonstrated that veterans who were unemployed and with greater levels of disability were more likely to use VA relative to non-VA outpatient health care services.[35] Findings from the first years of OEF and OIF demonstrated that the proportion of enrollees with serious mental illness in VHA was greater than that in private insurance plans or the Military Treatment System, and comparable to the proportion among Medicaid recipients; the proportion of those with depression was greater in the VA than any of the other coverage systems.[36] Finally, findings that PTSD predicted use of VHA services among Vietnam-era veterans[37] were consistent with recent unpublished findings that PTSD and other mental health conditions predicted VHA use among OEF and OIF veterans. The findings reported here were consistent with the hypothesis that suicide rates were higher among veterans who received VHA services than among those who did not receive VHA services. The results did not, however, confirm the hypothesis that mental health enhancements led to decreases over time in suicide rates. We noted that VHA mental health enhancements continued beyond 2008, and further monitoring is needed to determine whether these enhancements led to decreases in suicide rates.

Our findings demonstrate important trends among veteran men younger than 30 years. First, suicide rates increased between 2005 and 2008 in the total population of young veteran men in the 16 states included in NVDRS. Although the mechanisms underlying this increase remain to be determined, it is important to note that this effect appeared to parallel the increases observed among active duty service members.[38,39] Second, as hypothesized, rates among young utilizers decreased relative to those among nonutilizers. In principle, this effect could occur for either of 2 reasons. First, it could result from selection factors, if over time, the young men who came to VHA for services were increasingly at lower risk for suicide. Alternatively, the relative decline among VHA utilizers could occur as a result of enhancements in access to effective treatments or if VHA services became more effective at preventing suicide. Given that mental health conditions are major risk factors for suicide,[21] the increasing prevalence of mental health conditions in male VHA utilizers younger than 30 years (Table 3) appeared inconsistent with the possibility that the relative decreases in suicide rates in the young men served by VHA could be because of the enrollment of patients at lower risk. Accordingly, it was likely that the observed decreases in suicide rates for young male utilizers were because of enhancements in the effectiveness of VHA services. The findings presented in Figure 2 could be explained by assuming that young veteran men represented a group for whom the outcomes of care were most sensitive to these enhancements, possibly as a reflection of the acuity of their mental health conditions.

There were multiple potential limitations involved with the data sources and the necessary assumptions for completing these analyses. Of course, study findings might not be generalizable to the entire United States or the entire VHA health care system, to the extent that the 16 NVDRS states were not representative of the nation or the VHA health system, for example, with respect to the geographic distribution of veterans and patterns of VHA utilization. Also, there were constraints related to measurement. Most concerning was the possibility that the NVDRS indicators of veterans status were derived from responses regarding whether decedents had ever served in the US Armed Forces. In some cases, positive responses might have included nonveterans (e.g., active duty personnel, National Guard members who were never activated or deployed), and negative responses might have failed to identify veterans (e.g., those with previous service in the Coast Guard or Public Health Services; veteran decedents whose survivors were unaware of their veteran status). This raised important concerns regarding study findings, as secular trends in suicide mortality among activity duty personnel could affect the assessment of trends in suicide mortality among veterans who did not utilize VHA services. Certainly further research is needed to address this concern. Finally, we noted 3 other sources of potential measurement error. First, the source of veteran population counts was based on census data, information from the Department of Defense, and updates estimated using actuarial methods. Given the recent increases in the number of veterans returning from Afghanistan and Iraq, there might have been greater imprecision in the veteran population estimates, particularly for younger veterans. Second, because it was not possible to directly match individuals who were counted as veteran suicides by NVDRS with the VHA data, the calculation of rates among veteran nonutilizers was perforce estimated; rates for utilizers and nonutilizers were calculated for the 16 states from the number of individuals identified by VHA as utilizers in these states and, for nonutilizers, by the total number counted by NVDRS minus the number identified by VHA. Third, although the NVDRS attributed individuals to states based on the location of their deaths, the VHA attributed veterans to states based on the location of the facility where they last received VHA services. Consequently, the different processes might have resulted in mismatches and noise or bias in the findings.

Mindful of these concerns, we noted that this study applied existing data to investigate pressing public health and health policy questions. Study findings offered new perspectives regarding suicide among veterans and differences in suicide rates between VHA utilizers and nonutilizers. The most significant findings might be the consistently higher rate of suicide among VHA utilizers aged 30–64 years and those 65 years and older and, among veterans younger than 30 years, the observed decreasing rates in VHA utilizers relative to nonutilizers between 2005 and 2008. Although definitive explanations for these findings will require additional research, the available evidence suggested that the increased rates in men aged 30–64 years and in elder populations might be because of the selective use of VHA services by individuals at increased risk, whereas among veterans younger than 30 years, the decreasing rates in VHA utilizers relative to nonutilizers might result from the ongoing enhancements in VHA mental health services.

ABOUT THE AUTHORS

All the authors are with the US Department of Veterans Affairs, Washington, DC. Ira R. Katz, John F. McCarthy, and Rosalinda V. Ignacio are with the VA Office of Mental Health Operations. Janet Kemp is with the VA Office of Suicide Prevention.

CONTRIBUTORS

I. R. Katz originated the analytic plan. I. R. Katz, J. F. McCarthy, and R. V. Ignacio conducted the analyses, interpreted the data, and wrote the article. All authors contextualized the findings, approved the final article, and take responsibility for the data integrity and accuracy of the analyses.

ACKNOWLEDGMENTS

This study was funded by the VA Office of Mental Health Services.

HUMAN PARTICIPANTS PROTECTION

This study was approved by the Ann Arbor VA Medical Center Institutional Review Board.

REFERENCES

1. Kaplan MS, Huguet N, McFarland BH, Newsom JT. Suicide among male veterans: a prospective population-based study. *J Epidemiol Community Health.* 2007;61:619–624.

2. McFarland BH, Kaplan MS, Huguet N. Datapoints: self-inflicted deaths among women with U.S. military service: a hidden epidemic? *Psychiatr Serv.* 2010;61:1177.

3. Miller M, Barber C, Azrael D, Calle EE, Lawler E, Mukamal KJ. Suicide among US veterans: a prospective study of 500,000 middle-aged and elderly men. *Am J Epidemiol.* 2009;170:494–500.

4. Institute of Medicine. *Deployment-Related Stress and Health Outcomes.* Vol 6. Washington, DC: National Academy Press; 2007.

5. Boscarino JA. External-cause mortality after psychologic trauma: the effects of stress exposure and predisposition. *Compr Psychiatry.* 2006;47:503–514.

6. Kang HK, Bullman TA. Risk of suicide among US veterans after returning from the Iraq or Afghanistan war zones. *JAMA.* 2008;300:652–653.

7. Maynard C, Boyko EJ. Datapoints: suicide rates in the Washington State veteran population. *Psychiatr Serv.* 2008;59:1245.

8. Kaplan MS, McFarland BH, Huguet N. Characteristics of adult male and female firearm suicide decedents: findings from the National Violent Death Reporting System. *Inj Prev.* 2009;15:322–327.

9. Kaplan MS, McFarland BH, Huguet N. Firearm suicide among veterans in the general population: findings from the National Violent Death Reporting System. *J Trauma.* 2009;67:503–507.

10. Kausch O, McCormick RA. Suicide prevalence in chemical dependency programs: preliminary data from a national sample, and an examination of risk factors. *J Subst Abuse Treat.* 2002;22:97–102.

11. Thompson R, Kane VR, Sayers SL, Brown GK, Coyne JC, Katz IR. An assessment of suicide in an urban VA Medical Center. *Psychiatry.* 2002;65:327–337.

12. Thompson R, Katz IR, Kane VR, Sayers SL. Cause of death in veterans receiving general medical and mental health care. *J Nerv Ment Dis.* 2002;190:789–792.

13. Desai RA, Dausey DJ, Rosenheck RA. Mental health service delivery and suicide risk: the role of individual patient and facility factors. *Am J Psychiatry.* 2005;162:311–318.

14. Zivin K, Kim HM, McCarthy JF, et al. Suicide mortality among individuals receiving treatment for depression in the Veterans Affairs health system: associations with patient and treatment setting characteristics. *Am J Public Health.* 2007;97:2193–2198.

15. Desai RA, Dausey D, Rosenheck RA. Suicide among discharged psychiatric inpatients in the Department of Veterans Affairs. *Mil Med.* 2008;173:721–728.

16. Mills PD, DeRosier JM, Ballot BA, Shepherd M, Bagian JP. Inpatient suicide and suicide attempts in Veterans Affairs hospitals. *Jt Comm J Qual Patient Saf.* 2008;34:482–488.

17. Desai MM, Rosenheck RA, Desai RA. Time trends and predictors of suicide among mental health outpatients in the Department of Veterans Affairs. *J Behav Health Serv Res.* 2008;35:115–124.

18. Ilgen MA, Downing K, Zivin K, et al. Exploratory data mining analysis identifying subgroups of patients with depression who are at high risk for suicide. *J Clin Psychiatry.* 2009;70:1495–1500.

19. McCarthy JF, Valenstein M, Kim HM, Ilgen M, Zivin K, Blow FC. Suicide mortality among patients receiving care in the Veterans Health Administration health system. *Am J Epidemiol.* 2009;169:1033–1038.

20. Pfeiffer PN, Ganoczy D, Ilgen M, Zivin K, Valenstein M. Comorbid anxiety as a suicide risk factor among depressed veterans. *Depress Anxiety.* 2009;26:752–757.

21. Ilgen MA, Bohnert AS, Ignacio RV, et al. Psychiatric diagnoses and risk of suicide in veterans. *Arch Gen Psychiatry.* 2010;67:1152–1158.

22. llgen, MA, Zivin K, Austin KL, et al. Severe pain predicts greater likelihood of subsequent suicide. *Suicide Life Threat Behav.* 2010;40:597–608.

23. Flood AM, Boyle SH, Calhoun PS, et al. Prospective study of externalizing and internalizing subtypes of posttraumatic stress disorder and their relationship to mortality among Vietnam veterans. *Compr Psychiatry.* 2010;51:236–242.

24. The President's New Freedom Commission on Mental Health. Achieving the Promise. Transforming Mental Health Care in America. *Final Report.* 2003. Available at: http://store.samhsa.gov/product/SMA03-3831. Accessed January 20, 2012.

25. Department of Veterans Affairs. *Administrative Data.* Washington, DC: Department of Veterans Affairs; 2011.

26. Veterans Health Administration. Enrollment Priority Groups. Available at: http://www.va.gov/healthbenefits/resources/priority_groups.asp. Accessed January 10, 2012.

27. Centers for Disease Control and Prevention, National Center for Health Statistics. National Death Index. Available at: http://www.cdc.gov/nchs/data_access/ndi/about_ndi.htm. Accessed January 10, 2012.

28. Centers for Disease Control and Prevention. National Violent Death Reporting System. Available at: http://www.cdc.gov/ViolencePrevention/NVDRS/index.html. Accessed January 10, 2012.

29. National Center for Injury Prevention, Control, Centers for Disease Control and Prevention. National Violent Death Reporting System Coding Manual Version 3. 2008. Available at: http://www.cdc.gov/violenceprevention/NVDRS/coding_manual.html. Accessed January 10, 2012.

30. National Center for Health Statistics, Centers for Disease Control and Prevention. Medical Examiners' and Coroners' Handbook on Death registration and Fetal Death Reporting (2003 Revision). Available at: http://www.cdc.gov/nchs/data/misc/hb_me.pdf. Accessed January 10, 2012.

31. National Center for Health Statistics, Centers for Disease Control and Prevention. Funeral Directors' Handbook on Death Registration and Fetal Death Reporting (2003 Revision). Availableat: http://www.cdc.gov/nchs/data/misc/hb_fun.pdf. Accessed January 10, 2012.

32. Department of Veterans Affairs. VetPop 2007. Available at: http://www.va.gov/VETDATA/Demographics/Demographics.asp. Accessed January 10, 2012.

33. Centers for Disease Control and Prevention. National Suicide Statistics at a Glance. Available at: http://www.cdc.gov/violenceprevention/suicide/statistics/aag.html. Accessed January 10, 2012.

34. Rosenheck R, Massari L. Wartime military service and utilization of VA health care services. *Mil Med.* 1993;158:223–228.

35. Elhai JD, Grubaugh AL, Richardson JD, Egede LE, Creamer M. Outpatient medical and mental healthcare utilization models among military veterans: results from the 2001 National Survey of Veterans. *J Psychiatr Res.* 2008;42:858–867.

36. Gibson TB, Lee TA, Vogeli CS, et al. A four-system comparison of patients with chronic illness: The Military Health System, Veterans Health Administration, Medicaid, and Commercial Plans. *Mil Med.* 2009;174:936–943.

37. Rosenheck R, Fontana A. Do Vietnam-era veterans who suffer from posttraumatic stress disorder avoid VA mental health services? *Mil Med.* 1995;160:136–142.

38. United States Army. Army Health Promotion, Risk reduction, and Suicide Prevention Report. 2010. Available at: http://www.army.mil/article/42934. Accessed January 10, 2012.

39. Department of Defense Task Force on the Prevention of Suicide by Members of the Armed Forces. Executive Summary. 2010. Available at: http://www.health.mil/dhb/downloads/TaskForce2010/Suicide%20Prevention%20Task%20Force_EXEC%20SUM_08-20-10%20v6.doc. Accessed January 10, 2012.

29

Suicide Among Patients in the Veterans Affairs Health System: Rural–Urban Differences in Rates, Risks, and Methods

John F. McCarthy, PhD, MPH, Frederic C. Blow, PhD, Rosalinda V. Ignacio, MS, Mark A. Ilgen, PhD, Karen L. Austin, MPH, and Marcia Valenstein, MD, MS

Objectives. Using national patient cohorts, we assessed rural–urban differences in suicide rates, risks, and methods in veterans.

Methods. We identified all Department of Veterans Affairs (VA) patients in fiscal years 2003 to 2004 (FY03–04) alive at the start of FY04 (n = 5 447 257) and all patients in FY06–07 alive at the start of FY07 (n = 5 709 077). Mortality (FY04–05 and FY07–08) was assessed from National Death Index searches. Census criteria defined rurality. We used proportional hazards regressions to calculate rural–urban differences in risks, controlling for age, gender, psychiatric diagnoses, VA mental health services accessibility, and regional administrative network. Suicide method was categorized as firearms, poisoning, strangulation, or other.

Results. Rural patients had higher suicide rates (38.8 vs 31.4/100 000 person-years in FY04–05; 39.6 vs 32.4/100 000 in FY07–08). Rural residence was associated with greater suicide risks (20% greater, FY04–05; 22% greater, FY07–08). Firearm deaths were more common in rural suicides (76.8% vs 61.5% in FY07–08).

Conclusions. Rural residence is a suicide risk factor, even after controlling for mental health accessibility. Public health and health system suicide prevention should address risks in rural areas.

Suicide among veterans is a national concern,[1,2] and suicide prevention is a priority for the US Department of Veterans Affairs (VA) health system, the Veterans Health Administration. The VA provides health services to approximately 5.5 million veterans each year, more than one fifth of all veterans. The VA serves a patient population with important suicide risk factors. Patients are predominantly male and older, and often have substantial physical morbidities, substance use problems, and mental illnesses.[3-5] Also, VA patients are more likely to reside in rural settings than is the general US population.[6,7] This trend is expected to continue because rural residents are overrepresented among military recruits. In 2005, although 7.6% of 18- to 24-year-old US residents lived in rural areas, 11.8% of 18- to 24-year-old military recruits were from these areas.[8] Research is needed to assess whether rural residence is associated with differential suicide rates and risks among the national population of VA patients.

Since the early 1970s, suicide rates among men in rural areas of the United States have exceeded those of urban men, and rural–urban differentials have increased for both genders.[9,10] Similar trends have been observed outside of the United States.[11-13] Elevated suicide rates in rural areas have been attributed to factors including geographic and interpersonal isolation, economic and social distress, and rural culture.[14] Rural populations are smaller and more dispersed, potentially limiting opportunities for social integration and social support. Geographic accessibility of mental health treatment resources is often diminished, with providers fewer and farther between. Economic declines may affect rural areas more drastically. Further, rural agrarian cultural values, which champion a strong work ethic, independence, and self-reliance, may inhibit treatment-seeking behavior.[15]

Previous research on suicide risks associated with veteran status among community residents produced mixed results.[16-20] Among male respondents to the US National Health Interview Survey, suicide risks between 1986 and 1997 for male veterans were found to be twice those of male nonveterans (adjusted hazard ratio [HR] for veterans = 2.04; 95% confidence interval [CI] = 1.10, 3.80), controlling for rurality of residence.[19] However, in an analysis of middle-aged and older men who participated in a large prospective cohort study from 1982 to 2004, which did not adjust for rurality, veteran status was not associated with suicide risk.[20] In their review, Kang and Bullman noted that "historically the rates of suicide among veterans in general have been lower than that of the US population."[18(p 760)] To date, however, few studies have adjusted for rurality,[19] and it is important to consider rural–urban differentials in risks among veterans.

Among VA patients, research suggested that suicide rates were greater than those in the general US population. Before the conflicts in Afghanistan and Iraq, and before recent VA health system initiatives, the standardized mortality ratio for suicides among male VA patients in 2001 was 1.66 compared with men in the general US population; for female patients, it was 1.87.[21] Elevated risks among VA patients might reflect the fact that they represent a treatment-seeking population with substantial medical and psychiatric morbidities and meeting eligibility requirements means testing, based on income thresholds, or military service-related disability status.[22]

Currently, little is known about rural–urban differences in suicide risks among VA health system users. However, if consistent with general trends in the United States,[9,10,14] suicide risks may well be greater for VA patients residing in rural areas compared with those in urban areas. Studies indicated that VA patients in rural areas had more physical comorbidities and worse health-related quality of life than those in suburban or urban areas,[23] and that they had reduced access to health services and fewer alternatives to VA care.[24] Access barriers might limit receipt of needed health services and continuity of care,[25] and this might exacerbate suicide risks.

Another factor that may relate to differential suicide risks is access to lethal means of suicide, notably firearms. Among suicide attempt methods, firearms have the highest case fatality rate (suicides/[suicides + nonfatal injuries due to self-harm]): 84% in the United States during 2002 to 2006.[26] In non-VA populations, method of suicide differs across rural–urban settings. State-level analyses indicated that higher firearm ownership was associated with increased rates of firearm suicides,[26] and suicide deaths among veterans were more likely to involve firearms than those among nonveterans.[19,28] Between 2002 and 2006, although firearms were the most common method among male suicide decedents in the United States (58%), poisoning was the most common method among female suicide decedents (39%).[26] To date, little is known regarding potential rural–urban differences in means of suicide among VA patients, overall or by gender.

The objectives of this study were to examine rural–urban differences in rates, risks, and methods of suicide among the population of individuals receiving services in the VA health system. We hypothesized that VA patients in rural areas and those residing farther from VA mental health facilities were at greater risk for suicide, and that method of suicide differed by rural–urban status. Further, we examined 2 periods of time to assess potential differences over time. Research in this area might inform health services organization and delivery and advance assessments of whether and how veteran status relates to suicide risks.

METHODS

Since 2005, the Veterans Health Administration has substantially expanded mental health services and developed programs designed to prevent suicide. We assessed suicide mortality in 2 periods: fiscal years 2004 to 2005 (FY04–05; October 1, 2003 to September 30, 2005) and FY07–08 (October 1, 2007, to September 30, 2008). Risks were assessed for 2 national patient cohorts. These consisted of: (1) VA patients with observation time in FY04–05, defined as all individuals with VA inpatient or outpatient encounters in FY03–FY04 who were alive at the start of FY04, and (2) VA patients with observation time in FY07–08, defined as all individuals with VA encounters in FY06–FY07 who were alive at the start of FY07. This was based on established approaches to defining VA patient cohorts for health system suicide surveillance,[4,21] and it assumed that patients seen in VA settings in the previous year continued to be in VA care and part of the at-risk patient population.

The days at risk for an observed suicide were identified as follows.[21] For individuals who had VA encounters in the FY before the first FY of the cohort observation period, risk time began on the first day of the first FY of the observation period (October 1, 2003, and October 1, 2006, respectively). For those individuals without VA encounters in the preceding year, risk time began on the day of their first use in the first FY of the observation period (i.e., FY04 or FY07, respectively). The risk period ended at death or the end of the cohort observation period (September 30, 2005, and September 30, 2008, respectively), whichever came sooner.

This project was reviewed and approved by the Ann Arbor VA human subjects committee, and a waiver of informed consent was obtained for this secondary data analysis.

Data Sources

The VA's National Patient Care Database (NPCD) was used to identify all individuals with VA inpatient or outpatient service encounters. Indicators of vital status and cause of death were based on National Death Index (NDI) search records. The NDI is regarded as the "gold standard" for mortality assessments,[29] including date and causes of death for all decedents in the United States, based on death certificates filed in state vital statistics offices. Using established approaches,[21] NDI records were searched for all individuals with VA encounters in FY03–04 or in FY06–07 and who did not have VA encounters in FY09 or FY10. That is, to avoid unnecessary searches, we excluded from the NDI searches individuals with health system contacts subsequent to the final suicide risk period. The NDI searches were based on patient social security number, name, date of birth, race/ethnicity, gender, and state of residence. Search results might include multiple records that were potential matches, and "true matches" were identified based on established procedures.[30]

Measures

Using indicators included in the NPCD, we identified age and gender for the 2 cohorts. Age was calculated as of October 1, 2003, for the FY04–05 risk cohort and as of October 1, 2006, for the FY07–08 risk cohort, using 3 age categories: 18 to 29, 30 to 64, and at least 65 years. Race/ethnicity indicators were not consistently available and were not included.

Psychiatric diagnoses were assessed based on *International Classification of Diseases, Ninth Revision, Clinical Modification*[31] diagnostic codes recorded in VA encounters during the baseline year. The psychiatric diagnoses examined were bipolar disorder, depression, posttraumatic stress disorder (PTSD), other anxiety disorders, schizophrenia/schizoaffective disorder, and substance use disorders (SUDs; alcohol use disorders or drug use disorders). These diagnoses were selected based on previously established links to suicide in existing literature.[4] These indicators were not mutually exclusive, because individuals could have diagnoses recorded for more than 1 condition.

Distance to nearest VA mental health provider was assessed as straight-line miles from the population centroid of the individual's zip code of residence, from their first VA encounter of the baseline year, to that of the nearest VA facility providing substantial mental health services. These facilities were medical centers or community-based outpatient clinics serving at least 500 unique patients and where at least 20% of outpatient visits were mental health visits.[32] We also identified the VA regional network (of 21 networks) where each patient had their last VA encounter in the baseline year. Rurality was assessed by categorizing patients' zip codes of residence as rural or urban based on criteria used by the VA Office of Rural Health, which are based on US Census categories. Veterans were categorized as residing in an urban area if they lived within a census-defined urban area (having a population density of at least 1000 people per square mile and surrounding areas have a density of at least 500 per square mile). Rural areas were defined as those areas that did not meet these criteria.

Using NDI data, we identified dates and causes of death. Suicide deaths were identified using the *International Classification of Diseases, Tenth Revision*,[33] codes X60–X84, Y87.0. Method of suicide was categorized as involving use of firearms (X72–X74); poisoning (X60–X69); hanging, suffocation, or strangulation (X70); and other methods. These categories reflect common methods of suicide in the United States.[34]

Statistical Analyses

Descriptive statistics were calculated for each risk cohort, overall and by rural–urban status. We used bivariate analyses to compare patient characteristics by rurality status, using t test, χ^2, and nonparametric median tests, as appropriate. In further bivariate analyses, we examined whether suicide decedents differed from other individuals in the analyses, in terms of distance to nearest VA mental health services, overall and stratified by rural–urban status.

In proportional hazards regression analyses, we evaluated rurality and VA mental health geographic accessibility as predictors of suicide, controlling for patient gender, age, psychiatric morbidities, and VA regional network. Consistent with previous work regarding distance to VA care,[32] we included a quadratic distance term to assess potential curvilinear effects of distance on suicide risks. Analyses included covariance sandwich estimators to adjust for the nested nature of the data, with individuals clustered within VA facilities (identified by 3-digit facility prefix codes.) To reduce multicolinearity, because distance and distance-squared are highly correlated, distance measures were centered around their mean. An initial analytic model examined the influence of rurality and distance to nearest VA mental health services. A supplemental analysis included interaction terms between rurality and the distance and the quadratic distance terms.

Also, for each cohort, we used the χ^2 test to assess differences in method of suicide, by rural–urban status and by categories of distance to nearest VA mental health facility ($<$ 15, 15–49, 50–99, $\geqslant$100 miles), overall and stratified by gender. All statistical analyses were completed using SAS (version 9; SAS Institute, Cary, North Carolina).

RESULTS

Approximately 35% of VA patients in the FY04–05 risk cohort and 36% of the FY07–08 risk cohort lived in rural areas (unpublished analyses by the authors indicated that among similarly defined users in FY01–02, rural patients accounted for 34.3% of individuals). By comparison, 21% of the US adult population resided in rural settings.[7]

Table 1 presents information regarding the 2 risk cohorts, overall and by rurality status. For each cohort, rural–urban differences were statistically significant ($P <$ .001) for each measure. For the FY07–08 risk cohort, VA patients in rural areas were more likely to be male (93.8% vs 89.1%) and older (mean [SD] age = 62.8 [14.9] vs 60.1 [16.8] years). In the FY07–08 risk cohort, rural patients were less likely than urban patients to have had a diagnosis of bipolar disorder, schizophrenia, or substance use disorders, and they were more likely to have had a diagnosis of depression, PTSD, and other anxieties. Median distance to nearest VA mental health provider was 46.0 miles for the FY04–05 cohort and 37.4 miles for the FY07–08 cohort. Median distance was substantially greater for patients in rural areas (71.1 vs 28.3 miles for the FY04–05 cohort; 54.6 vs 22.8 miles for the FY07–08 cohort); 29.4% of the FY07–08 cohort lived within 15 miles of a VA mental health facility compared with 26.7% of the FY04–05 cohort.

The crude suicide rate was 34.01 per 100 000 person-years for the FY04–05 cohort and 35.01 per 100 000 person-years for the FY07–08 cohort. Crude suicide rates were greater in rural areas than in urban areas (38.76 per 100 000 vs 31.45 per 100 000 person-years in the FY04–05 cohort, and 39.62 per 100 000 vs 32.44 per 100 000 person-years in the FY07–08 cohort).

Table 2 presents results from multivariable proportional hazards regression results for the FY04–05 and the FY07–08 cohorts. These analyses indicated that residence in a rural zip code was associated with an increased risk for suicide mortality (HR = 1.20; 95% CI = 1.11, 1.29 for the FY04–05 cohort;

Table 1. Characteristics of Veterans Affairs Patients by Cohort, Overall, and Rurality Status: Suicide Among Patients in the Veterans Affairs Health System: United States, 2003–2008

	FY04–05 Risk Cohort			FY07–08 Risk Cohort		
	All	Rural	Urban	All	Rural	Urban
Total no. (%)	5 447 257	1 896 234 (35)	3 539 893 (65)	5 709 077	2 033 819 (36)	3 669 917 (64)
Gender, no. (%)						
Male	4 956 763 (91.0)	1 781 069 (93.9)	3 166 165 (89.4)	5 181 769 (90.8)	1 907 523 (93.8)	3 269 689 (89.1)
Female	490 494 (9.0)	115 165 (6.1)	373 728 (10.6)	527 308 (9.2)	126 296 (6.2)	400 228 (10.9)
Age, y						
Mean (SD)	60.9 (15.53)	62.66 (14.22)	59.96 (16.11)	61.09 (16.20)	62.81 (14.92)	60.14 (16.79)
Median	61	64	60	61.00	63	60
18–29, no. (%)	211 194 (3.9)	45 757 (2.4)	164 670 (4.7)	296 484 (5.2)	72 307 (3.6)	223 798 (6.1)
30–64, no. (%)	2 794 872 (51.3)	928 725 (49.0)	1 859 568 (52.5)	2 962 162 (51.9)	1 015 212 (49.9)	1 943 567 (53.0)
≥ 65, no. (%)	2 441 191 (44.8)	921 752 (48.6)	1 515 655 (42.8)	2 450 431 (42.9)	946 300 (46.5)	1 502 552 (40.9)
Psychiatric condition, no. (%)						
Bipolar disorder	91 864 (1.7)	26 281 (1.4)	65 480 (1.8)	104 987 (1.8)	31 781 (1.6)	73 147 (2.0)
Depression	692 579 (12.7)	250 159 (13.2)	441 636 (12.5)	800 119 (14.0)	294 189 (14.5)	505 541 (13.8)
Other anxiety	250 974 (4.6)	94 809 (5.0)	155 851 (4.4)	306 879 (5.4)	115 876 (5.7)	190 804 (5.2)
PTSD	284 996 (5.2)	104 450 (5.5)	180 104 (5.1)	409 452 (7.2)	153 342 (7.5)	255 824 (7.0)
Schizophrenia	103 162 (1.9)	25 841 (1.4)	77 185 (2.2)	97 662 (1.7)	25 017 (1.2)	72 573 (2.0)
SUD	344 925 (6.3)	93 255 (4.9)	251 133 (7.1)	396 496 (6.9)	113 308 (5.6)	282 918 (7.7)
Risk days						
Mean (SD)	680.06 (125.69)	681.38 (126.51)	679.35 (125.26)	684.83 (122.17)	686.66 (122.17)	683.83 (122.17)

(continued on next page)

Table 1. (*continued*)

	FY04–05 Risk Cohort			FY07–08 Risk Cohort		
	All	Rural	Urban	All	Rural	Urban
Median	730	730	730	731	731	731
25% quartile	730	730	730	731	731	731
Distance to VA mental health care, mi						
Mean (SD)	84.64 (146.69)	94.21 (107.19)	78.99 (162.12)	72.45 (142.28)	76.50 (103.34)	69.69 (158.09)
Median	46.0	71.06	28.34	37.45	54.61	22.76
<15	1 452 655 (26.7)	110 333 (5.8)	1 341 979 (37.9)	1 679 315 (29.4)	169 282 (8.3)	1 509 682 (41.1)
15– <50	1 395 175 (25.6)	538 994 (28.4)	856 011 (24.2)	1 680 593 (29.4)	755 229 (37.1)	925 303 (25.2)
50– <100	1 154 539 (21.2)	605 181 (31.9)	549 239 (15.5)	1 250 521 (21.9)	659 535 (32.4)	590 941 (16.1)
≥100	1 430 037 (26.3)	640 083 (33.8)	788 027 (22.3)	1 092 593 (19.1)	449 150 (22.1)	641 577 (17.5)
Suicide[a]						
Suicide deaths, no.	3442	1371	2071	3744	1515	2229
Person-years of risk time, no.	10 121 503	3 537 435	6 584 068	10 694 415	3 823 541	6 870 875
Rate/100 000 person-years	34.01	38.76	31.45	35.01	39.62	32.44

Note. FY = fiscal year; PTSD = posttraumatic stress disorder; SUD = substance use disorder; VA = Veterans Affairs.

[a]For both risk cohorts, significant differences were observed by rurality for each suicide risk measure (*P* < .001). Rurality information was unavailable for 11 130 patients in the FY04–05 risk cohort (0.2%), including 6 suicide decedents, and for 5341 patients in the FY07–08 risk cohort (0.1%), including 1 suicide decedent. In reporting risk-time and rates, we excluded individuals with missing rurality data.

Table 2. Proportional Hazards Regression Analyses of Time to Suicide Death: Suicide Among Patients in the Veterans Affairs Health System, United Stated, 2003–2008

Focal Independent Variables	FY04–05 Risk Cohort		FY07–08 Risk Cohort	
	HR (95% CI)	P	HR (95% CI)	P
Distance to VA mental health facility[a]	1.001 (1.000, 1.001)	.171	1.000 (0.999, 1.001)	.698
Distance[a] squared	1.000 (1.000, 1.000)	.205	1.000 (1.000, 1.000)	.454
Rural residence	1.195 (1.107, 1.289)	< .001	1.223 (1.122, 1.334)	.001

Note. CI = confidence interval; FY = fiscal years; HR = hazard ratio; VA = Veterans Affairs. Models also included patient age, gender, psychiatric diagnosis indicators, and VA regional network.
[a]Centered.

HR = 1.22; 95% CI = 1.12, 1.33 for the FY07–08 cohort). Neither distance nor distance-squared were significant predictors. In separate analyses, we explored potential interactions between distance and rurality. These produced inconsistent results. For the FY04–05 cohort, although the interaction between distance and rurality was nonsignificant, the interaction between distance-squared and rurality was significant ($P < .01$); however, the exponentialized parameter estimate was only 1.0000016. For the FY07–08 cohort, neither interaction term was significant.

Race/ethnicity indicators were not included in the main analyses because of the high levels of missing data for these indicators. In sensitivity analyses, we investigated whether study findings differed when including available information for race/ethnicity and indicators of missing or unknown values. Results were consistent with main study findings, with increased risk associated with rural residence (FY04–05: HR = 1.10; 95% CI = 1.03, 1.19; FY07–08: HR = 1.16; 95% CI = 1.06, 1.26).

In separate sensitivity analyses that excluded individuals living more than 800 miles from VA mental health services (primarily VA patients residing in Alaska), distance measures reached statistical significance and were associated with slightly increased risks (FY04–05: HR = 1.002; 95% CI = 1.001, 1.002; $P < .001$; FY07–08: HR = 1.001; 95% CI = 1.000, 1.002; $P = .028$). We did not observe significant interactions with rurality.

Of the 3448 suicides for the FY04–05 cohort, 3334 (96.7%) were among men and 114 (3.4%) among women. For the FY07–08 cohort, there were 3745 suicides, with 3620 suicides among men (96.7%) and 125 among women (3.3%). In each cohort, the method of suicide differed significantly by rural–urban status (χ^2 = 97.2; P < .001, in FY04–05; χ^2 = 107.1; P < .001, in FY07–08) and by gender (χ^2 = 69.8; P < .001, in FY04–05; χ^2 = 110.1; P < .001, in FY07–08). Among male suicide decedents, method of suicide differed significantly by rural–urban status (χ^2 = 89.1; P < .001, in FY04–05; χ^2 = 84.4; P < .001, in FY07–08). Among female suicide decedents, we did not observe significant differences in method of suicide by rural–urban status.

Figure 1 shows percentage of categories of suicide methods for the FY07–08 cohort, by rurality and gender. Firearms were the most common method of suicide (68% of all suicides). Firearms were more common in rural than in urban areas (77% vs 61%). Firearm use was most common among male suicide decedents in rural areas (77%) and least common among urban women (35%). Poisoning was substantially more common among female suicide decedents (46%) than among male suicide decedents (13%). For both male and female suicide decedents, the percentage of suicides by firearms was greater in rural than in urban areas. Similar trends were observed for the FY04–05 cohort.

DISCUSSION

VA users were more likely than the general population to live in rural areas, with 35% or more VA users residing in rural areas during the study period. In

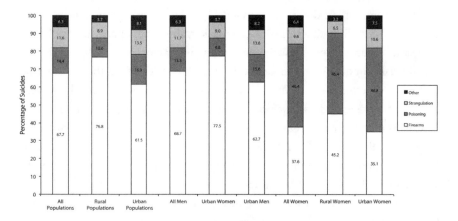

Figure 1. Percentage of Suicides among Veteran Affairs patients, by rurality, gender, and mechanism: fiscal years 2007-2008.

2 large national cohorts of individuals receiving services in the VA, residence in rural areas was associated with higher suicide rates and increased suicide risks after adjusting for important individual and contextual factors. Furthermore, rural individuals who died from suicide were more likely than urban decedents to die from firearms. Rural–urban differentials in rates and risks were fairly consistent between FY04–05 and FY07–08.

Study findings were consistent with recent studies that indicated greater suicide risks among individuals in rural settings.[9-13] This study contributed to the literature because it was specific to the entire patient population of the largest integrated health system in the United States, which provides care to a patient population that is at elevated risk for suicide,[21] and it included important demographic, clinical, and health system measures.

Moreover, although considerable previous work documented that greater distance to health system providers was associated with decreased health services utilization volume and continuity of care,[25] in this study, distance measures were not appreciably related to suicide risks. This finding suggested that elevated suicide risks observed among rural populations might have little to do with health system accessibility barriers and much to do with endemic contextual factors. Thus, this study demonstrated the need to better understand the nature of rurality as it relates to suicide risks, separate from its frequent association with decreased health system geographic accessibility.

Future studies should consider contextual factors that might underlie the observed rural–urban differentials in suicide risks.[14] For example, there might be unmeasured differences in socioeconomic status across patients residing in rural and urban settings.[35] Social environmental factors were associated with suicide risks among VA mental health patients.[36] Clearly, further research is needed to better understand rural–urban differences in health service treatment seeking and the sociocultural factors relating to suicide mortality.

Consistent with previous analyses,[26] method of suicide differed substantially by gender. Furthermore, rural residence was associated with greater use of firearms among suicide decedents, overall and for both genders. Firearm suicide mortality is a significant public health problem in rural areas.[37] Firearm ownership is greater in rural areas, and greater state-level firearm ownership has been associated with greater firearm suicide mortality.[27] Among suicide methods, firearms sadly have the highest case-fatality rates.[26] As Miller and Hemenway noted, "A suicide attempt with a firearm rarely affords a second chance."[38] Thus, greater access to lethal means may in part explain rural–urban differences in suicide mortality. This relationship suggests the importance of gun safety efforts and firearm awareness as part of suicide prevention efforts.

Public health and health care innovations are needed to address the elevated suicide risks in rural areas. The VA has pioneered health system suicide prevention initiatives, including 24-hour and web-based suicide prevention crisis lines (1-800-273-TALK), ongoing national monitoring, and support for development of suicide prevention programs.[16] Study findings suggested the importance of outreach efforts to enhance suicide prevention in rural settings, including access to mobile crisis teams and telehealth services. Health systems should seek to facilitate outreach, services integration, and access to emergency care services in rural settings.

Finally, the study findings had implications for future efforts to examine the suicide risks associated with veteran status. Increased risks among rural VA patients might result from unmeasured factors associated with rural residence.[14] Because veterans are disproportionately represented in rural settings and rurality is associated with increased suicide risk, studies examining the influence of veterans status on suicide mortality[18] should include adjustment for rural residence. In the absence of such adjustment, risks that are related to rurality might be misinterpreted as related to veteran status.

This large national multiyear study had several limitations. First, it was not possible to include some patient factors that might be related to suicide and might differ by rural–urban status, including patient income, race/ethnicity, and marital status. Second, it was not feasible to account for residential mobility among VA patients. Consequently, for patients with residential moves during the observation period, this might introduce measurement error in assessing distance to nearest VA mental health provider. Residential moves among VA patients were more common among individuals with psychiatric conditions that were associated with increased suicide mortality.[39] Finally, we noted that the recording of suicide deaths by medical examiners might differ systematically across rural and urban areas. Previous work suggested rural–urban variation in the prevalence of deaths of undetermined intent, and this might indicate measurement error in the identification of suicide deaths.[40]

Despite these limitations, the study findings provided substantial timely and important information regarding rural–urban differences in suicide rates, risks, and methods among the population of individuals receiving health care services in the US Department of Veterans Affairs health system. These findings supported continuing development of health care policy and health services and suicide prevention initiatives to address the suicide risks of veterans, with focused attention on rural settings.

ABOUT THE AUTHORS

All of the authors are with the Department of Veterans Affairs (VA), Office of Mental Health Operations, Serious Mental Illness Treatment Resource and Evaluation Center (SMITREC), Ann Arbor, MI.

CONTRIBUTORS

All authors contributed to developing the study design and analytic plan. R. V. Ignacio and K. L. Austin executed the analyses. J. F. McCarthy and M. Valenstein interpreted and contextualized the findings and wrote the article. All authors approved the article and take responsibility for the accuracy of the analyses.

ACKNOWLEDGMENTS

This study was funded by the VA Office of Mental Health Services.

We acknowledge and thank Ira R. Katz, MD, PhD, Senior Consultant, VA Office of Mental Health Operations, for comments regarding study design and presentation.

HUMAN PARTICIPANT PROTECTION

This study was approved by the Ann Arbor VA Medical Center Institutional Review Board.

REFERENCES

1. Institute of Medicine. *Reducing Suicide: A National Imperative*. Washington, DC: National Academies Press; 2004.

2. US Department of Health and Human Services. *The Surgeon General's Call to Action to Prevent Suicide*. Washington, DC: National Institutes of Health; 1999.

3. Agha Z, Lofgren RP, VanRuiswyk JV, Layde PM. Are patients at Veterans Affairs medical centers sicker? *Arch Intern Med.* 2000;160(21):3252–3257.

4. Ilgen MA, Bohnert ASBB, Ignacio RV, McCarthy JF, Valenstein MM, Kim HM, et al. Psychiatric diagnoses and risk of suicide in Veterans. *Arch Gen Psychiatry.* 2010;67(11):1152–1158.

5. Lambert MT, Fowler DR. Suicide risk factors among veterans: risk management in the changing culture of the Department of Veterans Affairs. *J Ment Health Adm.* 1997;24(3):350–358.

6. Hawthorne K. Statement to the Senate Committee on Veterans' Affairs. February, 26, 2009. Available at: http://veterans.senate.gov/ hearings.cfm?action=release.display&release_id=7fd5424b-eac7-4fd3-8e84- dda1a89daf80. Accessed January 1, 2011.

7. US Census Bureau. Geographic Comparison Table: United States–Urban/Rural and Inside/Outside Metropolitan Area. Available at: http://factfinder.census.gov/servlet/ GCTTable?_bm=y&-geo_id=01000US&-_box_head_nbr=GCT-P1&- ds_name=DEC_2000_SF1_U&-format=US-1. Accessed January 18, 2011.

8. Kane T. Who are the recruits? The demographic characteristics of U.S. military enlistment, 2003–2005. CDA06-09. Washington, DC: The Heritage Foundation.; October 26, 2006.

9. Kapusta ND, Zorman A, Etzerdorfer E, Ponocny-Seliger E, Jandl-Jager E, Sonneck G. Rural-urban differences in Austrian suicides. *Soc Psychiatric Psych Epidemiol.* 2008;43:311–318.

10. Singh GK, Siahpush M. Increasing rural-urban gradients in US suicide mortality, 1970-1997. *Am J Public Health.* 2002;92(7):1161–1167.

11. Levin KA, Leyland AH. Urban/rural inequalities in suicide in Scotland, 1981-1999. *Soc Sci Med.* 2005;60:2877–2890.

12. Middleton N, Gunnell D, Frankel S, Whitley E, Dorling D. Urban-rural differences in suicide trends in young adults: England and Wales, 1981-1998. *Soc Sci Med.* 2003;57:1183–1194.

13. Razvodovsky Y, Stickley A. Suicide in urban and rural regions of Belarus, 1990-2005. *Public Health.* 2009;123(1):27–31.

14. Hirsch JK. A review of the literature on rural suicide: risk and protective factors, incidence and prevention. *Crisis.* 2006;27(4):189–199.

15. Hoyt DR, Conger RD, Valde JG, Weihs K. Psychological distress and help seeking in rural America. *Am J Community Psychol.* 1997;25(4):449–470.

16. Bossarte R, Claassen CA, Knox K. Veteran suicide prevention: emerging priorities and opportunities for intervention. *Mil Med.* 2010;175(7):461–462.

17. Bruce ML. Suicide risk and prevention in veteran populations. *Ann N Y Acad Sci.* 2010;1208:98–103.

18. Kang HK, Bullman TA. Is there an epidemic of suicides among current and former U.S. military personnel? *Ann Epidemiol.* 2009;19(10):757–760.

19. Kaplan MS, Huguet N, McFarland BH, Newsom JT. Suicide among male veterans: a prospective population-based study. *J Epidemiol :Community Health.* 2007;61(7):619–624.

20. Miller M, Barber C, Azrael D, Calle EE, Lawler E, Mukamal KJ. Suicide among US Veterans: a prospective study of 500,000 middle-aged and elderly men. *Am J Epidemiol.* 2009;170:494–500.

21. McCarthy JF, Valenstein M, Kim HM, Ilgen M, Zivin K, Blow FC. Suicide mortality among patients receiving care in the Veterans Health Administration health system. *Am J Epidemiol.* 2009;169:1033–1038.

22. Department of Veterans Affairs. Fact Sheet 164–10: National Income Thresholds. Available at: http://www.va.gov/healtheligibility/Library/pubs/VAIncomeThresholds/VAIncomeThresholds.pdf. Accessed July 4, 2011.

23. Weeks WB, Kazis LE, Shen Y, et al. Differences in health-related quality of life in rural and urban veterans. *Am J Public Health.* 2004;94:1762–1767.

24. West A, Weeks WB. Physical and mental health and access to care among nonmetropolitan Veterans Health Administration patients younger than 65 years. *J Rural Health.* 2006;22(1):9–16.

25. McCarthy JF, Blow FC, Valenstein M, et al. Veterans Affairs Health System and mental health treatment retention among patients with serious mental illness: evaluating accessibility and availability barriers. *Health Serv Res.* 2007;42(3 Pt 1):1042–1060.

26. Centers for Disease Control and Prevention. Case Fatality Rate Among Persons Age 10 and Older, by Mechanism, United States, 2002-2006. Available at: http://www.cdc.gov/violenceprevention/suicide/statistics/case_fatality.html. Accessed January 28, 2011.

27. Price JH, Mrdjenovich AJ, Dake JA. Prevalence of state firearm mortality and mental health care resources. *J Community Health*. 2009;34:383–391.

28. Kaplan MS, McFarland BH, Huguet N. Firearm suicide among vterans in the general population: findings from the National Violent Death Reporting System. *J Trauma*. 2009;67(3):503–507.

29. Cowper DC, Kubal JD, Maynard C, Hynes DM. A primer and comparative review of major US mortality databases. *Ann Epidemiol*. 2002;12(7):462–468.

30. Sohn MW, Arnold N, Maynard C, Hynes DM. Accuracy and completeness of mortality data in the Department of Veterans Affairs. *Popul Health Metr*. 2006;4:2.

31. *International Classification of Diseases, Ninth Revision, Clinical Modification.* Hyattsville, Md: National Center for Health Statistics; 1980.

32. McCarthy JF, Blow FC. Older patients with serious mental illness: sensitivity to distance barriers for outpatient care. *Med Care*. 2004;42(11):1073–1080.

33. International Classification of Diseases. *10th Revision*. Geneva, Switzerland: World Health Organization; 1994.

34. Centers for Disease Control and Prevention. Percentage of Suicides Among Persons Ages 10 Years and Older, by Sex and Mechanism, United States, 2002-2006. Available at: http://www.cdc.gov/violenceprevention/suicide/statistics/mechanism01.html. Accessed July 4, 2011.

35. Page A, Morrell S, Taylor R, Dudley M, Carter G. Further increases in rural suicide among Australian adults: secular trends, 1979-2003. *Soc Sci Med*. 2007;65:442–453.

36. Desai RA, Dausey DJ, Rosenheck RA. Mental health service delivery and suicide risk: The role of individual patient and facility factors. *Am J Psychiatry*. 2005;162(2):311–318.

37. Branas CC, Nance ML, Elliott MR, Richmond TS, Schwab W. Urban-rural shifts in intentional firearm death: different causes, same results. *Am J Public Health*. 2004;94(10):1750–1755.

38. Miller M, Hemenway D. Guns and suicide in the United States. *N Engl J Med.* 2008;359(10):989–991.

39. McCarthy JF, Valenstein M, Blow FC. Residential mobility among patients in the VA health system: associations with psychiatric morbidity, geographic accessibility, and continuity of care. *Adm Policy Ment Health.* 2007;34(5):448–455.

40. Saunderson T, Haynes R, Langford IH. Urban-rural variations in suicides and undetermined deaths in England and Wales. *J Public Health Med.* 1998;20:261–267.

30

The Role of Pain, Functioning, and Mental Health in Suicidality Among Veterans Affairs Primary Care Patients

Kathryn M. Magruder, PhD, MPH, Derik Yeager, MBS, and Olga Brawman-Mintzer, MD

Objectives. We examined suicidality, pain, functioning, and psychiatric disorders among veterans in primary care by using both self-report and clinical measures of pain and mental health to determine correlates that might be clinically useful in primary care settings.

Methods. Data were from 884 Veterans Affairs patients enrolled in a regional 4-site cross-sectional study. Patients were administered measures that assessed functioning (including pain) and psychiatric disorders. Data were merged with medical records for clinical pain indicators.

Results. Overall, 9.1% (74 of 816) of patients indicated suicidal ideation, with those who were middle-aged, unemployed because of disability, had less than college education, and served in a warzone most likely to consider suicidality. Suicidal patients had worse functioning (measured by the Short Form-36) than did nonsuicidal patients in every domain, including bodily pain, and were more likely to meet criteria for a psychiatric diagnosis. However, when pain and mental health were jointly considered, only mental health (both psychiatric diagnosis and mental health functioning) was related to suicidality.

Conclusions. Although providers should be alert to the possibility of suicidality in patients with pain, they should be vigilant when patients have a psychiatric disorder or poor mental health.

Military veterans are more likely to commit suicide than nonveterans. Based on a large, nationally representative sample (n = 320 890), a recent publication reported that military veterans were twice as likely to commit suicide as nonveterans.[1] Chronic pain and depression—2 conditions not uncommon in Veterans Affairs (VA) medical settings—are leading contributing factors in deaths by suicide. A systematic literature review of pain and suicide, suicide attempts, and suicidal ideation revealed that patients with chronic pain had a 2-fold risk of death by suicide, a 14% prevalence of suicide attempts (compared with 5% without chronic pain), and a 20% prevalence of suicidal ideation.[2] The relationship between depression, as well as other psychiatric disorders, and suicidality is well established.[3-5] Older age and male gender are also highly related to suicide,[6] as are lower socioeconomic status[7,8] and unemployment[8]—all being predominant characteristics of the VA patient population.

In a study that analyzed data from the National Comorbidity Survey Replication sample, suicidal thoughts and behaviors were associated with self-reported medical conditions presumed to accompany pain (e.g., arthritis or rheumatism, chronic back or neck problems).[9] After controlling for mood and anxiety disorders, this association with pain-related conditions persisted for lifetime measures of suicidality (suicidal ideation, plan, or attempt); however, for current measures of suicidality, it only persisted for those who reported a suicide attempt. In a large study of VA service users, self-reported severe pain was predictive of subsequent suicide, even after controlling for physician-diagnosed psychiatric comorbidity.[10] Of note, this study used a single question from the Short Form-36 (SF-36) to measure pain severity.[11]

Although mental health settings are most often associated with detection and management of suicidal patients, primary care can potentially play an important part. Luoma et al. [12] found that 45% of those who committed suicide had contact with a primary care provider (PCP) in the month before suicide, thus highlighting the importance of PCPs in identifying and intervening with the 2% to 3% of primary care patients who display suicidal ideation.[6] The fact that pain is also very common in primary care patients and is one of the main reasons for seeking medical care[13,14] is further argument for including primary care clinics in planning for effective suicide prevention programs.

Interestingly, in the studies reviewed there was little attention given to functioning associated with pain. It might be that the functional limitations imposed by pain—as much as pain itself—might cause individuals to turn their thoughts to self-destruction. Furthermore, there was little attention to the relationship between pain and psychiatric distress (e.g., pain might cause symptoms of depression, and depression might exacerbate the sense of pain). Thus, our overall objective was to examine suicidality, pain, functioning, and psychiatric disorders among veterans in primary care, determining meaningful correlates that might prove to be clinically useful, especially in primary care settings.

METHODS

We used an existing dataset that was established from a random sample of primary care patients (consent rate 74%) drawn from 4 VA hospitals in 2 Southeast states. The parent study was approved by the institutional review boards of the 4 sites; our study was approved by the institutional review boards of the Medical University of South Carolina. The sampling and methods were described extensively in previous publications[5,15,16]; however, we provide a brief overview here. There were 1076 consenting patients (randomly sampled from the primary care rolls of 4 Veterans Integrated Service Network hospitals with an oversampling of women) for whom sociodemographic information and functioning status (SF-36) were collected at a primary care visit. Records of patients who completed the clinic interview were sent to Charleston, South Carolina, where trained clinicians contacted them via telephone for a longer interview, which included the Clinician Administered PTSD Scale (CAPS), considered the diagnostic "gold standard" for posttraumatic stress disorder (PTSD),[17] and the Mini International Neuropsychiatric Interview (MINI version 5.0.0)[18,19] to assess for mental and substance use disorders (*Diagnostic and Statistical Manual of Mental Disorders, Fourth Edition [DSM-IV]*[20] and *International Classification of Diseases-10 [ICD-10]* criteria[21]). The MINI also has a 6-item module that assesses suicidality and suggests a level of current suicide risk as low, moderate, or high. Using the electronic medical record, these data were merged with *ICD-9*[22] diagnoses. The medical record data covered the 12 months before and after the index clinic visit (a total of 24 months).

The dataset is unique in that all patients (not just those who screened positive) were administered the suicidality assessment as well as diagnostic instruments for common psychiatric disorders that include major depression or dysthymia, generalized anxiety disorder (GAD), PTSD, and substance use disorders (SUDs). Additionally, because the sample was drawn from active patient rolls, it did not overrepresent high utilizing patients.

The analytic dataset included all patients for whom we had suicidality (from the MINI), functional status, and psychiatric research diagnoses (from the MINI and CAPS). This resulted in data for 816 patients (82% of consenters).

We focused on the following variables: suicidality based on the MINI, psychiatric diagnoses based on the MINI, PTSD based on the CAPS, functioning status based on the SF-36 (including self-reported bodily pain based on the SF-36), pain conditions based on *ICD-9* codes, and overall medical morbidity based on the Charlson Comorbidity Index (CCI).

Variables

Sociodemographic variables.
Self-reported age, race, gender, educational attainment, employment status, warzone military service, and primary war era of service were collected at the time of the in-person interview.

Functioning variables.
All functioning variables were derived from the SF-36 Medical Outcomes Study (MOS) 36-Item Short-Form Health Survey, which was administered at the time of the in-person interview. The SF-36 is a self-reported, generic measure of functional health status that assesses 2 factors of analytically derived dimensions (physical health and mental health) with multiple subscales: physical functioning, role functioning limited by health, energy and fatigue, pain, general health, role functioning limited by emotional problems, emotional well-being, and social functioning.[23] The SF-36 discriminates severity of functional impairment across a variety of disease states, such as hypertension, arthritis, gastrointestinal disorders, myocardial infarction[24,25] and even PTSD.[26] The SF-36 raw scores were transformed to a 0 to 100 scale according to the formulas for scoring and transforming in the SF-36 Health Survey manual.[27]

Psychiatric diagnosis variables.
All psychiatric diagnoses were derived from MINI with the exception of PTSD, which was assessed by the CAPS. Our broad definition of major depressive disorder (MDD) could be satisfied by the presence of either MDD or

dysthymia. We also investigated GAD and SUDs to explore the relationship between these diagnoses and suicidal ideation.

The MINI (version 5.0.0) is comprised of closed questions (yes/no format) and measures *DSM-IV* (and *ICD-10*) mental diagnoses and conditions common in primary care. We selected the modules for: major depressive episode, dysthymia, suicidality, alcohol abuse and dependence, drug abuse and dependence, and GAD. For these modules, there were adequate to excellent psychometric properties for the selected disorders relative to the World Health Organization Composite International Diagnostic Interview (CIDI) and the Structured Clinical Interview-Patient (SCID-P).[18,19,23] With the CIDI as the gold standard, all sensitivities were $\geq$ 0.83; kappas (κ) were $\geq$ 0.73 except for GAD (0.36). Results were similar with SCID-P as the gold standard, with only current drug dependence having sensitivity of $<$ 0.50 and κ $<$ 0.50. Both inter-rater reliability (all $\geq$ 0.88) and test–retest reliability (all $\geq$ 0.78) were excellent.

Suicidality was based on MINI suicidality items. Indication of any single item suggested suicide risk, which could be classified as low, moderate, or high based on the number and pattern of affirmative responses.

The CAPS is a structured clinical interview developed at the National Center of Posttraumatic Stress Disorders in 1990 to rate the frequency and intensity of the 17 symptoms of PTSD outlined in the *DSM-IV* along with 5 associated features (guilt, dissociation, de-realization, depersonalization, and reduction in awareness of surroundings).[17,28,29] The CAPS has been shown to have strong inter-rater reliabilities (0.92–0.99) for each of the 3 PTSD symptom clusters (re-experiencing, avoidance, hyperarousal). The CAPS has a high degree of internal consistency (0.73–0.85), is highly correlated with the Mississippi Scale (0.70–0.91), Minnesota Multiphasic Personality Inventory-2 Keane PTSD subscale (0.77–0.84), and has good diagnostic utility compared with the SCID PTSD module.[28] It also has excellent correspondence with the PCL (area under the curve = 88.2%).[28] Magruder et al.[5] conducted a random sample of interviews (8%) by speaker phone to assess interrater reliability and found that raters were 100% concordant for PTSD diagnosis on the CAPS. Frequency and intensity information was collected for each of these symptoms within the context of lifetime and current (within the past month) patient experiences. Using the F1/I2 CAPS scoring rule, symptoms were coded as present if frequency was $\geq$ 1 and intensity was $\geq$ 2.[17] PTSD was established if patients satisfied *DSM-IV* criteria B, C, and D, and the duration of symptoms was more than 1 month.

Pain variables.

We measured pain in 2 different ways, self-reported bodily pain (SF-36) and pain-related medical diagnoses (ICD-9). We were particularly interested in the SF-36 subscale bodily pain, which is measured by 2 questions: "How much bodily pain have you had during the past 4 weeks?" and "During the past 4 weeks, how much did pain interfere with your normal work (including both work outside the home and housework)?" The responses to these items are normally used to create a single bodily pain variable scaled to range from 0 (poor functioning) to 100 (excellent functioning).[27] However, to understand better the involvement of both physical pain and functional impairment, we also considered the component questions of this subscale individually.

Medical comorbidity.

The CCI was used to measure medical comorbidity. The CCI is a measure of mortality risk determined from the presence or absence of specific medical comorbidities,[30] and reflects the relative burden of severe medical problems. The CCI was constructed from diagnostic information from fiscal years 2003 to 2005.

Analytic Approach

All patients were classified as being suicidal or not, and χ^2 analyses were calculated for simple comparisons of all categorical variables (sociodemographics, psychiatric diagnoses, pain diagnoses, and CCI). Generalized linear modeling was used to analyze SF-36 scales and subscales. Because many of the subscales on the SF-36 have non-normal distributions, we also ran analyses using the rank-sum test. Those variables that were statistically significant at $P < .1$ were retained for inclusion in the multivariable modeling procedures.

We made the decision to consider these remaining variables in 3 blocks: sociodemographics, psychiatric and functioning, and pain. This led to a series of logistic regression models that were then used to identify meaningful covariates and provide estimated odds ratios (ORs) for suicidality. As we developed these models, we retained variables that satisfied our criterion of $P < .1$ and tested for interaction effects among key variables. Because of their clinical relevance, we made the a priori decision to keep age, race, and gender regardless of their significance level. In the first suite of models, we analyzed only sociodemographic variables. Variables that met our criterion were retained in all subsequent models. The second suite of models included mental and physical health functioning, whereas the third suite focused on pain. The final model explored significant functioning, mental health, and pain variables derived from suites 2 and 3. The intent was to examine the effect of mental and physical health (without pain) on suicidality (suite 2), then look separately at the effect of pain (without mental and physical health variables) on suicidality (suite 3). The final model (suite 4) examined their presence together.

In each suite of statistical models, we tested interactive relationships among key independent variables through inclusion of interaction terms with the intention of preserving any significant interaction terms in all subsequent models.

RESULTS

Overall, 9.1% of patients (74 of 816) selected items indicating suicidal ideation, meaning that at least 1 of the MINI suicidality items was coded "yes"; by MINI scoring, these patients were classified as "suicide risk current." Of these, only 1 patient responded in a manner that indicated a high level of suicide risk; the remaining patients were classified as either moderate (n = 16) or low (n = 50) risk. Although the presence of suicidality was determined, suicide risk level was not available for 7 patients. We compared those at low risk with those at moderate or high risk. There were no significant differences between these groups in the sociodemographic variables and the functioning, pain, and psychiatric measures with 1 exception. There was a higher percentage of high-suicide-risk patients with PTSD than low- or moderate-risk patients (88% vs 52%). Based on these comparisons and in consideration of the small number of patients in the high and moderate risk categories (and because any level of suicide risk is clinically important), we grouped all patients with any suicide risk (n = 74) and considered them positive for suicidality.

Sociodemographic Characteristics

Table 1 shows the sociodemographic characteristics of our sample by suicidality status with simple χ^2 results based on a probability level of 0.05.

Table 1. Sociodemographic Characteristics by Suicidality: Veterans Integrated Service Network Hospitals, 1999–2001

Characteristic	Not Suicidal (n = 742), No. (%)	Suicidal (n = 74), No. (%)	χ^2 P
Age, y			.024
< 50	155 (90.1%)	17 (9.9%)	
50–64	279 (88.0%)	38 (12.0%)	
≥ 65	305 (94.1%)	19 (5.9%)	
Race			.887
White	455 (90.8%)	46 (9.2%)	
Non-White[a]	287 (91.1%)	28 (8.9%)	
Gender			.789
Male	622 (90.8%)	63 (9.2%)	
Female	119 (91.5%)	11 (8.5%)	
Education			.032
less than a high school diploma	144 (90.0%)	16 (10.0%)	
High School diploma	208 (92.0%)	18 (8.0%)	
Some college	255 (87.9%)	35 (12.1%)	
College degree or greater	135 (96.4%)	5 (3.6%)	
Employment			< .001
Working	264 (95.7%)	12 (4.4%)	
Not Working (retired)	270 (93.4%)	19 (6.6%)	
Not Working (disability)	208 (82.9%)	43 (17.1%)	
Warzone			.004
Served in warzone	321 (87.7%)	45 (12.3%)	
Did not serve in warzone	421 (93.6%)	29 (6.4%)	
War era			.35
World War II	92 (92.9%)	7 (7.1%)	
Korean War	140 (93.3%)	10 (6.7%)	
Vietnam War	431 (89.4%)	51 (10.6%)	
Persian Gulf War	79 (92.9%)	6 (7.1%)	
Site			.213
A	125 (92.6%)	10 (7.4%)	
B	175 (93.1%)	13 (6.9%)	
C	217 (91.6%)	20 (8.4%)	
D	225 (87.9%)	31 (12.1%)	

Note. HS = high school; MINI = Mini International Neuropsychiatric Interview. Suicidal was defined as any indication of suicidality by the MINI module C.
[a]93.7% of non-Whites are known to be of African American descent.

There were statistically significant differences in age (with those aged $\geq$ 65 years having the lowest prevalence of suicidality and those aged between 50 and 64 years having the highest); education (with those attaining at least a college degree having the lowest prevalence and those with some college having the highest), employment (with those not working because of disability having the highest prevalence and those working the lowest), and warzone exposure (with those exposed having a higher prevalence). There were no statistically significant differences by race, gender, war era, or site.

Functioning Status

We examined functioning status using SF-36 scores. For each of the subscales investigated (general health, mental health, vitality, physical functioning, social functioning, role physical, role emotional, and bodily pain), as well as the physical and mental health composite scores, suicidal patients had significantly worse functioning (Table 2). We also analyzed separately the 2 questions that make up the bodily pain scale, and as with the subscales, patients with suicidality were significantly worse on both. The results were unchanged after adjustments for age, gender, race, and education.

Psychiatric Diagnoses

We examined the presence of current psychiatric disorders (depression, including dysthymia; GAD; PTSD; and SUD), as measured by the MINI and CAPS (for PTSD; Table 3). In every category measured, patients meeting criteria for that disorder were much more likely to be suicidal. Not surprisingly, 79.7% of those who were suicidal were depressed compared with 17.8% of those who were not suicidal.

Pain-Related Diagnoses

We grouped patients according to whether they had an ICD-9 diagnosis related to back, chest, head, neurologic, musculoskeletal, or "other" pain (for groupings by diagnosis, see the data available as a supplement to the online version of this article at http://www.ajph.org). Suicidal patients were more likely than nonsuicidal patients to have head pain (21.6% vs 9.8%; $P = .002$) or musculoskeletal pain (78.4% vs 59.3%; $P = .001$); findings were not significant for back, neurologic, or "other" pain. Overall, 89.2% of patients

Table 2. SF-36 Functioning by Suicidality Status: Veterans Integrated Service Network Hospitals, 1999–2001

SF-36 Domain	Suicidal		Not Suicidal		Rank Sum P (unadjusted)	GLM P (adjusted)[b]
	Mean (SD)	Median	Mean (SD)	Median		
Physical functioning	43.9 (25.0)	45	61.1 (29.5)	65	.000	.000
Role: physical (continuous)	16.9 (30.4)	0	51.4 (42.4)	50	.000	.000
Role: emotional (continuous)	25.4 (34.0)	0	77.6 (37.7)	100	.000	.000
Bodily pain	35.9 (27.6)	25	60.5 (30.6)	62.5	.000	.000
Pain intensity (7 mo)[a]	3.7 (1.1)	4[a]	2.8 (1.2)	3[a]	.000	.000
Impairment due to pain (8 mo)[a]	3.5 (1.3)	4[a]	2.3 (1.4)	2[a]	.000	.000
General health (continuous)	55.3 (11.9)	55	59.1 (10.9)	60	.005	.005
Vitality	32.3 (20.6)	30	50.4 (24.8)	50	.000	.000
Social functioning (continuous)	49.2 (29.2)	45	77.9 (27.6)	90	.000	.000
Mental health (continuous)	46.1 (23.2)	48	77.5 (19.7)	84	.000	.000
Physical health (composite)	116.2 (52.8)	110	171.6 (66.2)	172	.000	.000
Mental health (composite)	152.9 (87.2)	135	283.4 (89.6)	310	.000	.000

Note. GLM = generalized linear model; SF-26 = Short Form-36.
[a]Raw score (neither reverse-scored nor transformed).
[b]Adjusted for age, race, gender, and education.

indicating suicidality received 1 or more pain diagnoses compared with 70.6% of patients with no suicidal ideation ($P = .001$; Table 4).

Charlson Comorbidity Index

As a measure of overall medical morbidity, we used ICD-9 codes to calculate a CCI for every patient. This index ranges from 0 to 2, with 0 the best and 2 the

Table 3. MINI and CAPS Psychiatric Diagnoses, by Suicidality: Veterans Integrated Service Network Hospitals, 1999-2001

	Not Suicidal (n = 742), No (%)	Suicidal (MINI module C; n = 74), No (%)	Total (n = 816), No (%)	χ^2 P
MDDbroad	132 (17.8%)	59 (79.7%)	191 (23.4%)	<.001
GAD	65 (8.8%)	33 (44.6%)	98 (12.0%)	<.001
PTSD[a]	54 (7.3%)	44 (59.5%)	98 (12.0%)	<.01
SUD	20 (2.7%)	7 (9.5%)	27 (3.3%)	.002
Any	185 (24.8%)	65 (87.8%)	249 (30.5%)	<.001

Note. CAPS = Clinician Administered PTSD Scale; GAD = generalized anxiety disorder; MDD = major depressive disorder; MINI = Mini International Neuropsychiatric Interview; PTSD = posttraumatic stress disorder; SUD = substance use disorder.
[a]CAPS diagnosis.

Table 4. Pain Diagnoses, by Suicidality Status: Veterans Integrated Service Network Hospitals, 1999-2001

Diagnosis	Not Suicidal (n = 742), No (%)	Suicidal (MINI module C; n = 74), No (%)	Total (n = 816), No (%)	χ^2 P
Back pain	173 (23.3%)	23 (31.1%)	196 (24.0%)	.136
Chest pain	97 (13.1)%	11 (14.9)%	108 (13.2%)	.664
Head pain	73 (9.8%)	16 (21.6%)	89 (10.9%)	.002
Neurologic pain	59 (8.0%)	9 (12.2%)	68 (8.3%)	.211
Musculoskeletal pain	440 (59.3%)	58 (78.4%)	498 (61.0%)	.001
Other pain types	82 (11.1%)	8 (10.8%)	90 (11.0%)	.950
Any pain	524 (70.6%)	66 (89.2%)	590 (72.3%)	.001

worst. There were no statistically significant differences between CCI distribution for suicidal versus nonsuicidal patients (Table 5); therefore, CCI was not included in multivariable analyses.

Table 5. Charlson Comorbidity Index by Suicidality: Veterans Integrated Service Network Hospitals, 1999–2001

	Not Suicidal (n = 742), No (%)	Suicidal (MINI module C; n = 74), No (%)	Total (n = 816), No (%)	χ^2 P
Charlson Index				.385
0	261 (35.2%)	32 (43.2%)	293 (35.9%)	
1	197 (26.6%)	17 (23.0%)	214 (26.2%)	
2	284 (38.3%)	25 (33.8%)	309 (37.9%)	
Total	742 (100%)	74 (100%)	816 (100%)	

Multivariable Analyses

Suite 1: Sociodemographics.

In our first analytic suite (Table 6) we explored the influence of socio-demographic variables on suicidality. ORs (adjusted for gender, race, education, employment, and warzone service) revealed that both middle-aged patients (50–64 years old; OR 2.42; 95% confidence interval [CI] = 1.22, 4.78) and younger patients (< 50 years old; OR 3.35; 95% CI = 1.34, 8.36) were more likely to indicate suicidality than were older patients (> 65 years). Patients with a college degree or greater were less likely to report suicidality than were patients with less than a college degree (OR 0.37; 95% CI = 0.14, 0.97). Patients who were either retired (OR 0.45 95% CI = 0.23, 0.90) or working (OR 0.19 [95% CI = 0.10, 0.39) were less likely to report suicidality than were patients who were not working because of disability. Patients who reported exposure to warzone military service were more likely to indicate suicidality than were unexposed patients (OR 3.00; 95% CI = 1.68, 5.29). Although patients indicating suicidality were more likely to be White, male, and not married, these differences were not significant in this suite. No significant interaction effects were found among the key variables in this model.

Suite 2: Sociodemographics, functioning, and psychiatric diagnoses.

In our first model, we used statistically significant and clinically relevant sociodemographic covariates as control variables in the presence of the 2 composite functioning scales. Only the mental health composite was statistically significant (OR 0.99; 95% CI = 0.99, 0.99). In our second model

Table 6. Odds of Suicidality From Multivariable Modeling, by Suite: Veterans Integrated Service Network Hospitals, 1999–2001

	Suite 1, OR (95% CI)	Suite 2, OR (95% CI)	Suite 3, OR (95% CI)	Suite 4, OR (95% CI)
Sociodemographics				
Age				
Middle vs older aged	2.42 (1.22, 4.78)	0.70 (0.30, 1.62)	1.70 (0.83, 3.46)	0.79 (0.35, 1.79)
Younger vs older aged	3.35 (1.34, 8.36)	0.72 (0.24, 2.16)	1.96 (0.75, 5.09)	0.72 (0.25, 2.10)
Race	1.31 (0.76, 2.26)	1.87 (0.95, 3.67)	1.56 (0.88, 2.77)	1.78 (0.94, 3.37)
Gender	0.85 (0.38, 1.90)	1.14 (0.44, 3.00)	1.18 (0.51, 2.76)	1.58 (0.63, 3.97)
Warzone	3.00 (1.68, 5.29)	1.47 (0.70, 3.07)	2.72 (1.50, 4.95)	1.92 (0.98, 3.76)
Employment				
Retired vs disabled	0.45 (0.23, 0.90)	0.56 (0.25, 1.25)	0.55 (0.27, 1.13)	0.64 (0.29, 1.39)
Working vs disabled	0.19 (0.10, 0.39)	0.50 (0.22, 1.13)	0.33 (0.16, 0.69)	0.43 (0.19, 0.95)
Marital status				
LWS vs single	1.80 (0.59, 5.45)	Dropped	Dropped	Dropped
SDW vs single	1.73 (0.54, 5.53)	Dropped	Dropped	Dropped
College education	0.37 (0.14, 0.97)	0.48 (0.17, 1.40)	0.43 (0.16, 1.16)	0.46 (0.16, 1.30)
Pain, functioning, and mental health				
SF-36 composite scores				
Physical health		Dropped		Dropped
Mental health		0.99 (0.99, 0.99)		0.99 (0.99, 0.99)
ICD-9 psychiatric diagnoses				
MDDb		4.40 (1.87, 10.36)		...[a]
GAD		2.13 (1.07, 4.23)		...[a]
PTSD		4.02 (1.95, 8.29)		...[a]
Any				7.58 (3.32, 17.31)

(continued on next page)

Table 6. (*continued*)

	Suite 1, OR (95% CI)	Suite 2, OR (95% CI)	Suite 3, OR (95% CI)	Suite 4, OR (95% CI)
SF-36 pain				
Severity (item 7)			Dropped	Dropped
Impairment (item 8)			1.44 (1.17, 1.77)	0.82 (0.62, 1.08)
Bodily pain			Dropped	Dropped
ICD-9 pain diagnoses				
Back pain			Dropped	Dropped
Chest pain			Dropped	Dropped
Head pain			1.83 (0.90, 3.71)	1.86 (0.84, 4.12)
Neurologic pain			Dropped	Dropped
Musculoskeletal pain			1.69 (0.90, 3.19)	1.95 (0.97, 3.91)
Other pain types			Dropped	Dropped

Note. GAD = generalized anxiety disorder; *ICD-9* = *International Classification of Diseases-9*; LWS = living with someone; MDDb = major despressive disorder broad definition (includes dysthymia); PTSD = posttraumatic stress disorder; SF-36 = Short Form 36; SUD = substance use disorder; SDW = separated, divorced, or widowed,

[a]Psychiatric diagnoses were collapsed into a single variable indicating the presence of any psychiatric diagnosis; this was done due to collinearity in the model.

(Table 6), we examined psychiatric diagnoses in the presence of the previously specified sociodemographic variables. Major depression (or dysthymia; OR 4.40; 95% CI = 1.87, 10.36), GAD (OR 2.13; 95% CI = 1.07, 4.23), and PTSD (OR 4.02; 95% CI = 1.95, 8.29) were related to suicidality. SUDs were not. In a combined model with both mental health composite score and psychiatric diagnoses (major depression, GAD, PTSD) each remained significant; there were no interactions. To simplify subsequent analyses and reduce the potential for collinearity, we created a variable indicating the presence of any psychiatric disorder. No significant interaction effects were found among the key variables in this model.

Suite 3: Sociodemographics and pain.

The first model in suite 3 (Table 6) examined the SF-36 bodily pain subscale in the presence of the sociodemographic covariates. This subscale was highly significant (OR 0.98; 95% CI = 0.97, 0.99). We then divided this subscale into its 2 component questions (pain severity and impairment because of pain), and only pain impairment was significant (OR 1.44; 95% CI = 1.17, 1.77). The next model tested sociodemographics and *ICD-9* pain categories and showed that musculoskeletal pain (OR 1.69; 95% CI = 0.90, 3.19) and head pain (OR 1.83; 95% CI = 0.90, 3.71) were related to suicidality. The final model in suite 3 combined sociodemographics, pain impairment, head pain, and musculoskeletal pain; all continued to reach our threshold (P < .10) for inclusion in subsequent models. No significant interaction effects were found among the key variables in this model.

Suite 4: Sociodemographics, functioning, psychiatric diagnoses, and pain.

In our final model (Table 6), we included our sociodemographic covariates as well as mental health functioning, the presence of any psychiatric diagnoses (major depression, dysthymia, GAD, PTSD, or SUD), pain impairment, and head and musculoskeletal pain. Only mental health functioning (OR 0.99; 95% CI = 0.99, 0.99) and psychiatric disorders OR 7.58; 95% CI = 3.32, 17.31) remained significant. No significant interaction effects were found among the key variables in this model.

DISCUSSION

Our findings indicated that VA patients reporting symptoms of suicidality had significantly different sociodemographic characteristics and clinical characteristics than nonsuicidal patients. Although many of our findings were not unexpected (e.g., high prevalence of psychiatric disorders among suicidal patients), some were new. In contrast to other published reports, we found that middle-aged veterans had the highest percentage of suicidal patients and elder patients the lowest. This might be a cohort-related phenomenon related to service era, or it might reflect variations in how VA accepts veterans for care over time. Nonetheless, it was clearly related to mental health because age-related findings became nonsignificant in the presence of psychiatric disorders. We expected to find higher rates of psychiatric problems and pain among suicidal patients; interestingly, the 2 are not often measured simultaneously. Furthermore, we incorporated both self-reported measures of pain and mental health (with the SF-36 scales), as well as independent measures (psychiatric diagnoses and *ICD-9* diagnoses associated with pain). Both methods were independently important in the separate models (suites 2 and 3) for defining a relationship with suicidality. However, when mental health and pain were considered jointly, pain—regardless of how measured—was no longer related to suicidality, but mental health (both presence of diagnoses as well as self-reported mental health functioning) was highly related. Thus, although PCPs should be alert to the possibility of suicidality in patients with chronic pain, they should be even more vigilant with their patients who have a psychiatric disorder, not only depression but also anxiety symptomatology, or importantly, poor mental health functioning.

Our study had a number of strengths, including the large random sample from primary care settings drawn from 4 regional hospitals, the use of both clinician and patient measures of pain, and the use of research-based psychiatric diagnoses to provide a consistent mental health assessment. Nevertheless, the study was limited in that it was cross-sectional; thus, we could only discuss association rather than causality. Additionally, we had only a regional sample of VA patients. We also measured suicidality and not suicide itself; however, suicidality was a clear risk factor for suicide that warrants clinical attention.

Our results had several policy implications. Presently, the US Preventive Services Task Force recommends neither for nor against screening for suicide in primary care; however, the VA might consider a different policy based on the higher prevalence of suicidality and suicide in veterans, unique patient characteristics, and more available and integrated mental health services. Pain-related diagnoses and pain functioning emerged as important factors related to suicidality, although that association did not persist in the presence of mental health problems. Nevertheless, Veterans Health Administration should strongly consider targeted screening for patients with pain-related diagnoses (particularly musculoskeletal and head pain). Suicide screening in pain clinics could be easily implemented, especially because many pain clinics already include behavioralists on the treatment team. Additionally, self-reported pain was related to suicidality, with pain-related functioning being more important than pain severity. Thus, providers should be careful to ask about pain-related functioning limitations. Presently, suicide screening in VA primary care clinics only occurs in the context of a positive mental health screening for either depression or PTSD. Because 20.2% of our suicidal patients did not meet criteria for depression or PTSD, the Veterans Health Administration should consider additional methods to identify these at-risk patients, which could include veterans reporting pain, veterans with pain-related diagnoses, or general screening in primary care.

ABOUT THE AUTHORS

Kathryn M. Magruder is with the Mental Health Service Line, Ralph H. Johnson VA Medical Center, Charleston, SC, and the Department of Psychiatry and Behavioral Sciences, Military Science Division, Department of Medicine, Biostatistics and Epidemiology Division, The Medical University of South Carolina, Charleston. Derik Yeager is with the Department of Psychiatry and Behavioral Sciences, Military Science Division, The Medical University of South Carolina, Charleston. Olga Brawman-Mintzer is with the Mental Health Service Line, Ralph H. Johnson VA Medical Center, Charleston, and the Department of Psychiatry and Behavioral Sciences, The Medical University of South Carolina, Charleston.

CONTRIBUTORS

K. M. Magruder and D. Yeager developed the statistical approach and conducted all statistical analyses. O. Brawman-Mintzer provided clinical guidance and interpretation of all clinical outcomes. All authors participated in the original conceptualization, collection, and compilation of background literature and synthesis of data; writing; and providing comments and corrections to various iterations of the article over time.

ACKNOWLEDGMENTS

This article is based upon work supported by the Department of Veterans Affairs, Veterans Health Administration, Office of Research and Development, Health Services Research and Development (VCR 99-010-2 and SHP 08-160).

Special thanks to our biostatistician, Rebecca Knapp, PhD, who helped address and answer specific statistical concerns brought up during the review process.

Note: The views expressed in this article are those of the authors and do not necessarily reflect the position or policy of the Department of Veteran Affairs or the US Government.

HUMAN PARTICIPANT PROTECTION

The present study was approved by the institutional review board of the Medical University of South Carolina.

REFERENCES

1. Kaplan MS, Huguet N, McFarland B, Newsom JT. Suicide among male veterans: a prospective population-based study. *J Epidemiol Community Health*. 2007;61:619–624.

2. Tang NK, Crane C. Suicidality in chronic pain: a review of the prevalence, risk factors and psychological links. *Psychol Med*. 2006;36(5):575–586.

3. Angst J, Angst F, Stassen HH. Suicide risk in patients with major depressive disorder. *J Clin Psychiatry*. 1999;60(suppl 2):57–62.

4. Ilgen MA, Bohnert AS, Ignacio RV, McCarthy JF, Valenstein MM, Kim HM, et al. Psychiatric diagnoses and risk of suicide in veterans. *Arch Gen Psychiatry*. 2010;67(11):1152–1158.

5. Magruder KM, Frueh BC, Knapp RG, et al. Prevalence of posttraumatic stress disorder in Veterans Affairs primary care clinics. *Gen Hosp Psychiatry.* 2005;27(3):169–179.

6. Gaynes BN, West SL, Ford CA, et al. Screening for suicide risk in adults: a summary of the evidence for the U.S. Preventive Services Task Force. *Ann Intern Med.* 2004;140(10):822–835.

7. Lorant V, Kunst AE, Huisman M, Costa G, Mackenbach J, EU Working Group on Socio-Economic Inequalities in Health. Socio-economic inequalities in suicide: a European comparative study. *Br J Psychiatry.* 2005;187:49–54.

8. Lewis G, Slogett A. Suicide, deprivation, and unemployment: record linkage study. *BMJ.* 1998;317:1283–1286.

9. Braden JB, Sullivan M. Suicidal thoughts and behavior among adults with self-reported pain conditions in the National Comorbidity Survey Replicaton. *J Pain.* 2008;9(12):1106–1115.

10. Ilgen MA, Zivin K, Austin K, et al. Severe pain predicts greater likelihood of subsequent suicide. *Suicide Life Threat Behav.* 2010;40(6):597–608.

11. Ware J Jr, Kosinski M, Keller SD. A 12-item short form health survey: construction of scales and preliminary tests of reliability and validity. *Med Care.* 1996;34:220–233.

12. Luoma JB, Martin CE, Pearson JL. Contact with mental health and primary care providers before suicide: a review of the evidence. *Am J Psychiatry.* 2002;159:909–916.

13. Smith BH, Hopton JL, Chambers WA. Chronic pain in primary care. *Fam Pract.* 1999;16:475–482.

14. Foley K. Dismantling the barriers: providing palliative and pain care. *JAMA.* 2000;283(1):115.

15. Magruder KM, Yeager DE, Knapp RG, Robinson RL. Is pain related to under-diagnosis of depression among primary care patients? Presented at: Institute on Psychiatric Services Meeting; October 11-14, 2007; New Orleans, LA.

16. Magruder KM, Yeager DE. Patient factors relating to detection of posttraumatic stress disorder in Department of Veterans Affairs primary care settings. *J Rehabil Res Dev.* 2008;45(3):371–381.

17. Blake DD, Weathers FW, Nagy LN, et al. A clinician rating scale for assessing current and lifetime PTSD: The CAPS-1. *Behav Therapist.* 1990;18:187–188.

18. Sheehan D, Lecrubier Y, Sheehan KH, Janavs J, Weiller E, Keskiner A, et al. The validity of the Mini International Neurospychiatric Interview (MINI) according to the SCID-P and its reliability. *Eur Psychiatry.* 1997;12:232–241.

19. Lecrubier Y, Sheehan DV, Weiller E, Amorim P, Bonora I, Sheehan KH, et al. The Mini Internationas Neurosphyciatric Interview (MINI). A short diagnostic structured interview: reliability and validity according to the CIDI. *Eur Psychiatry.* 1997;12:224–231.

20. *Diagnostic and Statistical Manual of Mental Disorders.* 4th ed. Washington, DC: American Psychiatric Association; 1994.

21. International Classification of Diseases. *10th Revision.* Geneva, Switzerland: World Health Organization; 1994.

22. International Classification of Diseases. *Ninth Revision.* Geneva, Switzerland: World Health Organization; 1980.

23. Sheehan DV, Lecrubier Y, Sheehan KH, et al. The Mini-International Neuropsychiatric Interview (M.I.N.I.): the development and validation of a structured diagnostic psychiatric interview for DSM-IV and ICD-10. *J Clin Psychiatry.* 1998;59(Suppl 20):22–33.

24. Stewart AL, Hays RD, Ware JE Jr. The MOS short-form general health survey. Reliability and validity in a patient population. *Med Care.* 1988;26:724–735.

25. Ware JE, Sherbourne CD. The MOS 36-item Short Form Health Survey (SF-36). I. Conceptual framework and item selection. *Med Care.* 1992;30:473–483.

26. Malik ML, Connor KM, Sutherland SM, Smith RD, Davidson RM, Davidson JR. Quality of life and posttraumatic stress disorder: A pilot study assessing changes in SF-36 scores before and after treatment in a placebo-controlled trial of fluoxetine. *J Trauma Stress.* 1999;12:387–393.

27. Ware JE, Kosinski M, Gandek B. SF-36® Health Survey Manual and Interpretation Guide. Lincoln, RI: Quality Metric Incorporated; 2000.

28. Weathers FW, Litz B. Psychometric properties of the Clinican-Administered PTSD Scale, CAPS-1. *PTSD Res Quart.* 1994:2–6.

29. Weathers FW, Ruscio AM, Keane TM. The psychometric properties of nine scoring rules for the Clinician Administered Posttraumatic Stress Disorder Scale. *Psychol Assess*. 1999;11(2):124–133.

30. Charlson M, Peterson JC. Medical comorbidity and late life depression: what is known and what are the unmet needs? *Biol Psychiatry*. 2002;52(3):226–235.

31

Differences Between Veteran Suicides With and Without Psychiatric Symptoms

Peter C. Britton, PhD, Mark A. Ilgen, PhD, Marcia Valenstein, MD, Kerry Knox, PhD, Cynthia A. Claassen, PhD, and Kenneth R. Conner, PsyD, MPH

Objectives. Our objective was to examine all suicides (n = 423) in 2 geographic areas of the Veterans Health Administration (VHA) over a 7-year period and to perform detailed chart reviews on the subsample that had a VHA visit in the last year of life (n = 381).

Methods. Within this sample, we compared a group with 1 or more documented psychiatric symptoms (68.5%) to a group with no such symptoms (31.5%). The groups were compared on suicidal thoughts and behaviors, somatic symptoms, and stressors using the χ^2 test and on time to death after the last visit using survival analyses.

Results. Veterans with documented psychiatric symptoms were more likely to receive a suicide risk assessment, and have suicidal ideation and a suicide plan, sleep problems, pain, and several stressors. These veterans were also more likely to die in the 60 days after their last visit.

Conclusions. Findings indicated presence of 2 large and distinct groups of veterans at risk for suicide in the VHA, underscoring the value of tailored prevention strategies, including approaches suitable for those without identified psychiatric symptoms.

Suicide is the eleventh leading cause of death in the United States and the fifth leading cause of years of potential life lost before age 65 years.[1] Prevention efforts must include a focus on veterans who use Veterans Health Administration (VHA) services.[2] The VHA is the largest health care system in the United States, and each year more than 1800 veterans using VHA services die by suicide,[3] representing 5% to 6% of all suicides in the United States annually. Moreover, compared with the general US population, rates of suicide in veterans using VHA services are estimated to be 1.66-times higher

(95% confidence interval [CI] = 1.58, 1.74) among men and 1.87-times higher (95% CI = 1.35, 2.47) among women.[3]

In a recent, national study of veterans who used VHA services, depression, bipolar disorder, posttraumatic stress disorder (PTSD), schizophrenia, and alcohol or drug use disorders were associated with increased risk of suicide,[4] which was congruent with findings in the general literature.[5,6] Interestingly, slightly less than half (i.e., 46.8%) of VHA patients who killed themselves were diagnosed with a mental disorder. The study was based on clinician diagnoses, and greater psychopathology would have undoubtedly been uncovered using research interviews. Nonetheless, the study indicated that a large proportion of VHA patients who killed themselves did not have documented (or recorded) symptoms of psychopathology.

Suicide decedents who receive psychiatric treatment differ from those who do not in demographics, diagnoses, and the type of stressors they experience,[7–9] suggesting that there are likely to be important differences between decedents with and without recorded psychiatric symptoms. These findings have implications for prevention and suggest the potential need for universal strategies to reduce risk for suicide in the group without documented psychiatric symptoms. Additionally, the differences between those with and without documented psychiatric symptoms are likely to extend to patterns of service use before death, with those reporting more symptoms making greater contact with the health care system and, thus, potentially having a shorter time to death after their last visit.

The purpose of our study was to compare 2 broad groups of users of VHA services who died by suicide, a group with clinician-documented psychiatric symptoms (i.e., depression, anxiety, alcohol use disorders, drug use disorders, schizophrenia, and mania) in the last year of life, and a group with no documented symptoms. Using systematic chart reviews, we examined differences in sociodemographic characteristics, suicide-related variables (i.e., received a suicide risk assessment, suicidal ideation, suicide plan, suicide attempt), treatment contacts (i.e., received care from a mental health professional), somatic symptoms (i.e., sleep, pain), and specific stressors (i.e., occupational, relational, housing, legal) in the last year of life and at the last visit (when data were available), as well as time to death after the last visit. We hypothesized that the medical records of the group with recorded symptoms would also be more likely to show suicide-related variables, somatic symptoms, and stressors. We also explored time to death in the 2 study groups.

METHODS

Participants were all 423 suicide decedents who received VHA services between fiscal years (FYs) 2000 and 2006 from either Veterans Integrated Service Network 2 (VISN 2; upstate New York and north central Pennsylvania, n = 130) or VISN 11 (central Illinois, Indiana, Michigan, and northwest Ohio, n = 293). Analyses focused on the 381 (90.07%) participants who received VHA services during the last year of life. The 42 (9.93%) decedents who were excluded from the analyses were more likely to be non-White (χ^2 = 13.60; P < .001) and younger (χ^2 = 13.60; P < .05) than those who were included.

Data Sources

Comprehensive information on patient factors and treatment utilization before suicide were obtained from 3 unique sources: (1) the VHA National Patient Care Database (NPCD) and other nationwide data resources available at the Austin Automation Center, (2) the National Center for Health Statistics (NCHS) National Death Index (NDI), and (3) information contained within the VHA Computerized Patient Record System (CPRS).

NPCD and NDI data.

Using linked data from the NPCD and the NDI, the VISN 11 Serious Mental Illness Training, Research, and Education Center (SMITREC) created a National Suicide Registry that contains information about suicide on all patients who used VHA services in FYs 2000 to 2007. The NPCD was used to identify all individuals who used VHA inpatient, residential, or outpatient services between FY 2000 through the end of FY 2007 and who did not have any record of VHA service use in FYs 2008 or 2009.

The NDI draws from US mortality data regarding dates and causes of death for all US residents. Data are derived from death certificates filed in state vital statistics offices and checked for accuracy by NCHS. NDI searches were conducted for all individuals identified by the NPCD search. The NDI data request protocol matched records using social security number, last name, first name, middle initial, date of birth, race/ethnicity, gender, and state of residence. Frequently, NDI searches yielded multiple records that were potential matches. In these instances, previously established procedures were used to ensure that the individuals identified by NPCD and NDI searches were the same person.[10] The

NDI is considered the "gold standard" for mortality assessment information because it has the greatest sensitivity in determining vital status among all available population-level sources of mortality data.[11]

CPRS data.

All clinical notes about care provided within the VHA system are recorded in the CPRS medical record. Notes can be written in free form or using templates, and typically include information about the patient's presenting problem and the type of care provided. CPRS data therefore provides information about symptoms (e.g., suicidal thoughts) or disorders that are noted in the narrative of notes and not limited to official templates that are tied to visit encounters, notations about patient stressors, or treatment plans.

Chart Reviews

Chart reviews were conducted at the Center of Excellence for Suicide Prevention located in VISN 2. They were used to extract data on documented symptoms of depression, alcohol use disorders, illicit drug use, prescription drug misuse, PTSD, mania, schizophrenia, sleep disturbance, and subjective pain. Note that symptoms were recorded whether there was a formal diagnosis, necessitating the use of chart reviews (as opposed to aggregate electronic data). Common stressors (e.g., marital or intimate relationship, employment, legal, housing) were also extracted from the charts.

One of the authors (M. V.) developed the chart review tool for a study of veterans treated for depression.[12] The tool systematically assesses care provided by the VHA in the year before suicide (last year codes) as well as during the last visit (last visit codes). For each patient record, we used 2 or more independent coders who, after initial coding, met to compare results and resolve discrepancies to create a consensus record for use in analyses. When a clear consensus could not be reached, the coding decisions were staffed at a weekly consensus conference. To assess the interrater reliability before consensus, we calculated weighted kappas among raters for both last year and last visit codes. Kappas were weighted to reflect the proportion of charts coded by each pair of raters. Landis and Koch's recommendations were used to classify kappas into poor ($\leq$ 0.40), moderate (0.41–0.60), substantial (0.60–0.79), and outstanding ($\geq$ 0.80) categories.[13]

Variables

Demographic characteristics.

Patients' age and gender are consistently available in VHA electronic treatment records.

Psychiatric symptoms.

Chart reviews assessed symptoms whether they reached a diagnostic threshold (e.g., depressive disorder) as well as symptoms (e.g., depressive symptoms), hereafter referred to as documented or recorded symptoms. These data were used to form the 2 study groups. Kappas for reliability between pairs of raters on documented symptoms were outstanding: depression (0.95 last year, 0.86 last visit), anxiety (0.89 last year, 0.91 last visit), alcohol use disorder (0.84 last year, 0.79 last visit), mania (0.89 last year, 0.97 last visit), psychosis (0.91 last year, 0.95 last visit), illicit drug use (0.92 last year, 0.81 last visit), and misuse of prescription drugs (0.80 last year, 0.82 last visit).

Treatment contacts.

Chart reviews were used to identify the specialization of the provider seen on the last visit (nonphysician and nonmental health, nonphysician and mental health, physician and nonmental health, or physician and mental health) to examine differences in the mental health treatment received by each group. The number of days between the last visit and death was also calculated to estimate the immediacy of risk between the 2 groups. The kappa for raters' reliability of specialization of the provider was outstanding: mental health provider (0.84 last visit).

Suicide-related variables.

Chart reviews were used to identify if a suicide risk assessment was conducted, and suicidal thoughts, plans, and previous attempts were recorded. History of suicide attempts was used because of the low number of documented suicide attempts in the year before death. Kappas for reliability of raters on suicide-related variables were substantial or outstanding: risk assessment (0.85 last year, 0.75 last visit), suicidal thoughts (0.85 last year, 0.75 last visit), suicidal plan (1.00 last year), and suicide attempts (0.82 last year); agreement on suicidal plan at the last visit was not given because it was rare.

Somatic symptoms.
Chart reviews also identified information on documented sleep and pain complaints. Sleep is a symptom of many psychiatric and physical disorders.[14-16] Previous work found that VHA patients with higher self-report of pain were at moderately increased risk for suicide.[17] Kappas for reliability of raters on somatic symptoms were substantial or outstanding: sleep (0.85 last year, 0.63 last visit) and pain (0.68 last year, 0.76 last visit).

Stressors.
Information about stressors was also obtained from the chart. Domains of interest included marital or intimate relationship, legal, housing, and occupational problems. Kappas for reliability between raters on somatic stressors were substantial or outstanding: marital or intimate relationship (0.75), legal (0.72), housing (0.82), and occupational (0.77).

Analyses

We compared the 2 study groups using the χ^2 test. For comparisons with sample sizes less than 5, we used the Fisher exact 2-sided test. Comparisons were made on demographic characteristics, treatment contacts (received care from a mental health professional), suicide-related variables (received a suicide risk assessment, presence of suicidal ideation, suicide plan, suicide attempt), somatic symptoms (presence of sleep or pain), and stressors (presence of occupational, relational, housing, legal) for the last year and last visit, when available.

Survival analyses compared days until death for the 2 study groups using Cox proportional hazard models, which can be used for uncensored data.[18,19] The day of last contact was treated as day 1 to account for the 4 deaths that occurred on the day of contact. Initial models included all demographic variables, which were removed from the models if they were associated at $P > .05$. Diagnosis violated the proportionality assumption. We therefore treated it as a time-varying covariate and calculated hazard ratios (HRs) over periods of time (i.e., 1–30, 31–60, 61–180, 181–365 days) within the same model. To examine the hazards of suicidal ideation, secondary analyses compared the association of suicidal ideation to time to death after controlling for documented symptoms and statistically significant demographic variables. Because suicidal ideation also violated the proportionality assumption, its HRs were calculated using the same strategy.

RESULTS

Analyses were based on the 381 patients who used services in the year preceding suicide. Of these veterans, 261 (68.5%) had clinician-documented symptoms and 120 (31.5%) had no recorded symptoms. Descriptive statistics indicated that there were differences in age and race/ethnicity between the 2 groups (see Table 1). Those with recorded symptoms were significantly more likely to receive a suicide risk assessment and report suicidal ideation and plans, the presence of occupational-, relational-, legal-, and housing-related stressors, as well as somatic symptoms such as chronic pain and sleep disturbance (see Table 2). Among those with documented symptoms, 91 of 198 (46.0%) who received a suicide risk assessment in the last year reported suicidal ideation, whereas no individuals without documented symptoms reported suicidal ideation.

The group with reported symptoms was significantly more likely to be seen by a mental health professional for the last visit, receive a suicide risk

Table 1. Demographics Among Veterans Health Administration Suicide Decedents, by Symptom Status: VISN 2 and VISN 11, 2000-2007

Characteristics	With Symptoms, No. (%)	Without Symptoms, No. (%)	χ^2	P
Total	261 (68.5)	120 (31.5)		
Gender			...	.091[a]
Male	251 (96.2)	119 (99.2)		
Female	10 (3.8)	1 (0.8)		
Race/ethnicity[b]			5.23	.022
White	220 (84.3)	89 (74.2)		
Minority	40 (15.3)	30 (25.0)		
Age, y			40.16	< .001
18–34	6 (2.3)	5 (4.2)		
35–54	61 (23.4)	10 (8.3)		
55–74	133 (51.0)	40 (33.3)		
> 75	61 (23.4)	65 (54.2)		
VISN center			0.01	0.909
VISN 2	83 (31.8)	37 (30.8)		
VISN 11	179 (68.6)	82 (68.3)		

Note. VISN = Veterans Integrated Services Network.
[a]One-sided Fisher exact test.
[b]Race/ethnicity was missing for 2 participants.

Table 2. Suicide-Related Variables, Somatic symptoms, and Stressors Among Veterans Health Administration Suicide Decedents, by Symptom Status: VISN 2 and VISN 11, 2000–2007

Variables	With Symptoms (n = 261), No. (%)	Without Symptoms (n = 120), No. (%)	χ^2	P
Last Year				
Suicide-related variables				
Assess suicidal ideation	198 (75.9)	25 (20.8)	102.56	< .001
Suicidal ideation	91 (34.9)	0	...	< .001[a]
Suicidal plan	47 (18.0)	0	...	< .001[a]
Suicide attempt (ever)	24 (9.2)	0	...	< .052[a]
Somatic symptoms				
Sleep	157 (60.2)	16 (13.3)	72.69	< .001
Pain	219 (83.9)	72 (60.0)	26.04	< .001
Stressors				
Occupational	89 (34.1)	5 (4.2)	38.85	< .001
Relational	66 (25.3)	1 (0.8)	...	< .001[a]
Housing	36 (13.8)	0	...	< .001[a]
Legal	36 (13.8)	1 (0.8)	...	< .001[a]
Last Visit				
Treatment contact: Psychiatric treatment	90 (34.5)	1 (0.8)	...	< .001[a]
Suicide-related variables				
Assess suicidal ideation	105 (40.2)	11 (9.2)	37.46	< .001
Suicidal ideation	15 (5.7)	0	...	.003[a]
Suicidal plan	3 (1.1)	0	...	.32[a]
Somatic symptoms				
Sleep	54 (20.7)	8 (6.7)	11.86	.001
Pain	98 (37.5)	44 (36.7)	0.03	.869

Note. VISN = Veterans Integrated Services Network.
[a]One-sided Fisher exact test.

assessment, and have recorded suicidal ideation and sleep complaints. There was no difference in documentation of chronic pain between the 2 groups at the last visit. Among those with recorded symptoms, 15 of 105 (14.3%) who received a suicide risk assessment at the last visit reported suicidal ideation. No individuals in the group without documented symptoms reported suicidal ideation at the last visit.

The 2 study groups differed in time to death after the last visit. Individuals with documented symptoms were almost 3 times as likely to die within 30 days of contact (HR = 2.95; 95% CI = 1.98, 4.39) and 74% more likely to die within 31 to 60 days of contact (HR = 1.74; 95% CI = 1.06, 2.85), but were not more likely to die after 60 days (61–90 days; HR = 1.32; 95% CI = 0.71, 2.43), 91 to 180 days(HR = 1.08; 95% CI = 0.64, 1.84), or 181 to 365 days (HR = 1.43;95% CI = 0.77, 2.65), after control for age cohort (HR = 1.20; 95% CI = 1.04, 1.38) and male gender (HR = 0.38; 95% CI = 0.21, 0.72). A survival curve was used to illustrate the difference in probability of death at any time point between these 2 groups (Figure 1).

Because of the potential importance of suicidal ideation, secondary analyses were conducted to compare time to death between those with documented suicidal ideation in their last year (n = 91) and those with no suicidal ideation (n = 290). Individuals with suicidal ideation were over twice as likely to die within 30 days of contact (HR = 2.19; 95% CI = 1.57, 3.05), but were not more likely to die after 30 days (31–60 days: HR = 1.75; 95% CI = 0.99, 3.08; 61–90 days: HR = 0.34; 95% CI = 0.08, 1.42; 91–180 days: HR = 0.80; 95% CI = 0.36, 1.78; 181–365 days: HR = 0.69; 95% CI = 0.26, 1.84), after control for documented symptoms (HR = 1.68; 95% CI = 1.32, 2.13), age

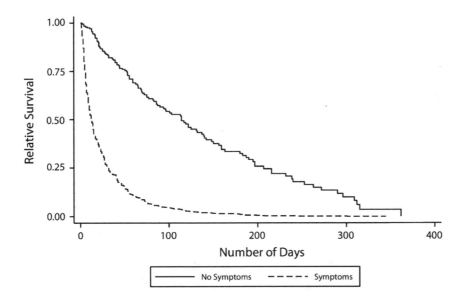

Figure 1. Suicide survival among Veterans Health Administration suicide decedents, by symptom status: VISN 2 and VISN 11, 2000-2007.

Note. VISN = Veterans Integrated Service Network.

cohort (HR = 1.24; 95% CI = 1.08, 1.43), and male gender (HR = 0.45; 95% CI = 0.24, 0.83). A survival curve was also used to illustrate the difference in probability of death at any time point between these 2 groups (Figure 2).

DISCUSSION

We examined differences in demographic characteristics, suicide-related variables, somatic symptoms, stressors, and time to death after the last visit between veteran decedents with documented symptoms in the last year of life (68.5%) and those with no such symptoms (31.5%).

As hypothesized, the group with recorded symptoms was more likely to receive a suicide risk assessment and to report suicidal ideation and a plan in the last year of life than was the group without such symptoms. Similarly, those with documented symptoms were also more likely to receive care from a mental health specialist, receive a suicide assessment, and report suicidal ideation at the last visit. Thus, the group with documented symptoms was

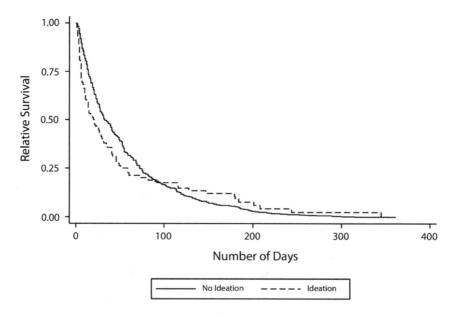

Figure 2. Suicide survival among Veterans Health Administration suicide decedents, by ideation status: VISN 2 and VISN 11, 2000–2007.

Note. VISN = Veterans Integrated Service Network.

more likely to be identified as being at high risk, providing the opportunity for intervention. These individuals might have required more intensive treatments that directly target suicide risk, such as cognitive therapy for suicide prevention[20] or dialectical behavioral therapy,[21,22] although the utility of such treatments with veterans remains to be demonstrated. The percentage of suicides with documented symptoms in the present study (68.5%) was considerably lower compared with that identified in postmortem psychological autopsy studies of suicide,[23,24] suggesting clinical underdetection and the potential value of increased screening and improved risk recognition. Additional universal strategies would also be of benefit,[25] particularly for patients who were not identified as having psychiatric symptoms despite screening efforts.

The group with recorded symptoms also had more documented somatic symptoms in the year before suicide and at the last visit than decedents without documented symptoms, with 1 exception. There was no difference in recorded chronic pain between the 2 subpopulations at the last visit. Previous research found an association between self-reported pain and risk for suicide in VHA patients.[17] Nonsymptomatic high-risk veterans might be more willing to disclose pain when they are distressed, suggesting that increased pain in veterans without reported symptoms might be indicative of increased risk. Alternatively, pain might be a risk factor for suicide that was mostly independent of psychiatric symptoms.[17] In addition, veterans with recorded symptoms also had more documented stressors than those with no symptoms, with occupational and relational stressors being the most prevalent. Research on the association of pain, occupational, and relational problems with suicide risk in veterans might identify important targets for selective interventions.

Individuals with documented symptoms were more likely to die by suicide within the first 60 days after contact, and those with suicidal ideation were more likely to die by suicide in the first 30 days. The associations among psychiatric problems, suicidal ideation, and time to death might have important implications for prevention efforts, with a history of greater psychiatric and suicidal symptoms indicating a need for more timely and intensive intervention. Caring letters, for example, were found to reduce risk for suicide for depressed inpatients who refused postdischarge treatment.[26] For veterans with documented symptoms, the data suggested the value of implementing such letters early in the course of treatment. Additionally, this finding further highlighted the need for intensive interventions that directly target suicide risk for veterans reporting suicidal ideation.

Over 30% of the sample had no reported symptoms, which indicates problems with detection, documentation, or the absence of critical variables in the chart review. Data suggested that decedents without documented symptoms were more likely to be racial/ethnic minorities than veterans with reported symptoms. Given the meager data, it was unclear if this finding represented a true difference in symptoms between at-risk minority and majority patients in the VHA or a problem of underdetection of symptoms in minority patients. Although our analyses focused on VHA patients who received VHA services in the last year of life, approximately 10% of the veterans who killed themselves did not receive any VHA treatment services in their last year, and racial and ethnic minorities were also overrepresented in this group. Outreach efforts that are tailored to racial and ethnic minorities may be needed to increase their utilization of potentially lifesaving services.

Since these data were collected, the VHA has implemented reliable and sensitive screens for depression,[27] alcohol misuse,[28] and PTSD.[29] The VHA has also mandated an annual suicide-risk assessment that is triggered when patients screen positive for psychiatric disorders or experience changes in treatment, such as hospitalization. Other changes include the mandated use of a standard Safety Plan with Veterans in those who are identified as being at high risk,[30] and the creation of a list of high-risk veterans whose care is overseen by suicide prevention coordinators located at each VHA medical center. These strategies are designed to reduce the number of at-risk veterans whose symptoms go undetected (most relevant to the study group without documented symptoms) and to provide intensive and potentially lifesaving treatment to those with clear indications of risk (most relevant to the study group without recorded symptoms). How these VHA initiatives might have changed the results obtained in this study is unclear, and is an important topic for future study. Regardless of the VHA's best efforts, it is inevitable that a subgroup of at-risk veterans will escape risk recognition efforts, and these patients (represented in the present study by those without documented symptoms) might benefit especially from universal prevention strategies aimed at general health promotion and safety.[25]

In our study, we used 2 strategies to minimize underdetection of psychopathology, first, by focusing on the year before death (rather than more distally) and, second, by coding psychiatric symptoms (rather than merely diagnoses). We identified a considerably higher percentage of suicides with psychopathology (68.5%) than that obtained in a recent cohort study of suicide among VHA patients (46.8%), which was extended more distally and relied on diagnoses,[4] suggesting that we were successful to some degree. Documentation in clinical records reflects interactions between patients and providers, and we presume that the group without documented symptoms in the present study (31.5%) contained individuals who did not experience or reveal symptoms in the last year of life (nonsymptom expression) as well as those who were symptomatic, but there were failures in clinical detection or documentation (symptom nonidentification). Psychological autopsy studies estimated that nearly 90% of suicide decedents had 1 or more psychiatric disorders.[23,24] Based on such data, it could be argued that the group without documented symptoms in the present study was overwhelmingly a case of nonidentification. However, it should be kept in mind that psychological autopsy studies focus on the last days and weeks of life, and there was a considerable time gap between the last appointment and the date of suicide in many patients in our study. As a result, a veteran's mental status and life circumstances at their last treatment visit did not necessarily reflect their experience near to the time of suicide.

There were some limitations to this study. The study sample was limited to VHA patients treated in the Midwest and Northeast, with unclear generalizability to VHA patients in other regions of the country. Data were based on chart reviews, and information about the reliability, validity, or completeness of the information contained in the charts was not available. Moreover, we could not control for clinician variability in documentation. Providers might be more or less prone to document symptoms generally, which might have contributed to our finding that a broad range of symptoms were elevated in 1 of the study groups. As mentioned, there were numerous suicide prevention practices instituted in the VHA since the suicides studied here occurred, making it unclear how the results might look with a more recent sample. There were additional limitations concerning the availability of potentially important variables. Data on health care services received outside of VHA were unavailable, chart reviews did not provide exhaustive coverage for all potential risk factors such as personality disorders, and some groups were underrepresented in the sample (e.g., female veterans). Despite these limitations, the study identified 2 large and rather different at-risk groups of veterans, suggesting the need for a broad suicide prevention strategy that extends from universal (i.e., health and safety promotion) to indicated (i.e., risk recognition and treatment) approaches.

ABOUT THE AUTHORS

Peter C. Britton, Kerry Knox, Cynthia A. Claassen, and Kenneth R. Conner are with the VISN 2 Center of Excellence for Suicide Prevention, Department of Veteran Affairs Medical Center, Canandaigua, NY, and the Center for the Study and Prevention of Suicide, Department of Psychiatry, University of Rochester School of Medicine and Dentistry, Rochester, NY. Mark A. Ilgen and Marcia Valenstein are with the VISN 11 Serious Mental Illness Treatment Resource and Evaluation (SMITREC), Department of Veteran Affairs Medical Center, Ann Arbor, MI, and the Department of Psychiatry, University of Michigan Medical School, Ann Arbor.

CONTRIBUTORS

P.C. Britton, M.A. Ilgen, M. Valenstein, K. Knox, C.A.Claassen, and K.R. Conner designed the study and authored the article. P.C. Britton conducted the analyses and took the lead on writing.

ACKNOWLEDGMENTS

This study was funded by the Department of Veterans Affairs (VA), VISN 2 Center of Excellence for Suicide Prevention.

The authors would like to thank Heather Walters for training the coders, Liam Cerveny, Suzanne Dougherty, Sharon Fell, Elizabeth Schifano, and Patrick Walsh for conducting the chart reviews, and Brady Stephens for creating and managing the database.

Note. The VA had no role in study design; in the collection, analysis and interpretation of data; in the writing of the article; or in the decision to submit the article for publication.

HUMAN PARTICIPANT PROTECTION

This study was approved by the Syracuse VA Medical Center Institutional Review Board.

REFERENCES

1. Centers for Disease Control and Prevention. Wisqars Injury Mortality Reports 1999-2006. 2009. Available at: http://www.cdc.gov.ezpminer.urmc.rochester.edu/ncipc/wisqars. Accessed September 25, 2009.

2. Blue Ribbon Report Group. Report of the blue ribbon work group on suicide prevention in the Veteran population. 2008. Available at: http://www.mentalhealth.va.gov/suicide_prevention/Blue_Ribbon_Report-FINAL_June-30-08.pdf. Accessed January 5, 2010.

3. McCarthy JF, Valenstein M, Kim HM, Ilgen M, Zivin K, Blow FC. Suicide mortality among patients receiving care in the Veterans Health Administration health system. *Am J Epidemiol.* 2009;169(8):1033–1038.

4. Ilgen MA, Bohnert AS, Ignacio RV, et al. Psychiatric diagnoses and risk of suicide in veterans. *Arch Gen Psychiatry.* 2010;67(11):1152–1158.

5. Harris EC, Barraclough B. Suicide as an outcome for mental disorders: a meta-analysis. *Br J Psychiatry.* 1997;170(3):205–228.

6. Nock MK, Borges G, Bromet EJ, Cha CB, Kessler RC, Lee S. Suicide and suicidal behavior. *Epidemiol Rev.* 2008;30:133–154.

7. Booth N, Owens C. Silent suicide: suicide among people not in contact with mental health services. *Int Rev Psychiatry.* 2000;12(1):27–30.

8. Law YW, Wong PW, Yip PS. Suicide with psychaitric diagnosis and without utilization of psychiatric services. *BMC Public Health.* 2010;10:431.

9. Lee HC, Lin HC, Liu TC, Lin SY. Contact of mental and non-mental healthcare providers prior to suicide in Taiwan: a population-based study. *Can J Psychiatry.* 2008;53(6):377–383.

10. Sohn MW, Arnold N, Maynard C, Hynes DM. Accuracy and completeness of mortality data in the Department of Veterans Affairs. *Popul Health Metr.* 2006;4:2.

11. Cowper DC, Kubal JD, Maynard C, Hynes DM. A primer and comparative review of major US mortality databases. *Ann Epidemiol.* 2002;12(7):462–468.

12. Valenstein M, Kim HM, Ganoczy D, et al. Higher-risk periods for suicide among VA patients receiving depression treatment: prioritizing suicide prevention efforts. *J Affect Disord.* 2009;112(1-3):50–58.

13. Landis JR, Koch GG. The measurement of observer agreement for categorical data. *Biometrics.* 1977;33(1):159–174.

14. Breslau N, Roth T, Rosenthal L, Andreski P, Sloane F. Sleep disturbance and psychiatric disorders: a longitudinal epidemiological study of young adults. *Biol Psychiatry.* 1996;39(6):411–418.

15. Léger D, Scheuermaier K, Philip P, Paillard M, Guilleminault C. SF-36: evaluation of quality of life in severe and mild insomniacs compared with good sleepers. *Psychosom Med.* 2001;63(1):49–55.

16. Léger D, Guilleminault C, Bader G, Levy E, Paillard M. Medical and socio-professional impact of insomnia. *Sleep.* 2002;25(6):625–629.

17. Ilgen MA, Zivin K, Austin KL, Bohnert AS, Czyz EK, Valenstein M, et al. Severe pain predicts greater likelihood of subsequent suicide. *Suicide Life Threat Behav.* 2010;40:597–608.

18. Cox DR. Regression models and life-tables. *J R Stat Soc [Ser A].* 1972;B34(2):187–220.

19. Cleves MA, Gould WW, Gutierrez RG, Marchenko Y. *An Introduction to Survival Analysis Using Stata.* 2nd ed. College Station, TX: Stata Press; 2008.

20. Brown GK, Ten Have T, Henriques GR, Xie SX, Hollander JE, Beck AT. Cognitive therapy for the prevention of suicide attempts: a randomized controlled trial. *JAMA.* 2005;294(5):563–570.

21. Koons CR, Robins CJ, Tweed JL, et al. Efficacy of dialectical behavior therapy in women veterans with borderline personality disorder. *Behav Therapy.* 2001;32(2):371–390.

22. Linehan MM, Comtois KA, Murray AM, et al. Two-year randomized controlled trial and follow-up of dialectical behavior therapy vs therapy by experts for suicidal behaviors and borderline personality disorder. *Arch Gen Psychiatry.* 2006;63(7): 757–766.

23. Cavanagh JTOO, Carson AJ, Sharpe M, Lawrie SM. Psychological autopsy studies of suicide: a systematic review. *Psychol Med.* 2003;33(3):395–405.

24. Yoshimasu K, Kiyohara C, Kazuhisa M. Suicidal risk factors and completed suicide: meta analyses based on psychological autopsy studies. *Environ Health Prev Med.* 2008;13(5):243–256.

25. Knox KL, Conwell Y, Caine ED. If suicide is a public health problem, what are we doing to prevent it? *Am J Public Health.* 2004;94(1):37–45.

26. Motto JA, Bostrom AG. A randomized controlled trial of postcrisis suicide prevention. *Psychiatr Serv.* 2001;52(6):828–833.

27. Kroenke K, Spitzer RL, Williams JBWW. The Patient Health Questionnaire-2: validity of a two item-depression screener. *Med Care.* 2003;41(11):1284–1292.

28. Bradley KA, Williams EC, Achtmeyer CE, Volpp B, Collins BJ, Kivlahan DR. Implementation of evidence-based alcohol screening in the Veterans Health Administration. *Am J Manag Care.* 2006;12(10):597–606.

29. Prins A, Ouimette P, Kimerling R, et al. The primary care PTSD screen (PC-PTSD): development and operating characteristics. *Prim Care Psychiatry.* 2003;9(1):9–14.

30. Stanley B, Brown GK. Safety planning: a brief intervention to mitigate suicide risk. *Cognitive and Behavioral Practice.* Available online April 15, 2011. Available at: http://www.sciencedirect.com/science/journal/aip/10777229. Accessed January 5, 2010.

32

Suicide Risk and Precipitating Circumstances Among Young, Middle-Aged, and Older Male Veterans

Mark S. Kaplan, DrPH, Bentson H. McFarland, MD, PhD, Nathalie Huguet, PhD, and Marcia Valenstein, MD, MS

Objectives. The purpose of this study was to evaluate the risk of suicide among veteran men relative to nonveteran men by age and to examine the prevalence of suicide circumstances among male veterans in different age groups (18–34, 35–44, 45–64, and ⩾ 65 years).

Methods. Data from the National Violent Death Reporting System (2003–2008) were used to calculate age-specific suicide rates for veterans (n = 8440) and nonveterans (n = 21 668) and to calculate the age-stratified mortality ratio for veterans. Multiple logistic regression was used to compare health status, stressful life events preceding suicide, and means of death among young, middle-aged, and older veterans.

Results. Veterans were at higher risk for suicide compared with nonveterans in all age groups except the oldest. Mental health, substance abuse, and financial and relationship problems were more common in younger than in older veteran suicide decedents, whereas health problems were more prevalent in the older veterans. Most male veterans used firearms for suicide, and nearly all elderly veterans did so.

Conclusions. Our study highlighted heightened risk of suicide in male veterans compared with nonveterans. Within the veteran population, suicide might be influenced by different precipitating factors at various stages of life.

As the 11th leading cause of death among Americans of all ages, suicide remains a serious public health problem, and reducing suicide is a national imperative.[1,2] The suicide of veterans has become a topic of intense public policy scrutiny in recent years. Until recently, most US studies indicated that both active-duty military personnel[3-5] and veterans[6] were at a lower risk for suicide than their demographically matched peers.

The increased risk of suicide recently observed among veterans of Operations Enduring Freedom and Iraqi Freedom has generated nationwide concern.[7,8] The Department of Veterans Affairs (VA) has drawn attention to the rising suicide rate among young veterans and declared the prevention of suicide to be a major priority.[9]

Lawmakers have also expressed concern about the heightened rate of veterans' suicides across the age spectrum.[10] For example, the House Committee on Veterans Affairs held a hearing entitled "The Truth About Veterans' Suicide" in May 2008,[11] and more recently, the Senate Committee on Veterans Affairs conducted a hearing entitled "Mental Health Care and Suicide Prevention for Veterans" in March 2010.[12] In his testimony before the House Committee in May 2008, the Secretary of Veterans Affairs[13] presented data showing that male veterans in the community had higher rates of suicide than did other men and that veterans aged 30 to 64 years had the highest rates.

According to the VA Office of the Inspector General, 1000 veterans who receive VA care and as many as 5000 of all veterans die by suicide every year.[9] In an analysis of suicide rates among male veterans and nonveterans in Washington state, which has large military bases and a substantial population of veterans, Maynard and Boyko[14] found that the 2006 suicide rate was higher among veterans in all age categories. Data from the 2007 Oregon Violent Death Reporting System revealed that the age-adjusted suicide rate was 45.7/100 000 among male veterans but 27.4/100 000 among nonveteran men.[15] McCarthy et al. [16] found that male (43/100 000) and female (10/100 000) VA patients had higher suicide rates than did nonveteran men (23/100 000) and women (5/100 000) in the general population, although these increases were likely due, in part, to health problems leading to VA use in addition to veteran status.

In a prospective follow-up study of 320 890 men who participated in the 1986 to 1994 National Health Interview Surveys, Kaplan et al.[17] showed that veterans were twice as likely (hazard ratio [HR] = 2.13; 95% confidence interval [CI] = 1.14, 3.99) to die of suicide as were male nonveterans in the general population. However, not all studies found that veterans were at increased risk for suicide. On the basis of a review of 13 studies of suicide risk among current and former military personnel, Kang and Bullman[6] noted that veterans historically had a lower risk of suicide than did the general population. Similarly, Miller et al.[18] found no connection between military service and suicide in a large (but not nationally representative) longitudinal study of middle-aged and elderly men.

The Blue Ribbon Work Group on Suicide Prevention in the Veteran Population[19] mentioned the conflicting evidence regarding the risk of suicide among veterans across age groups. Some evidence suggested that younger veterans[20] were more vulnerable to suicide than were their older counterparts. In the United Kingdom, Kapur et al.[21] found age differences in the rates of suicide and in the prevalence of contact with mental health professionals before death among veterans. They showed that British veterans younger than 24 years were at greater risk for suicide (vs nonveterans) but that fewer had been in contact with mental health professionals.[21] According to a recent analysis of data from Oregon, the rates of suicide for younger veterans have increased since 2005, whereas the rates for older veterans have declined.[15] The foregoing studies might offer conflicting evidence regarding the role of age in suicide among veterans because of different sampling methodologies and study designs (e.g., veterans of different eras, only VA health care users, and different follow-up periods) as well as possible misclassification (e.g., of persons on active duty or in reserve forces). An understanding of the precipitating circumstances associated with suicide can help clarify the situation and could lead to more efficacious clinical and community-based veteran suicide prevention interventions.

Our study was the first to examine suicide risk and precipitating circumstances among male veterans across different age groups in the general population. To address these aims, we used population-based data (1) to calculate the standardized mortality ratios (SMRs) of dying by suicide among male veterans by age group, and (2) to assess and compare suicide means as well as health status and stressful life events preceding suicide deaths among young, middle-aged, and older veterans. Our goal was to examine the precipitating suicide circumstances across age groups to determine variations across the life span. Information about age-associated precipitating circumstances might have important implications for developing national suicide prevention strategies.

METHODS

This study used restricted data for decedents aged 18 years and older from the 2003 to 2008 National Violent Death Reporting System (NVDRS). The NVDRS is a state-based active surveillance system that provides a detailed account of violent deaths that occur in the participating states. As of 2008, 16 states (Alaska, Colorado, Georgia, Kentucky, Maryland, Massachusetts, New Jersey, New Mexico, North Carolina, Oklahoma, Oregon, South Carolina, Rhode Island, Utah, Virginia, and Wisconsin) contributed data to the NVDRS.

The NVDRS includes all suicides, homicides, legal intervention deaths, unintentional firearm deaths, and undetermined deaths. The data were gathered from coroner or medical examiner records; police reports; death certificates; toxicology laboratories; crime laboratories; and Alcohol, Tobacco, Firearms and Explosives (ATF) firearm trace reports. The circumstances preceding suicide were derived from death investigations assembled by the coroner/medical examiner and law enforcement reports, based on on-scene investigations; information from next of kin and witnesses; autopsy examinations; postmortem toxicological testing; and, in some cases, contact with health care providers.[22]

Veteran status was ascertained with information obtained from national standardized death certificates. Veteran status was indicated on death certificates in the section "Ever served in US Armed Forces."[22] This death certificate item does not distinguish between military personnel currently serving on active duty, in the guard or reserves, or veterans who have separated from the service. In the present analysis, the term veteran denoted decedents who served in the US armed forces.

Pooled NVDRS data yielded 8440 veteran and 21 668 nonveteran (defined as decedents without US military service) male suicide decedents. Information on veteran status was missing or unknown for 9% of the suicide decedents. Suicide cases were identified using the *International Classification of Diseases-10th Revision*[23] codes X60-X84, and Y87.

Measures

Age was categorized into 4 commonly used groups: 18 to 34, 35 to 44, 45 to 64, and 65 years and older. Ages 18 to 24 and 25 to 34 years were collapsed into 1 group because there were very few significant differences in the circumstances preceding suicide between these 2 age groups. The variables of interest included mental health status, blood alcohol concentration (BAC), alcohol problems, suicidal behaviors, and life crises or events. The selection of variables of interest was based on evidence from previous studies that these factors were linked with suicidal behavior among veterans.[16,17,19–21,24–38]

Mental health status.

Mental health status was ascertained with 4 separate items ("perceived" depressed mood, diagnosed with a mental health problem, ever treated for a mental health problem, and current treatment of a mental health problem). First, family members or friends reported if the decedent or others perceived that he was depressed, sad, down, blue, or unhappy shortly before the suicide. Second, they provided information on whether the decedent had had a mental health diagnosis from his health care provider at the time of death. Third, current and past mental health treatment was assessed from evidence gathered at the scene or from family members or friends.

Suicidal behavior.

Family members or friends reported whether the suicide decedent disclosed his intention to complete suicide or had a history of suicide attempts.

Blood alcohol concentration.

The suicide decedent's blood was tested for the presence of alcohol, coded in terms of weight by volume, and then classified as BAC less than 0.08 grams per deciliter or 0.08 grams per deciliter or greater.

Alcohol and other drug problems.

Family members or friends reported whether the decedent perceived himself or was perceived by others to have an alcohol or substance abuse problem at the time of death.

Life events.

Family members or friends reported whether the decedent experienced a crisis within 2 weeks of the suicide or if a crisis was imminent. In addition, they were asked if the decedent experienced financial, physical health, job, intimate partner, or criminal or legal problems.

Suicide methods.

The coroner/medical examiner determined the method used to complete suicide. Suicide methods were dichotomized into firearm versus all other methods (i.e., a sharp or blunt instrument, poisoning, hanging, fall, drowning, fire or burns, a motor vehicle, or other).

Demographic characteristics.

Data included race (White or non-White), marital status (married or not married), region of residence (Northeast, Midwest, South, or West), and metropolitan status. Counties of death were assigned a rural–urban continuum code based on a classification system developed by the US Department of Agriculture Economic Research Service.[39] The continuum contains 9 categories and characterizes metropolitan counties by population size and nonmetropolitan counties by level of urbanization and adjacency to metropolitan areas. The categories range from "1" (counties in metropolitan areas of 1 million population or more) to "9" (completely rural counties or those with less than 2500 urban population, not adjacent to a metropolitan area). The 9 categories were then collapsed into 2 categories: metropolitan (codes 1 through 3) and nonmetropolitan (codes 4 through 9) status.

Analysis

To assess the risk of dying by suicide, we calculated SMRs and tested for their statistical significance. The SMR is the ratio of the observed number of veteran suicides to the expected number of suicides based on nonveteran suicide rates adjusted for race and calendar year. Veteran and nonveteran suicide rates were calculated with the number of decedents obtained from the NVDRS. Population estimates for those aged 18 and older who resided in the NVDRS states were based on VA veteran population estimates[40] and the American Community Survey (ACS) 2003 to 2008.[41] The ACS participants were asked "has this person ever served on active duty in the U.S. Armed Forces, military Reserves, or National Guard?" Those who responded "no, never served in the military" were considered nonveterans, and those who responded "yes, now on active duty" or "yes now training for Reserves/ National Guard" were classified as active duty military personnel.[42] Veteran population estimates included former and current military personnel (i.e., veterans, active duty personnel, National Guard, and Reserves). Veteran suicide rates were computed using population estimates that included current (derived from ACS data) and former (from the VA population data) military personnel. Nonveteran suicide rates were computed using ACS data.

The age-specific demographic characteristics were examined, and the prevalence of the precipitating suicide circumstances among the veteran decedents was estimated. Unadjusted age differences were assessed using logistic regression, with the youngest age group (18–34 years) used as the reference category. Next, a logistic regression was performed for each circumstance while adjusting for the effects of race, marital status, region of residence, and place of residence (urban–rural). Again, the youngest age group (18–34 years) was used as the reference category. All analyses were performed using the Statistical Package for the Social Sciences (SPSS; version 19.0; SPSS, Chicago, Illinois).

RESULTS

The risk of suicide among male veterans compared with nonveterans was statistically significantly greater in all age groups, except for those aged 65 years and older. Specifically, the SMRs for veterans aged 18 to 34, 35 to 44, 45 to 64, and 65 years and older were 1.26 ($P < .05$), 1.12 ($P < .05$), 1.04 ($P = .05$), and 0.98 ($P > .05$), respectively.

Table 1 presents the demographic characteristics of the veteran suicide decedents for all ages and in each age group. The findings showed that older veteran decedents were more likely to be White, married, and to have died in a rural area than were their younger counterparts.

Table 2 also shows that the antecedents of suicide appeared to be different across age groups. Unadjusted results had a similar pattern of findings as in the adjusted model for most of the circumstances and age groups.

In the adjusted model, compared with older veteran decedents, younger decedents were more likely to have had intimate partner problems as well as financial, legal, and occupational difficulties. Nearly 1 of every 2 younger veteran suicide decedents (aged 18–34 years) experienced relationship problems shortly before death. By contrast, older veteran decedents were more likely to have had health problems. It was interesting that the middle-aged veterans (aged 35–44) were more likely to have received a mental health diagnosis, whereas the older veterans (aged ≥ 65 years) were more likely to be

Table 1. Demographic and Geographic Characteristics of Young, Middle-Aged, and Older Male Veteran Suicide Decedents: National Violent Death Reporting System, 2003–2008

	Aged 18–34 Years (n = 845), %	Aged 35–44 Years (n = 1035), %	Aged 45–64 Years (n = 3266), %	Aged ⩾ 65 Years (n = 3294), %	All Ages
White (vs non-White)	80.2	86.9	93.6	97.3	92.3
Married (vs not married)	34.4	47.3	48.6	51.1	48.0
Region of residence					
Northeast	5.9	8.2	9.9	11.3	9.8
Midwest	5.1	9.7	8.1	6.4	7.3
South	62.5	54.8	52.5	55.0	54.7
West	26.5	27.3	29.6	27.4	28.1
Nonmetropolitan area (vs metropolitan)	19.6	19.4	25.2	27.2	24.7

suspected of being depressed at the time of death. For all age groups, depression was the most common diagnosis (> 70%). Posttraumatic stress disorder (PTSD) was reported in 7% of the younger veterans. Notable differences were also evident in relation to alcohol dependence (i.e., 14.9% and 6.2% among those aged 18–34 and ⩾ 65 years vs 23.8% and 24.3% among those aged 35–44 and 45–64 years, respectively). Evidence of acute alcohol use (BAC ⩾ 0.08) was present at the time of death in about one third of the younger veterans but in less than 10% of the elderly veterans.

The results also showed age differences in suicidal behaviors. Older and middle-aged men were less likely to have had a history of suicide attempts than were their youngest counterparts. Another notable difference was evident in relation to suicide methods. Firearm-related suicides were far more common among the older veterans (83.0%). Other variations across the 4 age groups were minor or did not form a clear or coherent pattern.

DISCUSSION

The risks of suicide (SMRs) among veterans were higher than among nonveterans across all age groups, except for the oldest veterans. Our estimates

Table 2. Suicide Risk and Precipitating Circumstances Among Young, Middle-Aged, and Older Male Veteran Suicide Decedents: National Violent Death Reporting System, 2003-2008

	Aged 18-34 Years, %	Aged 35-44 Years		Aged 45-64 Years		Aged ≥ 65 Years		All Ages
		%	AOR (95% CI)	%	AOR (95% CI)	%	AOR (95% CI)	
Mental health								
Ever treated for a mental health problem	29.8	36.3	1.25* (1.01, 1.53)	35.2	1.19 (1.00, 1.41)	25.1	0.72*** (0.60, 0.86)	30.9
Diagnosed with a mental health problem	33.7	41.1	1.29* (1.06, 1.58)	41.4	1.28* (1.08, 1.52)	30.6	0.79** (0.67, 0.94)	36.4
Current treatment of a mental health problem	24.4	28.8	1.15 (0.92, 1.43)	30.4	1.24* (1.03, 1.50)	21.9	0.79* (0.66, 0.96)	26.3
Current depressed mood	36.1	44.0	1.30** (1.07, 1.59)	45.2	1.33*** (1.13, 1.58)	48.1	1.52*** (1.29, 1.80)	45.3
Suicidal behaviors								
Disclosed intent to complete suicide	25.2	28.9	1.13 (0.90, 1.40)	26.3	0.98 (0.81, 1.18)	28.1	1.10 (0.91, 1.32)	27.2
Previous suicide attempts	16.6	19.8	1.12 (0.87, 1.44)	14.6	0.79* (0.63, 0.98)	6.9	0.33*** (0.26, 0.42)	12.4
Left a suicide note	29.5	32.6	1.17 (0.95, 1.45)	36.3	1.38*** (1.16, 1.65)	32.6	1.19 (0.99, 1.42)	33.7
Firearm suicide	61.3	53.4	0.78* (0.64, 0.95)	63.7	1.16 (0.98, 1.37)	83.5	3.51*** (2.92, 4.21)	69.9
Substance use								
Substance problem other than alcohol	14.7	14.4	0.99 (0.75, 1.31)	9.8	0.67** (0.52, 0.85)	0.9	0.05*** (0.03, 0.08)	7.4
Alcohol dependence	15.7	24.0	1.61*** (1.26, 2.06)	24.5	1.61*** (1.30, 2.00)	6.3	0.33*** (0.26, 0.42)	16.4
BAC ≥ 0.08	32.5	33.0	0.96 (0.75, 1.23)	27.9	0.75** (0.61 0.93)	8.8	0.17*** (0.13, 0.22)	22.5

(continued on next page)

VETERAN SUICIDE

Table 2. (continued)

Life events	Aged 18-34 Years, %	Aged 35-44 Years		Aged 45-64 Years		Aged ≥ 65 Years		All Ages
		%	AOR (95% CI)	%	AOR (95% CI)	%	AOR (95% CI)	
Crisis	38.3	35.8	0.88 (0.72, 1.07)	27.9	0.60*** (0.51, 0.71)	23.6	0.48*** (0.41, 0.58)	28.2
Financial problem	11.2	16.7	1.53** (1.16, 2.03)	16.7	1.48** (1.16, 1.88)	5.0	0.39*** (0.29, 0.52)	11.6
Health problem	5.3	11.7	2.41*** (1.66, 3.51)	26.8	6.43*** (4.62, 8.95)	66.7	36.09*** (25.92, 50.25)	38.4
Job problem	15.4	18.8	1.25 (0.97, 1.62)	15.8	0.97 (0.78, 1.22)	2.0	0.11*** (0.08, 0.15)	10.8
Criminal problem	13.5	17.4	1.38* (1.05, 1.81)	11.1	0.86 (0.67, 1.10)	1.9	0.14*** (0.10, 0.20)	8.5
Intimate partner problem	49.7	47.3	0.77* (0.63, 0.94)	25.8	0.27*** (0.23, 0.32)	8.6	0.07*** (0.06, 0.09)	24.1

Note: AOR = adjusted odds ratio; BAC = blood alcohol concentration; CI = confidence interval. Odds ratios were adjusted for race, marital status, metropolitan level, and region of residence. The age group 18-34 years was used as the reference category.

*P < .05; **P < .01; ***P < .001.

of suicide risks were consistent with those of other studies that found an increased risk of suicide among veterans,[15–18] but disagreed with the findings of Kang and Bullman[6] and Miller et al.[18] The present findings were based on current data, accounted for active duty or reserve military personnel, and might reflect recent changes in veterans' suicide rates. In addition, the large number of suicides in the present study provided substantial statistical power that might not have been available in earlier research.

Our results also demonstrated that the circumstances preceding suicide varied by age group. Although most veterans used firearms, older men were more likely to complete suicide with a firearm. This finding was consistent with that of Kaplan et al.,[20] who showed that older veterans were more likely to own and use a firearm than were younger veterans and nonveteran elderly men. This finding suggested that it is worthwhile for health care providers to probe for access to firearms among all depressed or suicidal older patients. In recognition of the problem of the availability and use of firearms, the VA adopted guidelines for VA providers to address the importance of means restriction in managing suicidal veterans.[43] These guidelines specify that rather than removing firearms, which might lead to conflict, a responsible person (e.g., family member) should safely store the weapons. The VA also initiated a Veteran Family Safety Program that provides free cable gunlocks at all VA Medical Centers for veterans and their family members. In the United States, many veterans are eligible for health care through the VA system. However, only a minority of veterans use VA programs,[44] although a higher percentage of veterans of Operation Enduring Freedom/Operation Iraqi Freedom (approximately 50%) have accessed services because of broader eligibility criteria. Thus, to address the needs of the broader veteran population, non-VA providers should be following these guidelines and might wish to address gun safety and storage issues.

Reports of relationship problems among younger veteran suicide decedents underscored the need for more extensive resources to assist veterans in coping with family concerns.[7] Those who work with veterans should consider moving beyond the standard "danger signs" of suicide risk (e.g., major depressive disorder or PTSD) and address the role that life crises play in triggering suicidal behavior. Therefore, interventions that focus on developing practical interpersonal skills could avert a suicidal crisis. Furthermore, Kapur et al.[21] recently observed that the main strategy used in the United Kingdom to date included the encouragement of appropriate help-seeking behavior once individuals left the armed forces. In the United Kingdom, all citizens, including veterans, are served through the National Health Service.

Many young veteran decedents had elevated BACs at the time of death. Nearly one third of the youngest veteran suicide decedents had a BAC $\geq$ 0.08. It is well accepted that acute alcohol use is associated with suicidal behavior, and some consider this relationship to be causal.[45] Other indicators of substance abuse were also elevated in the young and middle-aged veteran suicide decedents compared with the older veteran suicide decedents. For example, according to the NVDRS, evidence of alcohol dependence appeared more prevalent in the middle-aged than in the youngest and oldest groups. Earlier studies suggested that Vietnam-era veterans, now middle aged, were particularly vulnerable to substance abuse and other psychiatric conditions.[46-49] Specifically, several studies showed a relationship between PTSD and substance abuse problems among Vietnam veterans.[50,51] A question of some importance was whether substance abuse prevention and treatment programs that focus on young and middle-aged veterans could reduce suicide in this population. It should be noted that the VA currently has suicide prevention care managers at each facility who coordinate the care of suicidal VA users and work to ensure that evidence-based treatments are accessed and used.

Our study also pointed to the burden of physical health problems among older veterans who died by suicide. Physical health problems were associated with suicide in the general population[52-54]; however, further analyses of the NVDRS revealed that physical illness was more prevalent among older veterans than among nonveterans (data not shown). Although elderly veterans were more likely than younger veterans to be described as currently having a depressed mood, evidence of mental health treatment was less common among the older than the younger veterans. Consistent with earlier findings,[21] middle-aged and older veterans were less likely to have received treatment for mental health problems compared with nonveterans in the same age groups (data not shown). The lower prevalence of mental health problems reported among older veterans might be related to family members' lack of knowledge of the decedent's mental health status and treatment, or could be related to less contact with family or reluctance to divulge information on a diagnosis or treatment because of stigma. Suicide prevention programs for older veterans within the medical system might be more likely to be successful if they focus on primary (physical) health care rather than exclusively on mental health care.

This study made an important and unique contribution to the literature regarding the circumstances preceding suicide among male veterans of different age groups. The findings of our study added to knowledge of the role that life stressors play in suicide, including relationship and intimate partner problems among younger veterans, substance abuse among middle-aged veterans, and physical illness among older veterans. In addition, our results also showed that the use of firearms was the most common method of suicide among veterans of all ages (especially among older veterans). Of note, the rate and likelihood of firearm use were higher among veterans than among nonveterans in all age groups.[20]

The present study had some potential limitations. First, questions were raised about the accuracy of the designation of veteran status on death certificates. However, data from the National Mortality Followback Survey (NMFS) showed a high rate of agreement between death certificates and proxy-derived information regarding the decedent's military service ($\kappa = 0.91$; data not shown).[55] Second, veteran status on death certificates did not distinguish among service members who were on active duty, those who were in the National Guard or Reserves, and those who had been discharged. Further examination of the NMFS revealed that among those classified as veterans on the death certificates, only 10% of those aged 18 to 34 years, 5% of those aged 35 to 44 years, 0.7% of those aged 45 to 64 years, and 0.6% of those aged 65 years and older were on active duty or in the Reserves at the time of death. Of note, although the NMFS data suggested that veteran status on death certificates was valid, the data were gathered in 1993 and might or might not be relevant today. Third, the Blue Ribbon Work Group on Suicide Prevention in the Veteran Population[19] observed that veterans' deaths might be more accurately classified as suicides (and correspondingly less likely to be considered "undetermined" deaths) because there was generally more information available about veteran deaths than about nonveteran deaths. For example, veterans were likely to have health insurance, family support, and social support in the community (e.g., VA and veterans' organizations) and, thus, more likely than nonveterans to have collateral data. However, a supplementary analysis of the NVDRS revealed that the rates of "undetermined" deaths across age groups were nearly identical for veteran and nonveteran decedents. Fourth, not all coroners or medical examiners and law enforcement personnel routinely collected mental health, substance abuse, toxicology, and firearm information; thus, the prevalence of important circumstances associated with suicide cases might have been underestimated.[56] The collection of postmortem data was particularly difficult because some states have independent county coroner systems rather than a centralized medical examiner system.[57] However, 63% of the states participating in the NVDRS have a centralized state medical examiner system compared with only 15% of nonparticipating states.[58] Fifth, as noted earlier, many of the suicide circumstances were derived from proxy information and might be unreliable.[56,59] However, several studies using psychological autopsy data showed that proxy responses were valid.[60–63] Finally, this study was descriptive, and no causal inferences could be made.

Despite these limitations, data from the NVDRS had numerous strengths. First, the NVDRS is the only surveillance system for violent deaths in the United States. Second, the NVDRS collects information from multiple sources to characterize violent deaths as opposed to using only death certificates (which contain limited data). Third, the data on nearly all suicide deaths include precipitating circumstances. Finally, although the NVDRS states are not necessarily representative of the nation, the populations of these 16 states are similar in terms of gender, age, ethnic/racial composition, urban/rural characteristics, and overall suicide rates to the nation as a whole.

The evidence presented here indicated that the risk of dying by suicide was significantly higher among nonelderly male veterans than among male nonveterans. Although the results of our analysis showed that the relative risk of suicide (vs nonveterans) was generally higher for younger compared with older veterans, preventive interventions should reach a broad population, including different age groups and those who do not use VA health care services.[64] Our findings have important implications for the development and implementation of preventive interventions. Primary care and behavioral health providers both inside and outside the VA system need to be attentive to age-specific circumstances (in addition to signs of suicidal intent and access to firearms) that may lead to suicide. The use of highly lethal suicide methods, such as firearms, reduces the opportunity to intervene and rescue, and firearm access among high-risk populations needs to be addressed before crises develop.[65] Addressing the diversity of precipitating suicide circumstances across age groups may both advance causal theories related to suicide risk and result in more efficacious preventive interventions.

ABOUT THE AUTHORS

Mark S. Kaplan and Nathalie Huguet are with Portland State University, Portland, OR. Bentson H. McFarland is with Oregon Health and Science University, Portland. Marcia Valenstein is with the Department of Veterans Affairs Ann Arbor Health System and the University of Michigan, Ann Arbor.

CONTRIBUTORS

M. S. Kaplan, B. H. McFarland, and N. Huguet designed and conceptualized the study, analyzed and interpreted the data, and wrote the article. M. S. Kaplan and N. Huguet acquired the data. N. Huguet performed the statistical analysis. B. H. McFarland supervised statistical analysis. M. Valenstein contributed to the drafts and critical revisions of the article. All the authors approved the final draft.

ACKNOWLEDGMENTS

This research was supported by the American Foundation for Suicide Prevention. It used data from NVDRS, a surveillance system designed by the Centers for Disease Control and Prevention's (CDC) National Center for Injury Prevention and Control. The findings are based, in part, on the contributions of the 16 funded states that collected violent death data and the contributions of the states' partners, including personnel from law enforcement, vital records, medical examiners/coroners, and crime laboratories.

None of the authors has any interests that might be interpreted as influencing the research.

Note. The American Foundation for Suicide Prevention and the CDC had no role in the design and conduct of the study; in the analysis and interpretation of the data; or in the preparation, review, or approval of the article.

HUMAN PARTICIPANT PROTECTION

The Human Subject Review Committee at Portland State University reviewed and approved the project.

REFERENCES

1. Goldsmith SK, Pellmar TC, Kleinman AM, Bunney WE. *Reducing Suicide: A National Imperative.* Washington, DC: National Academies Press; 2002.

2. Nock MK, Borges G, Bromet EJ, Cha CB, Kessler RC, Lee S. Suicide and suicidal behavior. *Epidemiol Rev.* 2008;30(1):133–154.

3. Helmkamp JC. Suicides in the military: 1980-1992. *Mil Med.* 1995;160:45–50.

4. Shaffer D. *Suicide and Suicide Prevention in the Military' Forces; Report of a Consultation.* Washington, DC: Office of the Secretary of Defense; 1998.

5. Allen JP, Cross G, Swanner J. Suicide in the Army: a review of current information. *Mil Med.* 2005;170(7):580–584.

6. Kang HK, Bullman TA. Is there an epidemic of suicides among current and former U.S. military personnel? *Ann Epidemiol.* 2009;19(10):757–760.

7. Institute of Medicine (IOM). *Returning Home from Iraq and Afghanistan: Preliminary Assessment of Readjustment Needs of Veterans, Service Members, and Their Families.* Washington, DC: The National Academies Press; 2010.

8. Kuehn BM. Soldier suicide rates continue to rise: military, scientists work to stem the tide. *JAMA.* 2009;301(11):1111–1113.

9. Department of Veterans Affairs Office of Inspector General. *Implementing VHA's Mental Health Strategic Plan Initiatives for Suicide Prevention.* Washington, DC: Department of Veterans Affairs; 2007.

10. Hampton T. Research, law address veterans' suicide. *JAMA.* 2007;298(23):2732.

11. House Committee on Veterans' Affairs Hearing. The Truth About Veterans' Suicide, May 6 2008. Washington, DC: House of Committee on Veteran's Affairs. Available at: http://veterans.house.gov/hearings. Accessed April 20, 2009.

12. Senate Committee on Veterans' Affairs Hearing. Mental Health Care and Suicide Prevention for Veterans, March 3 2010, Washington, DC: Senate Committee on

Veterans' Affairs. Available at: http://veterans.senate.gov/hearings.cfm. Accessed April 20, 2009.

13. Peake JB. (Secretary of Veteran Affairs). The Truth about Veterans' Suicides before the House Committee on Veterans Affairs, June 5, 2008. Washington, DC: House of Committee on Veteran's Affairs. Available at: http://www.gpo.gov/fdsys/pkg/ CHRG-110hhrg43052/html/CHRG-110hhrg43052.htm. Accessed January 4, 2012.

14. Maynard C, Boyko EJ. Datapoints: suicide rates in the Washington State veteran population. *Psychiatr Serv.* 2008;59:1245.

15. Shen X, Millet L, Kohn M. Violent deaths in Oregon: 2005: Oregon Department of Human Services, Portland, Oregon; 2007. Available at: http://www.oregon.gov/ DHS/ph/ipe/nvdrs. Accessed April 20, 2009.

16. McCarthy JF, Valenstein M, Kim HM, Ilgen M, Zivin K, Blow FC. Suicide mortality among patients receiving care in the Veterans Health Administration Health System. *Am J Epidemiol.* 2009;169(8):1033–1038.

17. Kaplan MS, Huguet N, McFarland BH, Newsom JT. Suicide among male veterans: a prospective population-based study. *J Epidemiol Community Health.* 2007;61(7):619–624.

18. Miller M, Barber C, Azrael D, Calle EE, Lawler E, Mukamal KJ. Suicide among US veterans: a prospective study of 500,000 middle-aged and elderly men. *Am J Epidemiol.* 2009;170(4):494–500.

19. United States Department of Veterans Affairs. Report of the Blue Ribbon Work Group Report on Suicide Prevention in the Veteran Population, June 30 2008. Available at: http://www.mentalhealth.va.gov/suicide_prevention/ Blue_Ribbon_Report-FINAL_June-30-08.pdf. Accessed January 4, 2012.

20. Kaplan MS, McFarland BH, Huguet N. Firearm suicide among veterans in the general population: findings from the National Violent Death Reporting System. *J Trauma.* 2009;67(3):503–507.

21. Kapur N, While D, Blatchley N, Bray I, Harrison K. Suicide after leaving the UK armed forces–a cohort study. *PLoS Med.* 2009;6:e26.

22. Centers for Disease Control and Prevention. National Violent Death Reporting System (NVDRS) Coding Manual Revised [Online], 2008. National Center for Injury Prevention and Control, Centers for Disease Control and Prevention

(producer). Available at: http://www.cdc.gov/ncipc/pub-res/nvdrs-coding/vs2/default.htm. Accessed January 4, 2012.

23. *International Classification of Diseases. 10th Revision.* Geneva, Switzerland: World Health Organization; 1994.

24. Fontana A, Rosenheck R. An etiological model of attempted suicide among Vietnam theater veterans: prospective generalization to a treatment-seeking sample. *J Nerv Ment Dis.* 1995;183(6):377–383.

25. Kausch O, McCormick RA. Suicide prevalence in chemical dependency programs: preliminary data from a national sample, and an examination of risk factors. *J Subst Abuse Treat.* 2002;22(2):97–102.

26. Lehmann L, McCormick RA, McCracken L. Suicidal behavior among patients in the VA health care system. *Psychiatr Serv.* 1995;46(10):1069–1071.

27. Hartl TL, Rosen C, Drescher K, Lee TT, Gusman F. Predicting high-risk behaviors in veterans with PTSD. *J Nerv Ment Dis.* 2005;193(7):464–472.

28. Thompson R, Kane V, Cook JM, Greenstein R, Walker P, Woody G. Suicidal ideation in veterans receiving treatment for opiate dependence. *J Psychoactive Drugs.* 2006;38(2):149–156.

29. Tiet QQ, Ilgen MA, Byrnes HF, Moss RH. Suicide attempts among substance use disorder patients: steps towards a decision tree. *Alcohol Clin Exp Res.* 2006;30:998–1005.

30. Zivin K, Kim HM, McCarthy JF, et al. Suicide mortality among individuals receiving treatment for depression in the Veterans Affairs health system: associations with patient and treatment setting characteristics. *Am J Public Health.* 2007;97(12):2193–2198.

31. Jakupcak M, Conybeare D, Phelps L, et al. Anger, hostility and aggression among Iraq and Afghanistan war veterans reporting PTSD and subthreshold PTSD. *J Trauma Stress.* 2007;20(6):945–954.

32. Freeman TW, Roca V, Moore WM. A Comparison of chronic combat-related posttraumatic stress disorder (PTSD) patients with and without a history of suicide attempt. *J Nerv Ment Dis.* 2000;188(7):460–463.

33. Lish JD, Zimmerman M, Farber NJ, Kuzma MA, Plescia G. Suicide screening in a primary care setting at a Veteran's Affairs Medical Center. *Psychosomatics.* 1996;37:413–424.

34. Benda BB. Gender differences in predictors of suicidal thoughts and attempts among homeless veterans that abuse substances. *Suicide Life Threat Behav.* 2005;35(1):106–116.

35. Rodell DE, Benda BB, Rodell L. Suicidal thoughts among homeless alcohol and other drug abusers. *Alcohol Treat Q.* 2003;21:57–74.

36. Thoresen S, Mehlum L, Røysamb E, Tønnessen A. Risk factors for completed suicides in veterans of peacekeeping: repatriation, negative life events, and marital status. *Arch Suicide Res.* 2006;10(4):353–363.

37. MacLean A, Elder GH. Military service in the life course. *Annu Rev Sociol.* 2007;33:175–196.

38. Desai RA, Dausey DJ, Rosenheck RA. Mental health service delivery and suicide risk: the role of individual patient and facility factors. *Am J Psychiatry.* 2005;162(2):311–318.

39. United States Department of Agriculture Economic Research Service. Measuring rurality: Rural-urban continuum codes, 2003. Available at: http://www.ers.usda.gov/briefing/rurality/ruralurbcon. Accessed April 20, 2009.

40. United States Department of Veteran Affairs. Veteran Population 2007. Available at: http://www1.va.gov/vetdata. Accessed April 20, 2009.

41. United States Department of Commerce. Bureau of the Census. American Community Survey (ACS): Public Use Microdata Sample (PUMS), 2006. ICPSR22101-v1. Ann Arbor, MI: Inter-university Consortium for Political and Social Research; 2008.

42. US Census Bureau. 2007 American Community Survey (ACS) Questionnaire. Available at: http://www.census.gov/acs/www/SBasics/SQuest/SQuest1.htm. Accessed April 20, 2009.

43. Stanley B, Brown GK. *The Safety Plan Treatment Manual to Reduce Suicide Risk: Veteran Version.* Washington, DC: United States Department of Veterans Affairs; 2008.

44. National Center for Veterans Analysis and Statistics. (10/27/2008). VA benefits and health care utilization. Available at: http://www.va.gov/VETDATA/Pocket-Card/4X6_spring10_sharepoint.pdf. Accessed January 4, 2012.

45. Cherpitel CJ, Borges GL, Wilcox HC. Acute alcohol use and suicidal behavior: a review of the literature. *Alcohol Clin Exp Res.* 2004;28(Suppl 5):18S–28S.

46. Boudewyns PA, Woods MG, Hyer L, Albrecht WJ. Chronic combat-related PTSD and concurrent substance abuse: Implications for treatment of this frequent "dual diagnosis." *J Trauma Stress.* 1991;4(4):549–560.

47. Brooks MS, Laditka SB, Laditka JN. Long-term effects of military service on mental health among veterans of the Vietnam war era. *Mil Med.* 2008;173:570–575.

48. Boehmer TK, Flanders WD, McGeehin MA, Boyle C, Barrett DH. Post-service mortality in Vietnam veterans: 30-year follow-up. *Arch Intern Med.* 2004;164(17):1908–1916.

49. Goldberg J, Eisen SA, True WR, Henderson WG. A twin study of the effects of the Vietnam conflict on alcohol drinking patterns. *Am J Public Health.* 1990;80(5):570–574.

50. Boscarino J. Current excessive drinking among Vietnam veterans: a comparison with other veterans and nonveterans. *Int J Soc Psychiatry.* 1981;27(3):204–212.

51. McFall M, Fontana A, Raskind M, Rosenheck R. Analysis of violent behavior in Vietnam combat veteran psychiatric inpatients with posttraumatic stress disorder. *J Trauma Stress.* 1999;12(3):501–517.

52. Kaplan MS, McFarland BH, Huguet N, Newsom JT. Physical illness, functional limitations, and suicide risk: a population-based study. *Am J Orthopsychiatry.* 2007;77:56–60.

53. Conwell Y, Lyness JM, Duberstein P, et al. Completed suicide among older patients in primary care practices: a controlled study. *J Am Geriatr Soc.* 2000;48:23–29.

54. Conwell Y, Duberstein PR, Hirsch JK, et al. Health status and suicide in the second half of life. *Int J Geriatr Psychiatry.* 2010;25:371–379.

55. United States Department of Health and Human Services, National Center for Health Statistics. National Mortality Followback Survey, 1993. ICPSR version. Hyattsville, MD: U.S. Department of Health and Human Service; 2005.

56. Logan J, Hill HA, Black ML, et al. Characteristics of perpetrators in homicide-followed-by-suicide incidents: National Violent Death Reporting System–17 US States, 2003-2005. *Am J Epidemiol.* 2008;168(9):1056–1064.

57. Karch DL, Dahlberg LL, Patel N. Surveillance for violent deaths–National Violent Death Reporting System, *16 States, 2007. MMWR Surveill Summ.* 2010;59:1–50.

58. National Research Council. *Strengthening Forensic Science in the United States: A Path Forward.* Washington, DC: The National Academies Press, 2009.

59. Bossarte RM, Simon TR, Barker L. Characteristics of homicide followed by suicide incidents in multiple states, 2003-04. *Inj Prev.* 2006;12(Suppl 2):ii33–ii38.

60. Conner KR, Conwell Y, Duberstein PR. The validity of proxy-based data in suicide research: a study of patients 50 years of age and older who attempted suicide. II. Life events, social support and suicidal behavior. *Acta Psychiatr Scand.* 2001;104(6):452–457.

61. Conner KR, Duberstein PR, Conwell Y. The validity of proxy-based data in suicide research: a study of patients 50 years of age and older who attempted suicide. I. Psychiatric diagnoses. *Acta Psychiatr Scand.* 2001;104(3):204–209.

62. Brent DA, Perper JA, Moritz G, et al. The validity of diagnoses obtained through the psychological autopsy procedure in adolescent suicide victims: use of family history. *Acta Psychiatr Scand.* 1993;87(2):118–122.

63. Kelly TM, Mann JJ. Validity of DSM-III-R diagnosis by psychological autopsy: a comparison with clinician ante-mortem diagnosis. *Acta Psychiatr Scand.* 1996;94(5):337–343.

64. Bruce ML. Suicide risk and prevention in veteran populations. *Ann N Y Acad Sci.* 2010;1208:98–103.

65. Mann JJ, Currier D. Prevention of suicide. *Psychiatr Ann.* 2007;37(5):331–339.

33

Suicide Incidence and Risk Factors in an Active Duty US Military Population

Jeffrey Hyman, PhD, Robert Ireland, MD, Lucinda Frost, PsyD, and Linda Cottrell, MS

Objectives. The goal of this study was to investigate and identify risk factors for suicide among all active duty members of the US military during 2005 or 2007.

Methods. The study used a cross-sectional design and included the entire active duty military population. Study sample sizes were 2 064 183 for 2005 and 1 981 810 for 2007. Logistic regression models were used.

Results. Suicide rates for all services increased during this period. Mental health diagnoses, mental health visits, selective serotonin reuptake inhibitors (SSRIs), sleep prescriptions, reduction in rank, enlisted rank, and separation or divorce were associated with suicides. Deployments to Operation Enduring Freedom or Operation Iraqi Freedom were also associated with elevated odds ratios for all services in the 2007 population and for the Army in 2005.

Conclusions. Additional research needs to address the increasing rates of suicide in active duty personnel. This should include careful evaluation of suicide prevention programs and the possible increase in risk associated with SSRIs and other mental health drugs, as well as the possible impact of shorter deployments, age, mental health diagnoses, and relationship problems.

The rate of suicide among those serving in the military has been an increasing focus of concern for the respective Military Departments, Members of Congress, and Department of Defense (DoD) senior leadership. This has been of special concern for the US Army because their rate of completed suicides has markedly increased since 2006.[1] There has been a concerted effort by each Military Department to implement suicide prevention initiatives, especially those targeting early identification of manifest risk factors that may indicate a need for treatment. Self-recognition of indicators of distress and a willingness to seek help have also been emphasized. The Air Force Suicide Prevention program is an example. Initiated in the late 1990s, it is now listed as a best practice by the Centers for Disease Control.[2]

This study was initiated by the Secretary of the Army to examine potential risk factors associated with completed suicides. The goal was to determine what caused the marked increase in the rate of suicides in the Army between 2005 and 2007. The initial study population included the Marine Corp as a comparison population for the active duty Army. At the request of the Office of the Assistant Secretary of Defense for Health Affairs and the DoD Suicide Prevention and Risk Reduction Committee (SPARRC), the original study was expanded to include active duty Air Force and Navy personnel.

Before 2008, risk factor analyses for DoD completed suicides were performed for relatively small populations, primarily at the Military Department level using service-unique databases. Each department used a different data collection tool and information system. This made it extremely difficult to electronically merge the data for comparison or aggregate reporting. Available department level data were also subject to the statistical limitations that were associated with smaller populations and relatively rare events.

This study was the first to combine DoD standardized suicide data, DoD-wide personnel data including deployments and marital status, and DoD-wide medical data with diagnoses and medical treatments. The goal of this study was to use all available quantitative data to investigate a wide range of potential risk factors that might be associated with suicides and the increase of suicides among active duty military personnel.

METHODS

This was a cross-sectional study that included all individuals on active duty in the US military at any time during the years 2005 or 2007. The study sample size was 2 064 000 control and 183 case individuals in 2005 and 1 981 587 control and 223 case individuals in 2007.

Analysis

The study used a case–control analysis. The analysis was performed using Stata Statistical software (version SE 10; Stata Corp LP, College Station, Texas) and SAS software (version 9.1; SAS Institute Inc., Cary, North Carolina). For 2007, all study variables other than deployments and suicides were based on events that occurred between January 1, 2006, and December 31, 2007. Similarly, events for the 2005 cohort were included if they occurred between January 1, 2004, and 31 December 31, 2005. Deployments and deployed time in Operation Enduring Freedom or Operation Iraqi Freedom (OEF/OIF) were counted beginning on September 11, 2001 and ending December 31, 2005, and December 31, 2007, for the 2005 and 2007 cohorts, respectively.

Because this study included the entire population for each military service rather than samples, there were no inferences to be made from a sample to the underlying population. Accordingly, statistical measures such as P values and confidence intervals had no interpretation and were not reported. Odds ratios (ORs) and population attributable fractions (PAFs)[3] were used as effect measures. The formula used for PAF was PAF = pd((RR−1)/RR), where pd = the proportion of cases exposed to the risk factor, and RR was an estimate of the relative risk.

In the absence of reported P values, the reader must interpret the importance, or clinical significance, of these study results. This is no less the case when P values are reported because statistical significance often offers only limited insight into the clinical significance of study results.

ORs greater than 1.0 and PAFs greater than 0 suggested an increase in risk. In this study, we considered ORs of 1.5 and above to be meaningful.

Logistic regressions were limited to 3 independent variables because of the statistically small number of cases. The variables included were: any mental health diagnosis, number of deployments to OEF/OIF, and selective serotonin reuptake inhibitor (SSRI) prescriptions. These were chosen as the variables of greatest interest based on the univariate results.

Variables

The variable "mental health diagnosis" included all *International Classification of Disease-9th Revision-Clinical Modification* (*ICD-9-CM*) diagnosis codes in the Mental Disorders range of 290–319,[4] as well as suicide ideation and previous suicide attempts. Traumatic brain injury (TBI) diagnoses and tobacco dependency were excluded.

The variable "mental health visit" included all appointment encounters with a psychiatrist, psychologist, psychiatric nurse practitioner, or social worker who provided mental health services within the Military Healthcare System.

Because this variable included some encounters that were for administrative purposes, screenings, or psychoeducational prevention activities and were coded using V-codes, it modestly overestimated the number of mental health visits that were related to possible mental health issues. V-codes are *ICD-9* codes used to record factors influencing health or contact with health services other than diseases or injuries.[5]

The drug classes included in this study (based on the 5-digit generic code number)[6] were: mental health prescriptions, SSRI prescriptions, and sleep prescriptions.

RESULTS

The suicide rate increased for all services between 2005 and 2007. The increase was greatest for the Regular Army and National Guard. The rate decreased for the Army Reserve based on a very small number of case individuals, as shown in Table 1.

Table 1. Suicide Rates Among Active Duty Personnel, by Calendar Year: 2005 and 2007

	2005		2007		
	Population,[a] No.	Suicide Rate[b]	Population,[a] No.	Suicide Rate[b]	% Change
Army	916 411	11.56	875 621	16.37	41.56
Regular Army	583 617	12.43	595 496	17.87	43.71
National Guard	217 892	10.62	181 857	15.80	48.76
Army Reserve	114 907	7.08	98 268	4.78	-32.47
Marines	244 905	14.00	244 829	16.50	17.87
Navy	432 764	9.38	416 920	10.71	14.20
Air Force	470 103	9.27	444 440	9.83	6.03

[a]Includes those who were on active duty at any time during the year.
[b]Rates are per 100 000 person-years of active duty

Demographics

Tables 2 to 5 contain the study demographics and univariate findings for each service. In 2005, the mean year of birth for the active duty population ranged from 1975.2 to 1979.6. In 2007, the range was 1976.3 to 1981.7. In 2005, the percentage of the active duty population that was male ranged from 80.3 to 93.9. For 2007, the range was 79.9 to 93.8. In 2005, 35.7% of Marines and 52.8% of Air Force personnel had children. In 2007, the corresponding percentages were 29.6% and 47.6%, respectively. Similarly, 42.5% of Marines and 60.5% of Air Force personnel were married in 2007 compared with 42.8% and 60.1%, respectively, in 2007. Of the active duty Army, 36.3% were members of the Reserves and National Guard in 2005 compared with 6.7% for the Navy. In 2007, 32% of the active duty Army were Reserve or Guard personnel.

Suicide Risk

A mental health diagnosis was a very strong suicide risk factor, as seen in Tables 2 to 5 (also see Table A, available as a supplement to the online version of this article at http://www.ajph.org). Mental health visits, SSRIs, and sleep prescriptions also showed consistent associations, as did reduction in rank and separation or divorce. Deployments to OEF/OIF were associated with elevated ORs for all services in the 2007 population and for the Army in 2005. The Marines tended to demonstrate weaker associations in many risk factors than were seen in the other services, including the effects of deployments.

Deployments

Through 2007, the Army had the highest percentage of active duty personnel with any deployments to OEF/OIF, followed by the Marines, Navy, and Air Force, as shown in Tables 2 to 5.

Table B (available as a supplement to the online version of this article at http://www.ajph.org) shows that 1 or more OEF/OIF deployments was associated with an increased risk of suicide for all services in 2007. In some cases, those with more than 1 deployment had a somewhat smaller increase in ORs. In 2005, deployments to OEF/OIF were only associated with elevated ORs for the 3 Army components (Regular Army, Army Reserve, or National Guard).

Table 2. Demographics and Odds Ratios for Suicide for the Army (Including Army Reserve and National Guard): 2005 and 2007

	2005 Army			2007 Army		
	Not a Suicide (n = 916 329), %	Suicides (n = 82), %	OR	Not a Suicide (n = 875 507), %	Suicides (n = 114), %	OR
Mean year of birth	1975.2	1976.6	...	1977.4	1978.3	...
Gender (male)	85.20	96.34	4.57	85.06	96.49	4.83
Race						
White	69.17	73.17	1.00	70.80	81.58	1.00
Asian	5.11	2.44	0.45	5.31	2.63	0.43
Black	19.99	21.95	1.04	19.09	11.40	0.52
American Indian	0.84	1.22	1.38	0.90	0.88	0.85
Other	4.13	1.22	0.28	3.15	3.51	0.97
Unknown	0.76	0	...	0.75	0	...
Any children	51.10	48.78	0.91	46.68	48.25	1.06
Member category						
Regular	63.68	76.83	1.00	68.01	82.46	1.00
National Guard	23.78	17.07	0.60	20.77	14.91	0.59
Reserve	12.54	6.10	0.40	11.22	2.63	0.19
Marital status						
Divorced	6.03	10.98	1.00	6.34	2.63	1.00
Married	54.68	53.66	0.54	54.96	58.77	2.57
Single	39.01	35.37	0.50	38.55	38.60	2.41
Other	0.27	0	...	0.15	0	...
Marital change						

(continued on next page)

Table 2. (*continued*)

	2005 Army			2007 Army		
	Not a Suicide (n = 916 329), %	Suicides (n = 82), %	OR	Not a Suicide (n = 875 507), %	Suicides (n = 114), %	OR
Stay single	37.96	35.37	1.00	38.13	38.60	1.00
Stay married	43.93	41.46	1.01	44.14	42.11	0.94
Got married	10.57	12.20	1.24	10.75	16.67	1.53
Separated/divorced	2.83	6.10	2.31	2.65	1.75	0.65
Other	4.71	4.88	1.11	4.32	0.88	0.20
Rank						
Enlisted	85.28	91.46	1.00	84.78	89.47	1.00
Officer	14.71	8.54	0.54	15.21	10.53	0.66
Rank change						
Improvement	42.09	39.02	1.00	40.87	47.37	1.00
Reduction	2.26	2.44	1.14	2.38	5.26	1.91
No change	56.65	58.54	1.09	56.76	47.37	0.72
Mental health visit	19.86	37.80	2.45	25.73	47.37	2.60
Mental health diagnosis	13.50	29.27	2.14	18.20	40.10	3.01
Mental health prescription	17.27	23.17	1.44	20.18	35.09	2.14
TBI DoD	0.91	4.88	5.59	1.42	7.89	5.94
TBI AMSA	1.65	6.10	3.88	2.31	12.28	5.92

(continued on next page)

Table 2. (continued)

	2005 Army			2007 Army		
	Not a Suicide (n = 916 329), %	Suicides (n = 82), %	OR	Not a Suicide (n = 875 507), %	Suicides (n = 114), %	OR
PTSD diagnosis	1.33	2.44	1.86	2.31	9.65	4.51
Depression diagnosis	5.90	15.85	3.01	7.14	21.05	3.47
Substance misuse diagnosis	9.95	24.39	2.92	17.37	26.32	1.70
Suicide attempt	0.15	2.44	17.13	0.23	7.89	37.21
Ideation diagnosis	0.52	3.66	1.47	0.82	7.02	9.14
STD diagnosis	1.93	3.66	1.93	1.92	2.63	1.38
SSRI prescription	8.21	17.07	2.30	9.61	24.56	3.06
Sleep prescription	4.97	6.10	1.24	7.22	17.54	2.74
No. of deployments to OEF/OIF						
0	45.94	31.71	1.00	43.88	27.19	1.00
1	40.27	51.22	1.84	35.07	51.75	2.38
≥ 2	13.79	17.07	1.79	21.05	21.05	1.61

Note. AMSA = Army Medical Surveillance Activity; DoD = Department of Defense; OEF/OIF = Operation Enduring Freedom/Operation Iraqi Freedom; OR = odds ratio; PTSD = posttraumatic stress disorder; SSRI = selective serotonin reuptake inhibitor; STD = sexually transmitted disease; TBI = traumatic brain injury.

Table 3. Demographics and Odds Ratios for Suicide for the Marines: Suicide Incidence and Risk Factors in an Active Duty United States Military Population, 2005 and 2007

	2005 Marines			2007 Marines		
	Not a Suicide (n = 244 877), %	Suicide (n = 28), %	OR	Not a Suicide (n = 244 796), %	Suicide (n = 33), %	OR
Mean year of birth	1979.65	1980.14	...	1981.7	1983.2	...
Gender (male)	93.95	100	...	93.77	100	...
Race						
White	79.86	96.43	1.00	82.17	93.94	1.00
Asian	3.09	0	...	3.10	3.03	0.85
Black	11.60	3.57	0.25	10.65	3.03	0.25
Other	2.96	0	...	1.92	0	...
Any children	35.70	32.14	0.85	29.62	24.24	0.64
Member category						
Regular	86.62	89.29	1.00	89.13	100.00	...
National Guard	0.04	0.00	...	0.00	0.00	...
Reserve	13.34	10.71	0.78	10.87	0.00	...
Marital status						
Divorced	3.24	3.57	1.00	3.39	3.03	1.00
Married	42.48	46.43	0.99	42.76	42.42	1.11
Single	53.97	50.00	0.84	53.69	54.55	1.14
Other	0.32	0	...	0.16	3.03	...
Marital change						

(continued on next page)

Table 3. (continued)

	2005 Marines			2007 Marines		
	Not a Suicide (n = 244 877), %	Suicide (n = 28), %	OR	Not a Suicide (n = 244 796), %	Suicide (n = 33), %	OR
Stay single	52.86	50.00	1.00	53.40	54.55	1.00
Stay married	29.39	21.43	0.77	29.33	27.27	0.91
Got married	12.86	25.00	2.05	13.36	15.15	1.11
Separated/divorced	2.23	0	...	1.92	3.03	1.55
Other	2.66	3.57	1.42	2.00	0	...
Rank						
Enlisted	90.45	96.43	1.00	88.84	100	...
Officer	9.53	3.57	...	11.16	0	...
Rank change						
Improvement	55.46	42.86	1.00	57.01	72.73	1.00
Reduction	3.56	17.86	6.49	3.15	6.06	1.51
No change	40.99	39.29	1.24	39.84	21.21	0.42
Mental health visit	8.24	17.86	2.42	9.25	9.09	0.98
Mental health diagnosis	9.23	25.00	1.99	11.04	13.33	1.24
Mental health prescription	11.49	17.86	1.67	10.23	9.09	0.68
TBI DoD	1.18	7.14	6.43	1.34	15.15	13.10
TBI AMSA	2.21	14.29	7.39	2.53	18.18	8.57

(continued on next page)

Table 3. (*continued*)

	2005 Marines			2007 Marines		
	Not a Suicide (n = 244 877), %	Suicide (n = 28), %	OR	Not a Suicide (n = 244 796), %	Suicide (n = 33), %	OR
PTSD diagnosis	0.97	0	...	1.63	0	–
Depression diagnosis	3.52	7.14	2.11	3.94	3.03	0.76
Substance misuse diagnosis	6.13	21.43	4.17	8.41	18.18	2.42
Suicide attempt	0.14	7.14	53.28	0.16	12.12	84.27
Ideation diagnosis	0.56	3.57	6.57	0.70	3.03	4.43
STD diagnosis	1.25	3.57	2.94	1.26	3.03	2.45
SSRI prescription	5.05	14.29	3.14	5.92	0	...
Sleep prescription	2.83	7.14	2.64	4.03	3.03	0.74
No. of deployments to OEF/OIF						
0	51.36	60.71	1.00	47.73	42.42	1.00
1	32.16	28.57	0.75	30.02	33.33	1.25
≥ 2	16.48	10.71	0.55	22.25	24.24	1.23

Note. AMSA = Army Medical Surveillance Activity; DOD = Department of Defense; OEF/OIF = Operation Enduring Freedom/Operation Iraqi Freedom; OR = odds ratio; PTSD = posttraumatic stress disorder; SSRI = selective serotonin reuptake inhibitor; STD = sexually transmitted disease; TBI = traumatic brain injury.

Table 4. Demographics and Odds Ratios for Suicide for the Air Force: 2005 and 2007

	2005 Air Force			2007 Air Force		
	Not a Suicide (n = 470 066), %	Suicide (n = 37), %	OR	Not a Suicide (n = 444 403), %	Suicide (n = 37), %	OR
Mean year of birth	1974.22	1974.76	—	1976.25	1976.81	...
Gender (male)	80.26	89.19	2.03	79.94	100.00	...
Race						
White	77.52	83.78	1.00	77.09	72.97	1.00
Asian	3.03	2.70	0.82	3.43	2.70	0.83
Black	14.70	13.51	0.85	14.46	16.22	1.18
American Indian	0.64	0	...	0.68	2.70	4.17
Other	3.43	0	...	3.61	5.41	1.58
Unknown	0.69	0	...	0.71	0	...
Any children	52.77	51.35	0.95	47.60	51.35	1.16
Member category						
Regular	83.60	82.86	1.00	83.61	91.89	1.00
National Guard	10.70	5.71	0.54	10.86	2.70	0.23
Reserve	5.71	11.43	2.02	5.53	5.41	0.89
Marital status						
Divorced	7.24	13.51	1.00	7.44	8.11	1.00
Married	60.51	51.35	0.45	60.06	59.46	0.91
Single	31.78	35.14	0.59	32.13	32.43	0.93
Other	0.47	0		0.37	0	
Marital change						

(continued on next page)

Table 4. (*continued*)

	2005 Air Force			2007 Air Force		
	Not a Suicide (n = 470 066), %	Suicide (n = 37), %	OR	Not a Suicide (n = 444 403), %	Suicide (n = 37), %	OR
Stay single	30.90	32.43	1.00	31.79	32.43	1.00
Stay married	50.27	45.95	0.87	50.37	54.05	1.05
Got married	9.94	5.41	0.52	9.55	5.41	0.55
Separated/divorced	3.27	10.81	3.15	3.02	8.11	1.51
Other	5.62	5.41	0.92	5.27		
Rank						
Enlisted	80.66	91.89	1.00	80.50	83.78	1.00
Officer	19.34	8.11	0.37	19.49	16.22	0.80
Rank change						
Improvement	43.16	24.32	1.00	41.22	29.73	1.00
Reduction	1.24	13.51	19.39	1.20	2.70	3.13
No change	55.60	62.16	1.98	57.58	67.57	1.63
Mental health visit	20.58	45.95	3.28	23.46	48.65	3.09
Mental health diagnosis	12.97	48.57	2.53	14.44	37.10	3.49
Mental health prescription	20.26	48.65	3.73	23.44	35.14	1.77
TBI DoD	0.72	2.70	3.85	0.68	13.51	22.86
TBI AMSA	1.37	2.70	2.00	1.41	13.51	10.90

(continued on next page)

Table 4. (continued)

	2005 Air Force			2007 Air Force		
	Not a Suicide (n = 470 066), %	Suicide (n = 37), %	OR	Not a Suicide (n = 444 403), %	Suicide (n = 37), %	OR
PTSD diagnosis	0.37	2.70	7.40	0.54	5.41	10.57
Depression diagnosis	5.70	21.62	4.56	5.63	29.73	7.10
Substance misuse diagnosis	10.22	32.43	4.22	13.39	35.14	3.50
Suicide attempt	0.06	2.70	47.98	0.08	13.51	184.52
Ideation diagnosis	0.36	5.41	15.75	0.39	10.81	31.29
STD diagnosis	1.95	2.70	1.40	1.99	2.70	1.37
SSRI prescription	8.13	24.32	3.63	7.90	24.32	3.75
Sleep prescription	6.23	18.92	3.51	10.57	24.32	2.72
No. of deployments to OEF/OIF						
0	57.81	72.97	1.00	51.43	32.43	1.00
1	25.09	16.22	0.51	25.32	35.14	2.20
≥ 2	17.10	10.81	0.50	23.25	32.43	2.21

Note. AMSA = Army Medical Surveillance Activity; DOD = Department of Defense; OEF/OIF = Operation Enduring Freedom/Operation Iraqi Freedom; OR = odds ratio; PTSD = posttraumatic stress disorder; SSRI = selective serotonin reuptake inhibitor; STD = sexually transmitted disease; TBI = traumatic brain injury.

Table 5. Demographics and Odds Ratios for Suicide for the Navy: 2005 and 2007

	2005 Navy			2007 Navy		
	Not a Suicide (n = 432 728), %	Suicide (n = 36), %	OR	Not a Suicide (n = 416 881), %	Suicide (n = 39), %	OR
Mean year of birth	1975.79	1975.75	...	1977.67	1977.15	...
Gender (male)	85.05	97.22	6.15	84.76	87.18	1.22
Race						
White	67.59	75.00	1.00	66.36	76.92	1.00
Asian	5.97	8.33	1.26	6.32	2.56	0.35
Black	19.29	11.11	0.52	18.83	7.69	0.35
American Indian	3.22	5.56	1.56	4.14	7.69	1.60
Other	2.85	0	...	3.15	2.56	0.70
Unknown	1.07	0	...	1.21	2.56	1.83
Any children	50.00	33.33	0.50	44.15	46.15	1.08
Member category						
Regular	93.32	97.22	1.00	91.84	97.44	1.00
National Guard	0	0	...	0	0	...
Reserve	6.66	2.78	0.40	8.16	2.56	0.30
Marital status						
Divorced	3.71	5.56	1.00	3.67	5.13	1.00
Married	55.13	41.67	0.50	54.38	61.54	0.81
Single	40.76	52.78	0.86	41.58	33.33	0.57
Other	0.40	0	...	0.37	0	...
Marital change						

(continued on next page)

Table 5. *(continued)*

	2005 Navy			2007 Navy		
	Not a Suicide (n = 432 728), %	Suicide (n = 36), %	OR	Not a Suicide (n = 416 881), %	Suicide (n = 39), %	OR
Stay single	38.77	44.44	1.00	39.69	28.21	1.00
Stay married	42.88	36.11	0.73	43.20	51.28	1.67
Got married	12.08	5.56	0.41	11.09	10.26	1.30
Separated/divorced	2.69	8.33	2.70	2.51	7.69	4.31
Other	3.58	5.56	1.36	3.51	2.56	1.03
Rank						
Enlisted	85.42	88.89	1.00	84.91	84.62	1.00
Officer	14.58	11.11	0.73	15.04	15.38	1.03
Rank change						
Improvement	43.01	36.11	1.00	43.36	33.3	1.00
Reduction	2.30	2.78	1.44	2.12	7.69	4.72
No change	54.69	61.11	1.33	54.52	58.97	1.41
Mental health visit	12.99	16.67	1.34	13.79	33.33	3.13
Mental health diagnosis	11.89	19.44	1.69	12.88	37.25	4.01
Mental health prescription	15.39	19.44	1.33	15.99	25.64	1.81
TBI DoD	0.75	2.78	3.76	0.69	7.69	12.00
TBI AMSA	1.49	13.89	10.65	1.53	12.82	9.47

(continued on next page)

Table 5. (continued)

	2005 Navy			2007 Navy		
	Not a Suicide (n = 432 728), %	Suicide (n = 36), %	OR	Not a Suicide (n = 416 881), %	Suicide (n = 39), %	OR
PTSD diagnosis	0.50	0	...	0.72	0	...
Depression diagnosis	4.66	2.78	0.59	4.94	20.51	4.96
Substance misuse diagnosis	8.77	22.22	2.97	11.53	25.64	2.65
Suicide attempt	0.12	5.56	48.06	0.13	5.13	41.83
Ideation diagnosis	0.58	2.78	4.93	0.77	10.26	14.78
STD diagnosis	2.17	0	*	1.93	2.56	1.33
SSRI prescription	6.82	8.33	1.24	6.93	15.38	2.44
Sleep prescription	4.18	5.56	1.35	5.24	5.13	0.98
No. of deployments to OEF/OIF						
0	44.97	72.22	1.00	51.27	38.46	1.00
1	34.19	16.67	0.44	30.16	28.21	1.25
≥ 2	20.84	11.11	0.70	18.57	33.33	2.39

Note. AMSA = Army Medical Surveillance Activity; DOD = Department of Defense; OEF/OIF = Operation Enduring Freedom/Operation Iraqi Freedom; OR = odds ratio; PTSD = posttraumatic stress disorder; SSRI = selective serotonin reuptake inhibitor; STD = sexually transmitted disease; TBI = traumatic brain injury.

Between 2005 and 2007, the percentage of the study population with positive findings for either mental health visits, prescriptions, or, mental health diagnoses increased across all services, as shown in Table A. In 2007, approximately 61% of suicides in the Regular Army, 57% in the Air Force, 46% in the Navy, and 18% in the Marines had 1 or more of these findings. These exposures were a consistent risk factor. However, there was no association between the number of deployments through 2007 and the prevalence of a mental health diagnosis, as shown in Table C (available as a supplement to the online version of this article at http://www.ajph.org).

Suicide, SSRIs, and Sleep Medications

Of those who completed suicide, 17.5% of Army and 24% of Air Force personnel had a history of sleep prescriptions in 2007. More than 24% of Army and Air Force suicide completers also had previous SSRI prescriptions, as shown in Tables 2 to 5.

Sleep Medications, SSRIs, and Deployments

Table D (available as a supplement to the online version of this article at http://www.ajph.org) shows that through 2007, the use of sleep medications increased with the number of deployments for all services. SSRIs were more heavily prescribed by the Army than the other services. An association between prescriptions and deployments was only seen for the Army and Marines.

Logistic Regression Analysis

After adjustment, mental health diagnosis, deployments to OEF/OIF, and any SSRI prescriptions all showed a consistent association with suicide across all services during both study years, as seen in Table E (available as a supplement to the online version of this article at http://www.ajph.org). In 2005, the association with deployments was strongest for the Army Reserve and National Guard. SSRIs were associated with suicide risk in the Regular Army and the Air Force for both study years, and in the other services for 1 of the study years. A history of mental health diagnosis was also positively associated with suicide across all services in both study years. The association was strongest for the Army Reserve, National Guard, and the Air Force.

DISCUSSION

In univariate analyses, mental health diagnoses, especially TBI, posttraumatic stress disorder (PTSD) and depression, suicidal ideation, previous suicide attempts, mental health visits, and mental health prescriptions (especially SSRIs and sleep prescriptions) had relatively high ORs across all services. Separation or divorce also had generally elevated ORs.

The increase in suicide risk associated with deployments through 2005 was limited to the Army, especially the National Guard and Army Reserve. In 2007, all the services experienced an increase in risk associated with 1 or more deployments.

In multivariate models, there were consistent associations between a mental health diagnosis and suicide across all services during both study years. Deployments were consistently associated with suicides in 2007. In 2005, the association was primarily seen in the Army, especially the National Guard and Army Reserve. An elevated OR was associated with a history of SSRI prescriptions in 7 of the 10 logistic regression models.

The observed association between SSRIs and suicide are a concern. Population studies showed that SSRI use was associated with fewer suicides in both adolescents and for all ages of adult veterans.[7] In univariate analyses, SSRI prescriptions were consistently associated with elevated ORs of suicide. Prescriptions written at mobile medical facilities were generally not available for this study. The actual association between these drugs and suicide might be higher than the observed association because differential misclassification of exposure status would bias estimates of ORs toward the null.[8]

Conversely, it was also possible that the observed association might, in part, be an artifact if those with more severe mental health issues were more likely to receive the drugs. Because data on the severity of mental health conditions were not available to us, we were unable to investigate this.

Sleep prescriptions were also a potential cause for concern. However, this association must be evaluated in the context of operational risk management. For example, the Air Force approves their use for flight crews and support personnel at noisy bases to assure crew rest, reduce fatigue, and prevent accidents.

Relationship issues were frequently mentioned as major suicide risk factors.[9,10] Changes in marital status were the only relationship variables available for this study. Separation or divorce appeared to have a fairly consistent association with suicide. The strength of association was roughly comparable to 1 deployment. In addition to failed relationships, US military analyses consistently mentioned financial and legal problems, as well as substance misuse (usually alcohol) as significant risk factors.

The strengths of this study included the careful identification of case individuals through use of the SPARRC suicide data from the Office of the Armed Forces Medical Examiner, voluminous medical data, and detailed deployment histories.

Limitations

The major study weaknesses centered on the variables that were not available for analysis. These included legal and financial problems, job-related problems other than loss of rank, personal relationship issues other than separation or divorce, battle stress, unit relationships, and relationships with superiors, participation in suicide prevention training, and the nature of such training. There were also no data available on religion and the severity of mental health diagnoses. Data on medical encounters and prescriptions in theater at mobile facilities were incomplete.

The dose and duration of medication taken (as opposed to prescribed) was unknown, as were the identities of those who might have taken these drugs without a prescription. This study also did not investigate the existence of potential early adverse effects of SSRI use in those who died by suicide, including akathisia, anxiety, and psychomotor activation.[11]

Although the increasing number of active duty suicides represents a huge cost in lives lost, in statistical terms, the numbers were small, and this made multivariate analyses difficult. Many of the effect measure estimates might also be unstable (i.e., with some exposures, 1 additional suicide could have had a major effect on the outcome measures).

Accordingly, inferences based on the magnitude of the effect measures in this study should be made with care.[3] With a rare, multifactorial, pathological outcome (such as suicide), many of the univariate measures might be subject to varying levels of confounding. The possible presence of effect modification could not be assessed.

The reasons for the lower increase in risk with 2 or more deployments versus 1 deployment (observed in the Regular Army, National Guard, and Army Reserve) were unknown, and might represent the "healthy warrior" effect because of diminished likelihood of deployment if less fit.[12] Individuals might have been better prepared emotionally for a second deployment. They might also have received increased training, increased suicide prevention efforts, or encountered different stress levels in OEF/OIF.

The increase in prevalence of depression associated with multiple deployments that the Mental Health Advisory Team V[9] reported for the Army was not replicated in these results, and might be related to the Mental Health Advisory Team methodology using small convenience samples of combatants, as well as the absence of medical data being reported from mobile facilities in OEF/OIF or limited access to care. If this was the case, it was suggested that the mental health status of the active duty military (especially the Army) might be worse than what was reflected in this study.

The results from this study were generally in agreement with previous studies on suicide risk in this population and in other military populations. Between 1980 and 1992, active duty suicide rates were highest for the 17 to 24 years age group, for enlisted personnel, and for men.[13] Military suicide rates have traditionally been lower than those of the civilian population. This was demonstrated in the United Kingdom,[14] among military recruits,[15] in Canada,[16] and in the Army active duty population.[1]

Suicide rates in the active duty US military increased during and after the period covered by this study. The Army reported a rate of 20.2/100 000 in 2008, which was higher than the civilian rate for the first time since the Vietnam war.[18] The Navy also had an elevated suicide rate compared with the general population.[19] By January 2009, more soldiers died from suicide than from combat.[20]

An increase in mental illness associated with the stress and associated activities was also reported. Canadian military personnel in combat and peacekeeping experienced increases in PTSD and other mental disorders. A sizable portion of the mental health outcomes were attributable to the deployments.[21]

In a longitudinal study of an Army brigade combat team during OIF, the unit experienced a suicide rate of 58 per 100 000 person-years, based on a very small number of case individuals. Psychiatric disorders were the second most common nonbattle injury.[22] A study of Scottish soldiers in World War II also found an increase in suicide rates.[23]

We speculated that the increased risk associated with deployments in 2007 compared with 2005 resulted from the extended duration of the war and the increasing lengths of individual deployments for Army and Air Force personnel. The Army increased deployment lengths from 12 to 15 months in early 2007, and the Air Force increased them from 4 to 6 months. Marine deployment lengths remained at 7 months. In addition to increased levels of stress on the deployed service member, lengthened deployments also increased stress on families and partners, which may have contributed to failed relationships.

The findings regarding the Marine Corps were unexpected. They are the service that is closest to the Army in terms of ground combat experience. However, their increase in suicide rates between 2005 and 2007 was much lower than the increases seen in the Regular Army, National Guard, or Army Reserve.

Lower percentages of Marines had mental health visits, mental health diagnoses, or mental health prescriptions in 2005 and 2007. A higher percentage of Marines were single, and a much lower percentage had children. A lower percentage were separated or divorced. They also had lower increases in suicides associated with deployments to OEF/OIF. Their deployments to OEF/OIF were shorter than the Army's. In addition, a lower percentage of Marine suicide completers were deployed in 2007 than those of any other service.

It was not known if any of the observed differences in suicide trends in the Army and Marines resulted from self selection, differences in training or leadership, differences in suicide prevention programs, unmeasured sources of stress, or any of the other differences noted in this study.

Conclusions

Mental health diagnoses, deployments (especially in 2007), mental health visits, SSRIs and sleep prescriptions, reduction in rank, enlisted rank, and separation or divorce were found to be consistently associated with suicide. Additional research is needed to address the increasing rates of suicide in the active duty military population. This should include a careful evaluation of the effectiveness of suicide prevention programs and the possible increase in risk associated with SSRI and other mental health drugs.

Further studies are also needed to evaluate the possible impact of shorter deployments, age, mental health diagnoses, and relationship problems. The differences between services in the distribution of suicide risk factors and suicide rates should also be investigated. If unique protective factors can be identified in any of the services, they might be useful for risk mitigation in the entire active duty population.

ABOUT THE AUTHORS

Jeffrey Hyman is with Tricare Management Activity, Falls Church, VA. Robert Ireland is with the Office of the Assistant Secretary of Defense/(Health Affairs), Falls Church. Lucinda Frost is with Behavioral Health Program Policy Integration, Office of the Assistant Secretary of Defense/ (Health Affairs) Clinical and Program Policy, Falls Church. Linda Cottrell is with Kennell, Inc., Falls Church.

HUMAN PARTICIPANT PROTECTION

The study was granted Exempt Status from the Human Research Protection Office, Office of Research Protections, Army Medical Research and Material Command. A data use agreement was obtained from the Tricare Management Activity Privacy Office to allow access to their medical records and protected health information data.

REFERENCES

1. Army Health Promotion Risk Reduction and Suicide Prevention Report 2010. Available at: http://usarmy.vo.llnwd.net/e1/HPRRSP/HP-RR-SPReport2010_v00.pdf. Accessed February 15, 2011.

2. SAMHSA National Registry of Evidence-based Programs and Practices. Available at: http://www.nrepp.samhsa.gov/ViewIntervention.aspx?id=121. Accessed February 18, 2011.

3. Rockhill B, Newman B, Weinberg C. Use and misuse of population attributable fractions. *Am J Public Health*. 1998;88:15–19.

4. National Center for Health Statistics Centers for Disease Control and Prevention. Available at: http://www.cdc.gov/nchs/icd/icd9cm.htm. Accessed February 18, 2011.

5. *ICD-9-CM Expert for Hospitals.* Volumes 12 and 3. Sixth Ed. Eden Prarie, MN: Ingenix; 2006.

6. National Drug Data File (NDDF) Plus. San Bruno (CA): First Databank Inc. National Drug Data File (NDDF) Plus. Available at: http://www.firstdatabank.com/products/nddf. Accessed February 22, 2011.

7. Gibbons RD, Brown CH, Hur K, Marcus SM, Bhaumik DK, Mann JJ. Relationship between antidepressants and suicide attempts: an analysis of the Veterans Health Administration data sets. *Am J Psychiatry.* 2007;164:1044–1049.

8. Flegal KM, Keyl PM, Nieto FJ. Differential misclassification arising from nondifferential errors in exposure measurement. *Am J Epidemiol.* 1991;134:1233–1244.

9. Mental Health Advisory Team [MHAT] Report V Available at: http://www.armymedicine.army.mil/reports/mhat/mhat_v/mhat-v.cfm. Accessed on February 22, 2011.

10. American Association of Suicidology. Suicide in the USA Available at: http://www.suicidology.org/c/document_library/get_file?folderId=232&name=DLFE-159.pdf. Accessed on February 18, 2011.

11. Akagi H, Kumar TM. Lesson of the week: akathisia: overlooked at a cost. *BMJ.* 2002;324:1506–1507.

12. Hoge CW. Re: "Psychiatric diagnoses in historic and contemporary military cohorts: combat deployment and the healthy warrior effect." *Am J Epidemiol.* 2008;168:1095–1096, author reply 1096–1098.

13. Helmkamp JC. Suicides in the military: 1980-1992. *Mil Med.* 1995;160:45–50.

14. Fear NT, Ward VR, Harrison K, Davison L, Williamson S, Blatchley NF. Suicide among male regular UK Armed Forces personnel 1984-2007. *Occup Environ Med.* 2009;66:438–441.

15. Scoville SL, Gubata ME, Potter RN, White MJ, Pearse LA. Deaths attributed to suicide among enlisted U.S. Armed Forces recruits 1980-2004. *Mil Med.* 2007;172:1024–1031.

16. Belik SL, Stein MB, Asmundson GJ, Sareen J. Are Canadian soldiers more likely to have suicidal ideation and suicide attempts than Canadian civilians? *Am J Epidemiol.* 2010;172(11):1250–1258.

17. Gibbons RD, Brown CH, Hur K, et al. Early evidence on the effects of regulators' suicidality warnings on SSRI prescriptions and suicide in children and adolescents. *Am J Psychiatry.* 2007;164(9):1356–1363.

18. Lizette Alvarez. "Suicides of Soldiers Reach High of Nearly 3 Decades". *The New York Times.* January 29, 2009;Sect A:19.

19. Kang HK, Bullman TA. Is there an epidemic of suicides among current and former US military personnel? *Ann Epidemiol.* 2009;10:757–760.

20. Bell NS, Harford TC, Amoroso PJ, Hollander IE, Kay AB. Prior health care utilization patterns and suicide among US Army soldiers. *Suicide Life Threat Behav.* 2010;40:407–415.

21. Sareen J, Belik SL, Afifi TO, et al. Canadian military personnel's population attributable fractions of mental disorders and mental health service use associated with combat and peacekeeping operations. *Am J Public Health.* 2008;12:2191–2198.

22. Belmont PJ, Goodman GP, Waterman B, DeZee K, Burks R, Owens BD. Disease and nonbattle injuries sustained by a US Army Brigade Combat Team during Operation Iraqi Freedom. *Mil Med.* 2010;175:469–476.

23. Henderson R, Stark C, Humphry RW, Selvaraj S. Changes in Scottish suicide rates during the Second World War. *BMC Public Health.* 2006;6:167.

34

Suicidal Behavior in a National Sample of Older Homeless Veterans

John A. Schinka, PhD, Katherine C. Schinka, MA, Roger J. Casey, PhD, MSW, Wes Kasprow, PhD, and Robert M. Bossarte, PhD

Objectives. We examined self-reported suicidal behavior of older homeless veterans to establish frequencies and predictors of recent suicidal behaviors, and their impact on transitional housing interventions.

Methods. We analyzed the records of a national sample of 10 111 veterans who participated in a transition housing program over a 6-year period, ending in 2008.

Results. Approximately 12% of homeless veterans reported suicidal ideation before program admission; 3% reported a suicide attempt in the 30 days before program admission. Older homeless veterans exhibiting suicidal behavior had histories of high rates of psychiatric disorders and substance abuse. Regression analyses showed that self-report of depression was the primary correlate of suicidal behavior. Suicidal behavior before program entry did not predict intervention outcomes, such as program completion, housing outcome, and employment.

Conclusions. Suicidal behavior was prevalent in older homeless veterans and was associated with a history of psychiatric disorder and substance abuse. Self-reported depression was associated with these behaviors at the time of housing intervention. Despite the association with poor mental health history, suicidal behavior in older homeless veterans did not impact outcomes of transitional housing interventions.

Across all age groups, suicide is the 11th leading cause of death and seventh leading cause of death among men.[1] Historically, the rate of suicide has been highest in the elderly, and the rate among older men is approximately 7 times that among women. Suicide attempts among the elderly are more likely to be lethal than among younger age groups. This finding has been attributed to declines in physical condition, making survival less likely, social isolation reducing the probability of successful rescue, and suicide attempts that are more carefully planned.[2] Several factors constitute notable risk factors for suicide among the elderly.[3] These include the presence of physical health factors, alcohol abuse, stressful life events, social isolation, and Axis I psychiatric disorders (especially depressive disorders). In interviews with surviving relatives of older suicide victims, Duberstein et al.[4] found that being unmarried, unemployed, financially disabled, and having a psychiatric disorder were the most common factors. Suicidal ideation is typically, but not always, a precursor to suicide attempts or self-harm and provides an estimate of the population that is usually considered to be at immediate risk. In analyses of data from the Canadian Community Health Survey, Corna et al.[5] reported relatively low general population rates (slightly more than 2%) of suicidal ideation occurred in the past year. Estimates of lifetime suicide ideation and attempts among a nationally representative sample of US adults suggested a similar presence. Results from analyses of data obtained from the 2008 National Survey of Drug Use and Health reported that 3.7% of adults thought about suicide in the past 12 months, and 0.5% reported a suicide attempt.[6]

Because US veterans are predominantly older individuals with substantial medical morbidities, high levels of substance abuse and mental illness, and increased knowledge of and access to firearms,[7–9] it is not surprising that some research reported that male veterans were at approximately twice the risk for suicide than male nonveterans.[10] However, the associations between history of military service and risk for suicide are not clear.[11] For example, subsequent studies of male veterans in the general population failed to identify increased risk among middle-aged and elderly males.[12] Among veterans receiving care from the Veterans Health Administration (VHA), suicide risk for men and women combined across all age groups was estimated to be 66% higher than that observed in the general population.[13] For male veterans, the risk in age groups 50 to 70 years was 56% to 108% greater than that in the general male population. The frequency of suicidal ideation also appeared to be higher in veterans receiving VHA health services. In a study of older veterans receiving services in Veterans Affairs (VA) primary care clinics, Ayalon et al.[14] found that 5% of veterans reported suicidal ideation in the 2 weeks before assessment. Notably, this same study found that poorer cognitive functioning contributed to the occurrence of suicidal ideation.

From the standpoint of health risk, a particularly vulnerable group of veterans are those that are homeless. The most recent estimates[15] indicate that approximately one seventh of the adult homeless population consists of veterans. Current point-in-time population estimates suggest that 75 000 or more veterans are homeless on any given night, and about twice as many experience homelessness at some point during the course of a year. Veteran status is associated with increased risk for homelessness; a larger percentage of veterans are homeless than in either the general population or the population living in poverty. Studies of homeless veterans revealed exceptionally high rates of significant psychiatric disorders, alcohol and drug abuse, and chronic medical conditions.[16] These factors are potentiated by the impact of aging in the veteran population. Current estimates show that more than 20% of homeless veterans are aged 55 years or older. Thus, cognitive decline because of aging and possible early onset of degenerative dementias adds to the cumulative impact of health risks in older homeless veterans. Although it is anticipated that the increasing health vulnerability produced by these risk factors increases morbidity and reduces life expectancies because of all-cause mortality, few studies have approached these issues in a programmatic manner. Much of what we know about homeless suicidal behavior is based on data from the Access to Community Care and Effective Services and Supports (ACCESS) program.[17] The ACCESS program provided clinical mental health services to 7224 individuals in 15 cities across the country. All participants were homeless adults with evidence of serious mental illness who self-reported a suicide attempt in the 30 days before admission to the program or a 2-week period of persistent serious thoughts of suicide in the same 30-day period. In the aged 55 years and older ACCESS group, 3.5% of participants reported a suicide attempt, and 19.0% reported persistent suicidal ideation in this 30-day period.[18] Roughly equivalent estimates were obtained in studies of veterans. In a sample of 34 245 veterans (mean age = 46.6 years) who sought treatment of substance abuse or psychiatric disorders, 3.4% of veterans reported an attempted suicide in the month before seeking services.[19] A similar study of 600 veterans (mean age = 56.3 years) who sought treatment of substance abuse at a Midwestern VA revealed that 40.0% reported current suicidal ideation as determined by an established cutoff score on a suicidal ideation self-report scale.[20]

The limited research to date suggests that older homeless veterans may be at substantively greater risk for suicidal behavior than are individuals in the general population. We attempted to expand the research literature on suicidal behavior in this target group by reporting analyses of self-reported suicidal behavior (ideation and attempts) in a large sample of older homeless veterans admitted into a nationwide VA housing intervention program. The data set allowed us to provide estimates of the frequencies of recent suicidal behaviors, predictors of suicidal behaviors, and the impact of suicidal behaviors on interventional outcomes.

METHODS

Data for this study were provided by the VA Northeast Program Evaluation Center and consisted of de-identified records of veterans aged 55 years and older who were admitted into, and discharged from, the VA Grant and Per Diem (GPD) program during federal fiscal years 2003 to 2009. The GPD program provides grants to community-based providers to acquire and renovate facilities to create furnished housing for veterans. The program also funds per diem to defray operational expenses and the cost of supportive services, which may include vocational, substance abuse, and educational interventions. The GPD program provides housing support for up to 2 years and is designed as a transitional program leading to permanent housing. Community-based providers differ in terms of the requirements for admission and the mix of services provided. Homeless veterans typically enter the GPD program from the street or a shelter, but may move into GPD programs directly from a hospital, halfway house, or other short-term housing situations. To examine predictors and sequelae of suicidal behaviors, we limited our analysis to records of completed first admissions; that is, the first admission occurring on or after the first day of fiscal year 2003 (October 1, 2002) with a discharge on or before September 30, 2008. The dataset was composed of the records of completed first admissions for 10 111 unique veterans who had complete data on suicidal behavior variables.

The analyses were based on data from 2 sources of information. The first source was Form X, which is a comprehensive structured interview administered by program staff to veterans at the time of admission to specialized VA homeless service programs. Form X captures sociodemographic, psychosocial, health, housing, and employment information (e.g., recent work history). Form X contains 2 items that require "yes/no" responses for the experience of "serious thoughts of suicide" and for "suicide attempt" in the previous 30 days. The second source was Form D, an administrative form that captures basic information at the point of discharge from the GPD program (e.g., reason for discharge, work status). In this dataset, Form X was administered no more than 14 days before admission and no more than 5 days after admission.

Preliminary analyses provided descriptive statistics for the sample as a whole, including the frequencies of serious suicidal ideation and suicide attempt. Independent groups were then created on the basis of responses to the Form X suicidal ideation and suicide attempt questions. Participants who responded positively to either of the suicidal behavior questions comprised the suicidal behavior (SUI-BEH) group. The remaining participants constituted the negative suicide behavior (SUI-NEG) group. Descriptive statistics and group comparisons were then conducted on variables in the following domains: demographic characteristics, medical and psychiatric history, work and financial support, and treatment outcomes. Additional variables included suspected diagnoses in several categories (e.g., mood disorder, combat posttraumatic stress syndrome [PTSD]). These diagnoses were not based on formal diagnostic interview or medical records, but were the clinical judgment impressions of staff based on Form X responses and behavior during the Form X interview. Chi-square statistics were calculated to determine significant differences between groups on categorical variables. Independent-sample t tests were used to examine differences on continuous variables. When the Levene test for homogeneity of variance was significant, the examination of mean differences was adjusted accordingly.

Because of the large sample size, we anticipated that many analyses would produce results that would be considered significant by examination of P values. To aid in meaningful interpretation of results, we calculated effect sizes for all t test and χ^2 analyses. The Cohen[21] d was computed to provide an effect size for the t test. Following the convention offered by Cohen, we interpreted absolute values for d of 0.2, 0.5, and 0.8, indicating small, medium, and large effect sizes, respectively. Absolute values for d that were less than 0.2 were designated as meaningless, regardless of levels of statistical significance for the t test. We calculated Cramer's φ to provide an effect size estimate for χ^2 analyses.[22] φ is a measure of association between 2 binary variables and is similar to the Pearson correlation coefficient in its interpretation.[23] Again following a convention offered by Cohen,[21] we interpreted absolute values for

φ of 0.10, 0.30, and 0.50 as indicating small, medium, and large effect sizes, respectively. Absolute values for φ that were less than 0.10 were designated as meaningless, regardless of levels of statistical significance for the χ^2 statistic. Because we focused interpretation of statistical results on effect sizes, we did not correct P values for the number of analyses that were conducted (e.g., by employing Bonferroni adjustments).

Logistic regression analysis was used to identify predictors of suicidal ideation and suicide attempt. In these analyses, predictor variables (e.g., demographic variables, psychiatric history variables) were all allowed to enter the analysis at step 1, using a stepwise forward method of entry with a significant Wald χ^2 test as a criterion for determining entry (at $P < .05$) and removal (at $P > .1$). A second set of logistic regression analyses, using the same procedure, was directed at determining predictors of intervention outcomes (program completions, length of stay, housing on discharge, employment on discharge). In these analyses, suicidal ideation and suicide attempt were treated as predictor variables. In all logistic regression analyses, we calculated the McKelvy–Zavoina index per the recommendation of DeMaris.[24] This index also serves as a measure of effect size, with an explanation of 1% of the variance in the dependent variable considered to be the lower boundary of a small meaningful effect.[21] All analyses were carried out using SPSS (version 19.0; SPSS Inc., Chicago, Illinois).

RESULTS

The sample as a whole had a mean (SD) age of 59.4 (4.8) years and was uniformly male (98.1%) and unmarried (95.1%). A slight majority of participants were White (54.1%), and a minority (34.1%) had been exposed to combat fire during their military service. The majority (81.0%) were referred by outreach staff or community agencies, and almost all (95.7%) completed their Form X interviews at a community site (e.g., shelter, housing provider) rather than at a VA facility. A majority of participants reported positive histories of alcohol or drug abuse (77.7%) and psychiatric disorders (57.9%). Almost half of the sample (48.6%) had histories positive both for alcohol or drug abuse and for psychiatric disorders; 13.1% had no history of either. Serious thoughts of suicide in the 30 days before program admission were reported by 1267 (12.1%) participants. A suicide attempt in the 30 days before program admission was reported by 275 (2.7%) participants. A total of 1267 (12.5%) reported either suicidal ideation or attempt and comprised the SUI-BEH group. The remaining 8844 participants comprised the SUI-NEG group. Group membership was not related to whether Form X was completed before or after admission to the housing program ($\chi^2 = 3.48$; $P > .05$). Table 1 provides descriptive statistics and the results of t-tests and χ^2 analyses of comparisons of the SUI-BEH and SUI-NEG groups.

Demographic and Background Characteristics

Examination of demographic characteristics revealed several significant differences between the SUI-BEH and SUI-NEG groups. SUI-BEH participants were slightly older, more frequently White, more likely to be married, and more likely to report being under fire in combat during their military service. The SUI-BEH participants were less likely to have worked in the 30 days before admission, but no less likely to have had full-time employment in the past 3 years. VA pension support was significantly more common in the SUI-BEH group, but there were no differences between the 2 groups on non-VA support. Notably, significant differences between groups on demographic and background variables were all characterized by effect sizes that failed to reach a level of meaningful interpretation.

Health, Substance Use, and Mental Health Variables

Numerous comparisons between veterans in the SUI-BEH and SUI-NEG groups in measures of health, alcohol and substance use, and mental health were conducted, and all produced significant differences. An effect of medium size was obtained for serious depression in the 30 days before admission, in which the SUI-BEH group reported twice the rate of the SUI-NEG group. Small effect size differences showing higher frequencies were found for current drug abuse, current psychiatric problems, history of hospitalization for psychiatric disorder, and use of psychiatric medications in the 30 days before admission. The SUI-BEH group had greater frequencies than the SUI-NEG group for the reported presence of a serious medical problem, current and past alcohol abuse, previous hospitalization for alcohol abuse, past drug abuse, previous hospitalization for drug abuse, and use of VA health services in the

Table 1. Characteristics and Outcomes in a National Sample of Homeless Veterans: United States, 2003–2008

	Condition		Statistical Tests			
Variable	Negative for Suicidal Behavior (n = 8844), Mean ±SD or No. (%)	Positive for Suicidal Behavior (n = 1267)	t or χ^2 [a]	df	P	d or φ[b]
Demographics/background						
Age, y	59.55 ±4.89	58.64 ±3.85	7.54	1904	<.001	0.19
Caucasian	4720 (53.4)	750 (59.2)	15.14	1	<.001	0.039
Married	411 (4.6)	81(6.4)	7.29	1	.007	0.027
Combat fire	2966 (33.5)	478 (37.7)	8.66	1	.003	0.029
Full-time work, past 3 y	2487 (28.1)	330 (26.0)	2.37	1	.123	-0.015
Any work, past 30 d	1536 (17.4)	156 (12.3)	20.32	1	<.001	-0.045
VA SC/NSC pension	2684 (30.3)	458 (36.1)	17.40	1	<.001	0.041
Non-VA support	3051 (34.5)	414 (32.7)	1.63	1	.201	-0.013
Health/substance use/mental health						
No. of medical problems	2.69 ±1.88	3.41 ±2.05	-11.70	1587	<.001	0.38
Days drinking in past 30 d	3.64 ±7.71	5.89 ±9.34	-8.198	1523	<.001	0.28
Days intoxicated in past 30 d	2.21 ±6.19	3.94 ±7.91	-7.483	1491	<.001	0.27
Days used drugs in past 30 d	1.90 ±5.81	3.55 ±7.79	-7.274	1473	<.001	0.27
Days used multidrugs in past 30 d	0.73 ±3.58	1.55 ±5.26	-5.351	1436	<.001	0.22
Serious medical problem	5406 (61.4)	935 (74.2)	77.83	1	<.001	0.088
Current alcohol abuse	2925 (33.1)	580 (45.8)	79.60	1	<.001	0.089
Past alcohol abuse	5579 (63.1)	916 (72.4)	41.07	1	<.001	0.064
Ever hospitalized for alcohol abuse	3893 (44.2)	665 (52.7)	32.31	1	<.001	0.057
Current drug abuse	2113 (23.9)	465 (36.8)	95.96	1	<.001	0.097
Past drug abuse	3992 (45.2)	711 (56.15)	53.18	1	<.001	0.073
Ever hospitalized for drug abuse						

(continued on next page)

Table 1. (*continued*)

Variable	Condition		Statistical Tests			
	Negative for Suicidal Behavior (n = 8844), Mean ±SD or No. (%)	Positive for Suicidal Behavior (n = 1267)	t or χ^2 [a]	df	P	d or φ [b]
Current psychiatric problem	3064 (34.7)	549 (43.4)	36.31	1	< .001	0.060
Ever hospitalized for psychiatric problem	4256 (48.2)	1114 (88.1)	706.61	1	< .001	0.265
	2533 (28.7)	802 (63.4)	604.14	1	< .001	0.245
Used VA services in past 6 mo	5939 (67.3)	1000 (79.1)	71.80	1	< .001	0.084
Serious depression in past 30 d	3644 (41.2)	1190 (93.9)	1232.22	1	< .001	0.349
Psychiatric medications in past 30 d	2980 (33.8)	868 (68.8)	573.61	1	< .001	0.238
Diagnostic impressions						
Alcohol abuse	4844 (54.8)	819 (64.6)	43.75	1	< .001	0.066
Drug abuse	3362 (38.0)	626 (49.4)	60.18	1	< .001	0.077
Schizophrenia	346 (3.9)	86 (6.8)	22.34	1	< .001	0.047
Other psychotic disorder	319 (3.6)	101 (8.0)	53.01	1	< .001	0.072
Mood disorder	3187 (36.0)	845 (66.7)	434.30	1	< .001	0.207
Combat PTSD	1316 (14.9)	300 (23.7)	63.85	1	< .001	0.079
Treatment outcomes						
Days in program	150.73 ±168.78	135.94 ±147.31	3.27	1778	.001	0.09
Complete program	5206 (58.9)	748 (59.0)	0.014	1	.907	0.001
Has residence at discharge	4559 (51.5)	653 (51.5)	0.000	1	.995	0.000
Employed at discharge	1803 (20.4)	256 (20.2)	0.023	1	.881	-0.001

Note. df = degree of freedom; NSC = not service-connected; PTSD = posttraumatic stress disorder; SC = service connected; VA = Veterans Affairs.

[a] t test for means ±SD and χ^2 for number (%).

[b] d for mean ±SD and φ for number (%).

previous 6 months. However, these differences did not reach the level of a meaningful effect.

Diagnostic Impressions and Treatment Outcomes

High frequencies of diagnoses of alcohol and drug abuse, schizophrenia and other psychotic disorders, mood disorders, and combat PTSD were suspected by homeless program staff in both the SUI-BEH and SUI-NEG veterans. Suspected diagnoses were significantly more common in the SUI-BEH group, but only achieved status of a small effect for mood disorder.

A small majority of both SUI-BEH and SUI-NEG veterans finished homeless intervention programs, with program stays that averaged approximately 5 months. There were no differences between the groups in program completion or in length of program stay. Approximately one half of all veterans had a permanent residence on discharge; there was no difference between groups in this outcome. There was no difference between the SUI-BEH and SUI-NEG groups in frequency of employment on discharge—less than one quarter of the veterans had a positive status on this outcome measure.

Predictors of Suicidal Behavior

On the basis of the univariate analyses results and the literature on homeless veterans, the following predictors were used in conducting the logistic regression analysis for presence of suicidal behavior: race (White vs non-White), any employment in the 30 days before admission, number of reported medical problems, days drinking in the 30 days before admission, days of drug use in the 30 days before admission, report of serious depression in the 30 days before admission, and diagnostic impression of mood disorder by program staff. Table 2 presents the results of this analysis. Six predictor variables made significant contributions to the prediction of suicidal behavior, together explaining 26.9% of the variance in risk for suicidal behavior. However, the only variable that made a meaningful contribution was the report of serious depression in the 30 days before admission to the program, which alone explained 24.9% of the variance in risk and accounted for 93% of the predictive ability of the 6-variable model.

Table 2. Logistic Regression Analysis for Presence of Suicidal Behavior in National Sample of Homeless Veterans: United States, 2003–2008

Significant Predictors	OR (95% CI)	P	Increase in McKelvy–Zelvoina R^2
Serious depression in previous 30 d	16.66 (13.09, 21.22)	< .001	24.9
Mood disorder	1.53 (1.34, 1.76)	< .001	0.07
Days of drug abuse in past 30 d	0.98 (0.97, 0.98)	< .001	0.05
No. of medical problems	0.93 (0.90, 0.96)	< .001	0.03
Race	1.34 (1.17, 1.53)	< .001	0.03
Days of drinking in past 30 d	0.99 (0.98, 1.00)	.003	0.02

Note. CI = confidence interval; OR = odds ratio.
McKelvy–Zelvoina R^2 provides an estimate of the percent of variance in the outcome measure explained by the predictor variable (e.g., 0.6 = 0.6 of 1%; 10.3 = 10.3%).

Predictors of Treatment Outcomes

Table 3 presents the results of logistic regression analyses conducted to predict treatment outcome, using program completion, housing status, and employment status as outcome variables. On the basis of previous analyses and research, the following predictors were used: number of days drinking in the 30 days before program admission, number of days using drugs in the 30 days before program admission, history of hospitalization for alcohol abuse, history of hospitalization for drug abuse, history of hospitalization for psychiatric disorder, race (White vs non-White), number of days worked in the 30 days before program admission, VA financial support, number of reported medical problems, and presence of suicidal behavior. Suicidal behavior was not a significant predictor for any of the outcome variables. There were several significant predictors for each of the outcome variables and, in general, previous hospitalizations for any reason and number of days drinking in the month before program admission explained variance in outcomes across the 3 outcome measures. For the program completion and housing status outcome variables, the best predictor for each analysis explained less than 1% of the variance in the outcome measure, and the set of significant predictors in each analysis explained only approximately 1% of the variance. For the employment status outcome variable, the VA financial support predictor explained 5% of the variance in outcomes. Approximately 25% of veterans not receiving VA

Table 3. Logistic Regression Analyses Examining 3 Program Intervention Outcome Variables in a National Sample of Homeless Veterans: United States, 2003–2008

Significant Predictors	OR (95% CI)	P	Increase in McKelvy–Zelvoina R^2
Outcome: complete program			
Past hospitalization for drug abuse	1.25 (1.15, 1.36	< .001	0.6
VA financial support	1.20 (1.10, 1.31)	< .001	0.3
Past hospitalization for psychiatric disorder	1.14 (1.04, 1.24)	.004	0.1
No. of days drinking in the 30 d before program admission	0.99 (0.99, 1.00)	.007	0.1
Outcome: homeless at discharge			
No. of days drinking in the 30 d before program admission	0.99 (0.98, 0.99)	< .001	0.5
No. of days employed in the 30 d before program admission	1.01 (1.01, 1.02)	< .001	0.2
Past hospitalization for alcohol abuse	1.16 (1.07, 1.26)	< .001	0.1
No. of days using drugs in the 30 d before program admission	0.99, (0.98, 0.99)	.001	0.1
Race	1.09 (1.00, 1.18)	0.04	0.1
Outcome: employed at discharge			
VA financial support	3.05 (2.67, 3.48)	< .001	5.0
No. of days drinking in the 30 d before program admission	1.02 (1.02, 1.03)	< .001	0.9
No. of days employed in the 30 d before program admission	0.98 (0.97, 0.99)	.001	0.2
No. of reported medical problems	0.96 (0.94, 0.99)	.001	0.1
Past hospitalization for drug abuse	0.84 (0.76, 0.94)	.005	0.1
Past hospitalization for psychiatric disorder	1.13 (1.01, 1.27)	.027	0.1

Note. CI = confidence interval; OR = odds ratio; VA = Veterans Affairs. Analyses used forward stepwise method of entry with Wald. McKelvy–Zelvoina R^2 provides an estimate of the percent of variance in the outcome measure explained by the predictor variable (e.g., 0.6 = 0.6 of 1%; 10.3 = 10.3%).

financial support were employed on discharge. In contrast, only 10.1% of veterans receiving such support were employed on discharge. No other predictor variable explained as much as 1% in incremental variance for this analysis.

DISCUSSION

In these analyses, we examined the frequency of recent suicidal behavior in a large sample of older homeless veterans admitted to a transitional housing intervention program. Older individuals have historically been at high risk for suicide relative to other age groups, and older men are particularly at risk. There is evidence to suggest that risk among veterans is enhanced, and we hypothesized that suicidal behavior might be especially prevalent among homeless older veterans because of the cumulative vulnerability resulting from substance abuse, mental illness, poor health, and limited access to health care. Our descriptive analyses suggested that suicidal behavior was quite common in older homeless veterans seeking to enter housing intervention programs. Approximately 12% of our large national sample reported suicidal ideation before program admission. Although this was substantially higher than estimates of 12-month prevalence of suicide ideation among the general population, this rate was substantially lower than that reported by Benda[20] for a small sample of substance-abusing veterans and might reflect differences in assessment methodology. Our suicidal ideation variable was based solely on responses to a single question, whereas the smaller sample of Benda[20] was based on a psychometric cutoff for a multi-item Likert scale. Approximately 3% of our sample reported a suicide attempt in the 30 days before program admission. This result was quite consistent with the 30-day prevalence reported previously for older homeless individuals (3.48%) by Desai et al.[18] and for veterans seeking treatment of substance abuse or psychiatric disorders (3.4%) by Tiet et al.[19]

Consistent with previous research on the elderly,[3] we found that older veterans with suicidal behavior had more problematic histories than older veterans without such behavior, as indicated by significant differences in measures of physical health, alcohol and substance use, and mental health. Most of these differences were questionably meaningful, but current serious depression in combination with a current psychiatric problem and history of hospitalization for psychiatric disorder appeared to be a key pattern of pathology characterizing suicidal behavior in older homeless veterans. There did not appear to be any differences in housing intervention outcomes based on the presence of suicidal behavior at the time of program admission.

We used logistic regression analysis to address the relative importance of demographic, background, health, and mental health variables on predicting the presence of suicidal behavior at the time of program admission. Although numerous significant predictors were identified, the importance of a report of recent serious depression was the sentinel variable. Logistic regression analyses were also used to examine the relative importance of suicidal behavior preceding program admission to program intervention outcomes. In essence, these analyses addressed the question of whether suicidal behavior had a negative impact on outcomes. These analyses identified a number of significant, but questionably meaningful predictors of outcome, but none included suicidal behavior as a significant predictor.

Limitations

We noted several caveats with regard to the results. Although Form X captures fairly comprehensive information at program intake, data for suicidal behavior is captured from only 2 questions, and the presence of serious depression is assessed with only a single question. There are no available data on the reliability of these questions. Given our findings, future research on characteristics of homeless veterans at point of entry into homeless housing programs should employ any one of several reliable multi-item self-report instruments for the assessment of suicidal ideation and depression.

A critical issue was whether the groups with and without suicidal behavior were comparable on important variables not addressed in this study. One particularly important confounding factor could have been the receipt of mental health services before program entry that might have ameliorated suicidal behaviors. Data were not available to address this issue specifically, but we noted that the large majority of veterans in the sample were referred by community agencies, and virtually all veterans were administered Form X in the community rather than in a VA health care setting. These findings suggested that no veterans in either group were actively receiving mental health treatment in VA health care facilities at the time of program admission.

Conclusions

The results of this study added evidence to the small body of literature documenting the increased prevalence of suicidal behavior in homeless veterans and extended previous research by illuminating the characteristics of older homeless veterans. Consistent with previous studies, older homeless veterans exhibiting suicidal behavior were found to have histories character-ized by high rates of psychiatric disorders and substance abuse. A particularly strong finding was the significance of the relationship between suicidal behavior and self-reported serious depression in the period before program admission. Notably, the presence of suicidal behavior was not found to have an impact on short-term intervention outcomes, such as program completion, housing outcome, and employment. Future studies of older homeless veterans would be most valuable if they employed longitudinal approaches to determine the significance of suicidal behavior on long-term homelessness, long-term housing intervention outcomes, health care access, health status, and mortality. Such studies would allow the development of informed policies for identifying, treating, and protecting veterans with suicidal behavior in VA housing programs.

ABOUT THE AUTHORS

John A. Schinka and Roger C. Casey are with the Veterans Affairs (VA) National Center on Homelessness Among Veterans, Washington, DC. John A. Schinka is also with the Department of Psychiatry, University of South Florida, Tampa. Katherine C. Schinka is with the Department of Psychology, Kent State University, Kent, OH. Roger C. Casey is also with the Department of Community and Family Health, University of South Florida. Wes Kasprow is with the VA Northeast Program Evaluation Center, West Haven, CT. Robert M. Bossarte is with the VA Center of Excellence, Canandaigua, NY.

CONTRIBUTORS

J. A. Schinka conceptualized the project, conducted analyses, and contributed to writing the article. K. C. Schinka assisted in conceptualizing the project, conducted the literature review, and participated in writing the article. R. J. Casey contributed to abstracting the data and interpretation of findings. W. Kasprow conducted data abstracting and assisted in the analysis. R. Bossarte assisted in interpretation of findings and editing the article.

ACKNOWLEDGMENTS

This research was supported by the National Center on Homelessness Among Veterans, Department of Veterans Affairs.

HUMAN PARTICIPANT PROTECTION

An institutional review board of the Department of Veterans Affairs determined that approval was not required.

REFERENCES

1. Centers for Disease Control and Prevention [Internet]. National Suicide Statistics at a Glance. Available at: http://www.cdc.gov/violenceprevention/suicide/statistics/aag.html. Accessed February 1, 2011.

2. Conwell Y. Suicide in later life: a review and recommendation for prevention. *Suicide Life-Threat Behav.* 2001;31(suppl):32–47.

3. Conwell Y, Duberstein PR, Caine ED. Risk factors for suicide in later life. *Biol Psychiatry.* 2002;52:193–204.

4. Duberstein PR, Conwell Y, Conner KR, Eberly S, Caine ED. Suicide at 50 years of age and older: perceived physical illness, family discord, and financial strain. *Psychol Med.* 2004;34:137–146.

5. Corna LM, Cairney J, Streiner DL. Suicide ideation in older adults: relationship to mental health problems and service use. *Gerontologist.* 2010;50:785–797.

6. National Institute for Mental Health [Internet]. Prevalence of Suicidality Among U.S. Adults by Age and Sex in 2008. Available at: http://www.nimh.nih.gov/statistics/pdf/NSDUH-Suicidality-Adults.pdf. Accessed February 1, 2011.

7. Agha Z, Lofgren RP, VanRuiswyk JV, Layde PM. Are patients at Veterans Affairs medical centers sicker? A comparative analysis of health status and medical resource use. *Arch Intern Med.* 2000;160(21):3252–3257.

8. Lambert MT, Fowler DR. Suicide risk factors among veterans: risk management in the changing culture of the Department of Veterans Affairs. *J Ment Health Adm.* 1997;24(3):350–358.

9. Hankin CS, Spiro A 3rd, Miller DR, Kazis L. Mental disorders and mental health treatment among US Department of Veterans Affairs outpatients: the Veterans Health Study. *Am J Psychiatry.* 1999;156(12):1924–1930.

10. Bossarte RM, Claassen CA, Knox KL. Evaluating evidence of risk for suicide among Veterans. *Mil Med.* 2010;175:703–704.

11. Miller M, Barber C, Azreal D, Calle EE, Lawler E, Mukamal KJ. Suicide among US veterans: a prospective study of 500,000 middle-aged and elderly men. *Am J Epidemiol.* 2009;170:494–500.

12. Kaplan MS, Huguet N, McFarland BH, Newsom JT. Suicide among male veterans: a prospective population-based study. *J Epidemiol Community Health.* 2007;61(7):619–624.

13. McCarthy JF, Valenstein M, Kim HM, Ilgen M, Zivin K, Blow FC. Suicide mortality among patients receiving care in the Veterans Health Administration health system. *Am J Epidemiol.* 2009;169:1033–1038.

14. Ayalon L, Mackin S, Arean PA, Chen H, McDonel Herr EC. The role of cognitive functioning and distress in suicidal ideation in older adults. *J Am Geriatr Soc.* 2007;55:1090–1094.

15. Khadduri J, Culhane DP, Cortes A. *Veteran Homelessness: A Supplemental Report to the 2009 Annual Homeless Assessment Report to Congress.* Washington, DC: US Department of Housing and Urban Development & Department of Veterans Affairs; 2010.

16. Kushel MB, Vittinghoff E, Haas JS. Factors associated with the health care utilization of homeless persons. *JAMA.* 2001;285:200–206.

17. Randolph F, Blasinsky M, Leginsky W, Parker LB, Goldman HH. Creating integrating service systems for homeless persons with mental illness: the ACCESS program. Access to Community Care and Effective Services and Supports. *Psychiatr Serv.* 1997;48:369–373.

18. Desai RA, Liu-Mares W, Dausey DJ, Rosenheck RA. Suicidal ideation and suicide attempts in a sample of homeless people with mental illness. *J Nerv Ment Dis.* 2003;191:365–371.

19. Tiet QQ, Finney JW, Moos RH. Recent sexual abuse, physical abuse, and suicide attempts among male veterans seeking psychiatric treatment. *Psychiatr Serv.* 2006;57:107–113.

20. Benda BB. Discriminators of suicide thoughts and attempts among homeless veterans who abuse substances. *Suicide Life Threat Behav.* 2003;33:430–442.

21. Cohen J. *Statistical Power Analysis for the Behavioral Sciences.* 2nd ed. London: Routledge Academic; 1988.

22. Lipsey M, Wilson D. *Practical Meta-Analysis.* London: Sage Publications, Inc.; 2000.

23. Cohen P, Cohen J, West SG, Aiken LS. *Applied Multiple Regression/Correlation Analysis for the Behavioral Sciences.* 3rd ed. London: Routledge Academic; 2002.

24. DeMaris A. Explained variance in logistic regression: A Monte Carlo study of proposed measures. *Sociological Methods and Research.* 2002;31:27–74.

35

Veterans and Suicide: A Reexamination of the National Death Index–Linked National Health Interview Survey

Matthew Miller, MD, ScD, Catherine Barber, MPA, Melissa Young, MPH, Deborah Azrael, PhD, Kenneth Mukamal, MD, MPH, and Elizabeth Lawler, DSc

Objectives. We assessed the risk of suicide among veterans compared with nonveterans.

Methods. Cox proportional hazards models estimated the relative risk of suicide, by self-reported veteran status, among 500 822 adult male participants in the National Death Index (NDI)–linked National Health Interview Survey (NHIS), a nationally representative cohort study.

Results. A total of 482 male veterans died by suicide during 1 837 886 person-years of follow-up (76% by firearm); 835 male nonveterans died by suicide during 4 438 515 person-years of follow-up (62% by firearm). Crude suicide rates for veterans and nonveterans were, respectively, 26.2 and 18.8 per 100 000 person-years. The risk of suicide was not significantly higher among veterans, compared with nonveterans, after adjustment for differences in age, race, and survey year (hazard ratio = 1.11; 95% confidence interval = 0.96, 1.29).

Conclusions. Consistent with most studies of suicide risk among veterans of conflicts before Operation Iraqi Freedom/Operation Enduring Freedom, but in contrast to a previous study using the NDI-linked NHIS data, we found that male veterans responding to the NHIS were modestly, but not significantly, at higher risk for suicide compared with male nonveterans.

In 2008, then Secretary of the Department of Veterans Affairs, James Peake, established the Blue Ribbon Working Group on Suicide Prevention to assess suicide risk among the veteran population.[1] The group issued 8 key findings, the first of which was that the literature was contradictory regarding whether veterans were at higher risk for suicide compared with nonveterans.

The contradiction was traced to a single survey-based cohort study, published in 2007 by Kaplan et al,[2] which found a greater than 2-fold increased risk of suicide among veterans compared with nonveterans. By contrast, the other studies[3-6] found that suicide risk among veterans as a whole was not higher than that among age-, gender-, and race-matched members of the general population.

Kaplan et al.'s study[2] differed in 2 important ways from the other work cited by the Working Group.[3-6] First, Kaplan et al. [2] relied on self-report to assess veteran status, whereas the other studies ascertained veteran status from databases maintained by the Department of Defense. Second, relative risk estimates in Kaplan et al.[2] were based on direct comparisons of suicide incidence among veterans to incidence among nonveterans, whereas other studies used standardized mortality ratios (SMRs) that tended to bias veteran risk toward the null because veterans and nonveterans were both included in the comparison group. Two additional studies were published after the Working Group released its findings. The first, a military cohort study,[7] assessed suicide risk among veterans who served in Operation Iraqi Freedom/ Operation Enduring Freedom (OIF/OEF) and who separated from the military before 2006 (i.e., before the unprecedented increase in suicide incidence among soldiers).[8] The second study [9] tracked mortality among male respondents in the Cancer Prevention Study. Both studies failed to find evidence of differential suicide risk attributable to veteran status.

Our study reexamines the question of whether veterans were at increased risk for suicide using public data from the National Health Interview Survey (NHIS; 1986–2000) that have been linked to the National Death Index (NDI) through 2006—the same data source used in the study by Kaplan et al.,[2] now available for several additional years of baseline interviews and mortality follow-up. Like the previous NHIS–NDI study, the present study was limited to pre-OIF/OEF veterans. Because access to firearms is a risk factor for suicide,[10,11] and because veterans are more likely to own firearms than are nonveterans,[12] the present study examined not only the relation between veteran status and overall suicide risk, as did the original NHIS–NDI study, but also whether any such risk was differentially related to firearm versus nonfirearm suicide.

Because our primary findings were discrepant with those reported by Kaplan et al.,[2] we conducted sensitivity analyses that restricted data to the survey years (1986–1994) and mortality follow-up (through 1997) used in the study by Kaplan et al.[2] Covariates included in these comparative analyses were, by design, the same as those used by Kaplan et al.[2]

METHODS

The study population consisted of 500 822 men, aged 18 years and older, who participated in the NHIS between 1986 and 2000. The NHIS, conducted through the National Center for Health Statistics (NCHS), has been collecting health information on a representative sample of noninstitutionalized civilians in the United States since 1957. Sampling and interviewing are continuous throughout each year. The NHIS uses a multistage probability sampling design that selects primary sampling units from approximately 1900 geographic areas (a county, a small group of contiguous counties, or a metropolitan statistical area) and then samples households within each unit. Face-to-face household interviews are conducted with members of selected households, with response rates of over 90% each year.[13]

The NCHS linked NHIS data with the NDI by matching participants older than 18 years from the date of interview through December 2006 using 12 weighted criteria: social security number, first and last names, middle initial, race, gender, marital status, birth date (day, month, and year), and state of birth and residence.[14]

The linked NHIS–NDI file was used to determine the main outcome of the study: death by suicide. Secondary analyses examined the relation between veteran status and suicide by method.

Respondents were identified as veterans if they answered affirmatively to the questions: "Did you ever serve on active duty in the Armed Forces of the United States?" (NHIS 1986–1996) or "Have you ever been honorably discharged from active duty in the US Army, Navy, Air Force, Marine Corp, or Coast Guard?" (NHIS 1997–2000). Women were excluded from the analytic sample because so few female respondents identified themselves as veterans.

Covariates from baseline interviews that were used in the previous NHIS–NDI study were included in sensitivity analyses in the present study to allow for direct comparison with previous findings. These include age group, race, marital status, living arrangement, education, employment status, region of residence, self-rated health status, body mass index (BMI; defined as weight in kilograms divided by the square of height in meters), family income, and interval since last doctors visit

SUDAAN statistical software program (version 9.0; Research Triangle Park, NC) was used to perform weighted analyses that took into account the multistage sample design employed by the NHIS in the collection of these data. Weighted Cox proportional hazards models were used to estimate the relative hazard of suicide among veterans compared with nonveterans. Primary models were adjusted for age, race, and survey year (dummy variables each covering 3 calendar years). Respondents were censored at death by any cause; survivors were censored at the end of the study window, December 31, 2006. Time to death was measured from the midpoint of the quarter (i.e., 3-month period) of the interview to the exact date of death.

RESULTS

Veterans made up 30% of the sample, were considerably older (72% were aged 45 years and older vs 29% of nonveterans), and more likely to be White (90% vs 83%). Other baseline differences between veterans and nonveterans were greatly attenuated within age-strata (Table 1).

Suicide Rates by Veteran Status

A total of 482 male veteran participants died by suicide during 1 837 886 person-years of follow-up (364 by firearms [76%] and 118 by other methods), and 835 male nonveterans died by suicide during 4 438 515 person-years of follow-up (519 by firearms [62%] and 316 by nonfirearm methods). Crude suicide rates for male veterans and nonveterans were 26.2 and 18.8 per 100 000 person-years, respectively. The risk of suicide was not significantly higher among veterans compared with nonveterans, after adjustment for differences in age, race, and survey year (hazard ratio [HR] = 1.11; 95% confidence interval [CI] = 0.96, 1.29; Table 2).

The rate of firearm suicides was significantly higher among veterans (19.8/ 100 000 person-years) than among nonveterans (11.7/100 000 person-years); increased risk of firearm suicide persisted after adjusting for age, race, and

Table 1. Baseline Characteristics Among Male Respondents: National Health Interview Survey, 1986–2000

	Nonveteran (n = 351 689), Weighted %	Veteran (n = 149 133), Weighted %	Aged 18–44 Years[a]		Aged 45–64 Years[a]		Aged ≥ 65 Years[a]	
			Nonveterans (n = 245 025; Mean [SD] Age = 30.6 [7.5]), Weighted %	Veterans (n = 40 978; Mean [SD] Age = 35.8 [6.5]), Weighted %	Nonveterans (n = 73 847; Mean [SD] Age = 52.5 [5.6]), Weighted %	Veterans (n = 66 285; Mean [SD] Age = 54.6 [5.8]), Weighted %	Nonveterans (n = 32 817; Mean [SD] Age = 75.2 [6.8]), Weighted %	Veterans (n = 41 870; Mean [SD] Age = 71.6 [5.3]), Weighted %
Age			70.9	27.7	20.4	44.1	8.7	28.2
Race								
White	83.2	89.5	83.0	84.0	82.7	91.0	86.0	92.4
Non-White	16.8	10.5	17.1	16.0	17.3	9.0	14.0	7.6
Marital status								
Married	62.0	78.4	55.3	71.3	80.3	82.2	73.8	79.5
Widowed/divorced/separated	8.7	13.6	6.1	11.8	12.1	12.9	21.5	16.6
Never married or unknown	29.4	8.0	38.7	16.9	7.6	4.9	4.7	3.9
Education								
< 12 y	21.7	16.6	16.9	7.2	26.0	14.1	50.5	29.7
≥ 12 y	77.5	82.9	82.5	92.4	72.9	85.4	47.8	69.5
Unknown	0.8	0.6	0.7	0.3	1.1	0.5	1.7	0.8
Employment status								
Has job	78.7	64.5	85.9	90.3	80.5	77.2	15.8	19.3
Looking for work	2.9	1.8	3.5	3.4	1.8	1.7	0.2	0.3
Has no job	18.3	33.8	10.5	6.3	17.6	21.2	84.0	80.4
Unknown	0.10	0.02	0.11	0.02	0.09	0.03	0.03	0.01

(continued on next page)

Table 1. (continued)

	Nonveteran (n = 351 689), Weighted %	Veteran (n = 149 133), Weighted %	Aged 18-44 Years[a]		Aged 45-64 Years[a]		Aged ≥ 65 Years[a]	
			Nonveterans (n = 245 025; Mean [SD] Age = 30.6 [7.5]), Weighted %	Veterans (n = 40 978; Mean [SD] Age = 35.8 [6.5]), Weighted %	Nonveterans (n = 73 847; Mean [SD] Age = 52.5 [5.6]), Weighted %	Veterans (n = 66 285; Mean [SD] Age = 54.6 [5.8]), Weighted %	Nonveterans (n = 32 817; Mean [SD] Age = 75.2 [6.8]), Weighted %	Veterans (n = 41 870; Mean [SD] Age = 71.6 [5.3]), Weighted %
Region								
Northeast	20.6	19.6	20.1	16.8	21.6	19.9	21.8	21.8
Midwest	24.6	24.6	24.7	25.0	24.0	24.9	25.5	23.8
South	34.3	35.2	34.0	36.7	35.2	34.5	34.7	34.6
West	20.6	20.7	21.3	21.5	19.3	20.7	18.0	19.8
Place of residence population								
≥ 1 000 000	40.7	35.9	41.4	36.2	40.4	36.3	36.0	34.8
250 000-999 999	23.1	25.5	23.4	26.6	22.5	25.3	22.5	24.9
≤ 250 000	36.1	38.6	35.2	37.2	37.1	38.4	41.5	40.3
Health status								
Poor	9.6	15.2	5.0	6.2	16.3	14.4	31.5	25.3
Good	90.1	84.5	94.7	93.5	83.4	85.3	68.1	74.3
Unknown	0.3	0.3	0.3	0.3	0.3	0.3	0.4	0.3
Activity limitations								
Not limited	86.7	77.7	91.7	88.4	80.3	79.1	61.2	65.1
Limited	13.3	22.3	8.3	11.6	19.7	20.9	38.8	34.9

(continued on next page)

Table 1. *(continued)*

	Nonveteran (n = 351 689), Weighted %	Veteran (n = 149 133), Weighted %	Aged 18-44 Years[a]		Aged 45-64 Years[a]		Aged ≥ 65 Years[a]	
			Nonveterans (n = 245 025; Age = 30.6 [7.5]), Mean [SD] Weighted %	Veterans (n = 40 978; Age = 35.8 [6.5]), Mean [SD] Weighted %	Nonveterans (n = 73 847; Age = 52.5 [5.6]), Mean [SD] Weighted %	Veterans (n = 66 285; Age = 54.6 [5.8]), Mean [SD] Weighted %	Nonveterans (n = 32 817; Age = 75.2 [6.8]), Mean [SD] Weighted %	Veterans (n = 41 870; Age = 71.6 [5.3]), Mean [SD] Weighted %
BMI category								
Underweight	4.2	2.6	4.4	2.6	2.6	1.9	5.8	3.7
Normal	34.0	30.7	36.2	34.6	25.7	27.7	34.8	31.5
Overweight	31.9	39.0	30.9	38.7	34.7	41.3	33.9	35.6
Obese	14.0	15.0	13.3	14.7	17.4	16.7	12.0	12.6
Missing	15.9	12.7	15.1	9.5	19.6	12.3	13.5	16.6
Family income, $								
< 20 000	26.2	22.5	24.8	21.4	20.4	15.6	50.7	34.5
≥ 20 000	70.4	74.0	72.2	76.5	75.5	81.1	43.9	60.3
Unknown	3.4	3.5	3.0	2.1	4.1	3.3	5.4	5.3
Doctor visits past 12 mo, no.								
< 10	92.4	88.3	94.6	92.9	89.4	89.2	81.4	82.4
≥ 10	7.3	11.3	5.1	6.8	10.2	10.4	18.0	17.0
Unknown	0.3	0.4	0.3	0.3	0.4	0.4	0.6	0.6

Note. BMI = body mass index (defined as weight in kilograms divided by the square of height in meters).

[a] To facilitate comparisons of baseline characteristics by veteran status, descriptive statistics are provided not only for veterans as a whole, but also by age groups because veterans during the study period were, in general, much older than nonveterans.

Table 2. Rates and Adjusted Hazard Ratios for Overall Suicide, Firearm Suicide, and Nonfirearm Suicide Among Male Respondents, According to Veteran Status: National Health Interview Survey, 1986–2000

	All Suicides		Firearm Suicides		Other Suicides	
	Veteran	Nonveteran (Ref)	Veteran	Nonveteran (Ref)	Veteran	Nonveteran (Ref)
Suicide rate/100 000 person-y	26.23	18.81	19.81	11.69	6.42	7.12
Crude HR (95% CI)	1.36 (1.19, 1.54)	1.00	1.63 (1.41,1.90)	1.00	0.89 (0.71, 1.13)	1.00
Adjusted HR[a] (95% CI)	1.11 (0.96, 1.29)	1.00	1.19 (1.01, 1.40)	1.00	0.97 (0.73, 1.29)	1.00

Note. CI = confidence interval; HR = hazard ratio. A total of 482 male veteran participants died by suicide during 1 837 886 person-years of follow-up (364 by firearm and 118 by other methods); 835 male nonveteran died by suicide during 4 438 515 person-years of follow-up (519 by firearm and 316 by nonfirearm methods).
[a]Adjusted for age (as a continuous variable), race, and survey year.

survey year (HR = 1.19; 95% CI = 1.01, 1.40). Veterans and nonveterans did not differ significantly in their risk of suicide by nonfirearm methods.

Sensitivity Analyses

Sensitivity analyses restricted to the survey and follow-up years used in the original NHIS–NDI study[2] produced HRs similar to those obtained using the longer study period (Table 3). In the restricted study period analysis, there were 209 suicides among 106 166 male veterans and 298 suicides among 220 993 nonveteran men. The age- and race-adjusted suicide risk among male veterans over this abbreviated study period was modestly, but not significantly, higher among veterans than among nonveterans (HR = 1.21; 95% CI = 0.97, 1.50). Models that included all the covariates used in the previous NHIS study ("extensively" adjusted models) showed a significantly elevated suicide risk among veterans compared with nonveterans (HR = 1.33; 95% CI = 1.03, 1.71). When age was entered into the extensively adjusted model as a continuous variable, rather than as the categorical age groupings used by Kaplan et al.,[2] the HR and significance associated with veteran status were attenuated further (HR = 1.23; 95% CI = 0.96, 1.58). Additional sensitivity analyses that excluded persons with missing values for baseline covariates produced results virtually identical to those presented in Table 1.

DISCUSSION

Consistent with retrospective cohort studies that used standardized mortality ratios to measure suicide risk among veterans relative to the general population,[5,7,15–17] and with 1 of 2 previous survey-based cohort studies of suicide risk among veterans,[9] we found that the risk of suicide among male veterans was modestly, but not significantly, higher than that among age-, race-, and period-matched male nonveterans (HR = 1.11; 95% CI = 0.96, 1.29). By contrast, our results were at odds with those reported by Kaplan et al.,[2] who, using the same underlying data source as the present study, found a 2-fold increased risk of suicide among male veterans compared with male nonveterans (adjusted HR = 2.13; 95% CI = 1.14, 3.99).

Sensitivity analyses restricted to the same years of survey administration and mortality follow-up as in the study by Kaplan et al.[2] produced relative risk estimates similar to those we observed over our entire study period—but

Table 3. Suicide Rates and Hazard Ratios Among Male Respondents, According to Veteran Status: National Health Interview Survey, 1986-1994

	Veterans, No.	Nonveterans, No.	Firearm Suicides, Unweighted %		Person-Years of Follow-Up		Suicide Rate[a]		Crude HR (95% CI)	HR (95% CI) Adjusted for Age (Continuous) and Race	Multivariable Adjusted HR (95% CI)[b]
			Veterans	Nonveterans	Veterans	Nonveterans	Veterans	Nonveterans			
Current reanalysis	106 166	220 993	209 (77%)	298 (59%)	735 744	1 542 018	28.4	19.3	1.50 (1.23,1.84)	1.21 (0.97, 1.50)	1.33 (1.03, 1.71)
Kaplan et al.[2]	104 026	216 864	197 (77%)	311 (59%)	NA[c]	NA[c]	NA[c]	NA[c]	NA[c]	NA[c]	2.13 (1.14, 3.99)

Note. CI = confidence interval; HR = hazard ratio; NA = not available. Study period restricted to years analyzed in the original study by Kaplan et al.[2] (i.e., deaths through December 31, 1997). Multivariate models that used all 11 covariates in the study by Kaplan et al.,[2] but characterized age as a continuous variable, produced an attenuated HR of 1.23 (95% CI = 0.96, 1.58).

[a]Suicide rate was suicides per 100 000 person-years.

[b]Multivariate analysis included the covariates as described in the original study by Kaplan et al.[2]: age at the time of the interview (18–44, 45–64, and ≥ 65 years), race (White or non-White), marital status (married; widowed, separated or divorced; never married), living arrangement (alone or with others), education (< 12 years, ≥ 12 years, or unknown), employment status (has job, looking for work, has no job, unknown), region of residence (Northeast, Midwest, South, or West), self-rated health status (good—defined as excellent, very good or good; poor—defined as fair or poor, or unknown), body mass index (underweight, normal, overweight, obese, or missing), family income (< $20 000, ≥ $20 000, or unknown), and interval since last doctors visit.

[c]Data omitted because Kaplan et al.[2] did not provide person-years of follow-up or crude suicide rates by veteran status.

considerably more modest than the 2-fold risk ratio reported by Kaplan et al.[2] Our attempts to replicate the study by Kaplan et al.[2] were unsuccessful, despite baseline data that appeared very similar (e.g., total male suicides 508 vs 507; veterans constituted 15.7% of all respondents; and 32% of all male respondents in our analysis vs 15.7% of all respondents in the study by Kaplan et al.[2]). Attempts to replicate the findings of Kaplan et al.[2] produced 95% CIs with standard errors much smaller than those reported in that study and, importantly, did not include the point estimate they reported. Although Kaplan et al.[2] analyzed the restricted-use mortality data, whereas we used the public-use file, it was unclear why the 2 files yielded such contrasting findings.

Salient differences between our primary analyses and those in the previous NHIS–NDI study were that the present study covered more person-years of follow-up, observed more than twice as many suicides (1317 vs 508), adjusted for period effects by including indicator variables, and adjusted for age as a continuous variable (the previous study controlled for age using 3 broad age groupings). In addition, whereas we reported both crude suicide rates and age- and race-adjusted suicide risk among veterans and nonveterans, Kaplan et al.[2] reported only multivariable HRs that adjusted for several characteristics ascertained years after separation from the military. Consequently, although we could report that (1) the crude suicide rate among our veterans (26.2/100 000 person-years) was similar to that reported in previously cited retrospective military cohort studies,[3–6] and (2) the age- and race-adjusted suicide risk was not significantly higher among veterans compared with nonveterans, no such comparison could be ascertained from data published by Kaplan et al.[2]

Although veterans in our study were not at significantly elevated risk for suicide, they were significantly more likely to die by suicide involving firearms. Male veterans are more likely than are male nonveterans to live in homes with firearms,[12] and the presence of firearms in the home is a well-recognized risk factor for suicide.[10,11,18–24] As such, suicide rates among veterans, although not significantly higher than those among male nonveterans, might be higher than they would be if veterans were no more likely than nonveterans to live in homes with firearms. This counterfactual possibility was consistent with all studies of current, active duty military personnel before the current conflict in Iraq and Afghanistan, which consistently found evidence of a "healthy warrior effect" for suicide among military personnel (i.e., markedly lower suicide rates compared with the age-, race- and gender-matched civilian population).[25-34]

Our findings should be interpreted with several limitations in mind. First, we did not have information about deployment during wartime or combat-related injuries, aspects of exposure that might be relevant to suicide risk.[4,7] Second, as in other cohort studies, suicides were identified on the basis of death certificates. Although death certificate data are believed to underreport suicide, death certificates have nevertheless been widely accepted as a valid mortality source for epidemiological research on suicide.[35,36] Third, all veterans in our study were men, most were identified at a time remote from military service, and all had separated from the military before the unprecedented rise in suicide rates among soldiers of the OIF/OEF era. Our findings did not, therefore, address the risk of suicide among women veterans, veterans of the recent conflicts in Iraq and Afghanistan, or veterans recently separated from military service—a period that some,[3] but not all,[7,15] previous studies suggested might be one of heightened suicide risk.

Despite these limitations, and in view of consistent evidence of a "healthy warrior" effect for suicide risk among military personnel of every conflict before,[25-34] but not including, the recent conflict in Iraq and Afghanistan,[8] findings from the present study underscore the need for population-based suicide prevention policies that focus on (1) cohorts of veterans likely to be at greatest risk, such as those recently returning from Iraq and Afghanistan, and (2) suicide risk factors observed commonly among veterans, such as combat-related injuries and easy access to firearms, rather than on the notion that veteran status per se is a risk factor for suicide.

ABOUT THE AUTHORS

Matthew Miller, Catherine Barber, and Deborah Azrael are with the Department of Health Policy and Management, Harvard Injury Control Research Center, Harvard School of Public Heath, Boston, MA. Melissa Young and Elizabeth Lawler are with the Massachusetts Veterans Epidemiology Research and Information Center (MAVERIC), Boston. Kenneth Mukamal is with the Department of Medicine, Beth Israel Deaconess Medical Center, Boston.

CONTRIBUTORS

M. Miller designed the study, interpreted the data, and drafted and revised the article. M. Young and E. Lawler obtained and analyzed the data. All co-authors participated substantially in interpreting the data and revising the drafts.

ACKNOWLEDGMENTS

This material and the effort by M. Young and E. Lawler was based upon work supported by the Department of Veterans Affairs, Veterans Health Administration, Office of Research and Development, VA Clinical Science Research and Development Service. This material was also the result of work supported with resources and the use of facilities at the VA Boston Healthcare System, Boston, MA, and the resources of the VA Cooperative Studies Program. Funding for M. Miller, C. Barber, and D. Azrael was provided, in part, by the Joyce and Bohnett Foundations.

HUMAN PARTICIPANT PROTECTION

The Boston Veterans Health Administration Institutional Review Board approved this study.

REFERENCES

1. US Department of Veterans Affairs. Report of the Blue Ribbon Work Group on Suicide Prevention in the Veteran Population. Washington, DC: Department of Veteran Affairs; 2008.

2. Kaplan MS, Huguet N, McFarland BH, Newsom JT. Suicide among male veterans: a prospective population-based study. *J Epidemiol Community Health*. 2007;61(7): 619–624.

3. Boehmer TK, Flanders WD, McGeehin MA, Boyle C, Barrett DH. Postservice mortality in Vietnam veterans: 30-year follow-up. *Arch Intern Med*. 2004;164(17):1908–1916.

4. Bullman TA, Kang HK. The risk of suicide among wounded Vietnam veterans. *Am J Public Health*. 1996;86(5):662–667.

5. Kang HK, Bullman TA. Mortality among US veterans of the Persian Gulf War. *N Engl J Med.* 1996;335(20):1498–1504.

6. Watanabe KK, Kang HK. Military service in Vietnam and the risk of death from trauma and selected cancers. *Ann Epidemiol.* 1995;5(5):407–412.

7. Kang HK, Bullman TA. Risk of suicide among US veterans after returning from the Iraq or Afghanistan war zones. *JAMA.* 2008;300(6):652–653.

8. Kuehn BM. Soldier suicide rates continue to rise: military, scientists work to stem the tide. *JAMA.* 2009;301(11):1111–1113.

9. Miller M, Barber C, Azrael D, Calle EE, Lawler E, Mukamal KJ. Suicide among US veterans: a prospective study of 500,000 middle-aged and elderly men. *Am J Epidemiol.* 2009;170(4):494–500.

10. Brent DA. Firearms and suicide. *Ann N Y Acad Sci.* 2001;932:225–239; discussion; 239–240.

11. Miller M, Hemenway D. The relationship between firearms and suicide: a review of the literature. *Aggress Violent Behav.* 1999;4(1):59–75.

12. Centers for Disease Control and Prevention (CDC). *Behavioral Risk Factor Surveillance System Survey Data.* Atlanta, GA: US Department of Health and Human Services, CDC; 2003.

13. CDC. National Health Interview Survey. Questionaires, Datasets, and Related Documentation. Available at: http://www.cdc.gov/nchs/nhis/nhis_questionnaires.htm. Accessed March 9, 2011.

14. Rogot E, Sorlie P, Johnson N. Probabilistic methods in matching census samples to the National Death Index. *J Chronic Dis.* 1986;39:719–734.

15. Kang HK, Bullman TA. Mortality among US veterans of the Persian Gulf War: 7-year follow-up. *Am J Epidemiol.* 2001;154(5):399–405.

16. Kang HK, Bullman TA. Is there an epidemic of suicides among current and former US military personnel? *Ann Epidemiol.* 2009;19(10):757–760.

17. Michalek JE, Ketchum NS, Akhtar FZ. Postservice mortality of US Air Force veterans occupationally exposed to herbicides in Vietnam: 15-year follow-up. *Am J Epidemiol.* 1998;148(8):786–792.

18. Cummings P, Koepsell TD, Grossman DC, Savarino J, Thompson RS. The association between the purchase of a handgun and homicide or suicide. *Am J Public Health*. 1997;87(6):974–978.

19. Kellermann AL, Rivara FP, Somes G, et al. Suicide in the home in relation to gun ownership. *N Engl J Med*. 1992;327(7):467–472.

20. Miller M, Azrael D, Hemenway D. Household firearm ownership and suicide rates in the United States. *Epidemiology*. 2002;13(5):517–524.

21. Miller M, Azrael D, Hepburn L, Hemenway D, Lippmann SJ. The association between changes in household firearm ownership and rates of suicide in the United States, 1981–2002. *Inj Prev*. 2006;12(3):178–182.

22. Miller M, Hemenway D, Azrael D. Firearms and suicide in the northeast. *J Trauma*. 2004;57(3):626–632.

23. Miller M, Lippmann SJ, Azrael D, Hemenway D. Household firearm ownership and rates of suicide across the 50 United States. *J Trauma*. 2007;62(4):1029–1034; discussion 1034–1025.

24. Wiebe DJ. Homicide and suicide risks associated with firearms in the home: a national case-control study. *Ann Emerg Med*. 2003;41(6):771–782.

25. Eaton KM, Messer SC, Garvey Wilson AL, Hoge CW. Strengthening the validity of population-based suicide rate comparisons: an illustration using US military and civilian data. *Suicide Life Threat Behav*. 2006;36(2):182–191.

26. Helmkamp JC. Suicides in the military: 1980-1992. *Mil Med*. 1995;160(2):45–50.

27. Helmkamp JC. Occupation and suicide among males in the US Armed Forces. *Ann Epidemiol*. 1996;6(1):83–88.

28. Helmkamp JC, Kennedy RD. Causes of death among US military personnel: a 14-year summary, 1980-1993. *Mil Med*. 1996;161(6):311–317.

29. Powell KE, Fingerhut LA, Branche CM, Perrotta DM. Deaths due to injury in the military. *Am J Prev Med*. 2000;18(3 Suppl):26–32.

30. Rothberg JM, Fagan J, Shaw J. Suicide in United States Army personnel, 1985-1986. *Mil Med*. 1990;155(10):452–456.

31. Rothberg JM, Jones FD. Suicide in the US Army: epidemiological and periodic aspects. *Suicide Life Threat Behav.* 1987;17(2):119–132.

32. Rothberg JM, McDowell CP. Suicide in United States Air Force personnel, 1981–1985. *Mil Med.* 1988;153(12):645–648.

33. Rothberg JM, Rock NL, Del Jones F. Suicide in United States Army personnel, 1981–1982. *Mil Med.* 1984;149(10):537–541.

34. Rothberg JM, Rock NL, Shaw J, Del Jones F. Suicide in United States Army personnel, 1983-1984. *Mil Med.* 1988;153(2):61–64.

35. Phillips DP, Ruth TE. Adequacy of official suicide statistics for scientific research and public policy. *Suicide Life Threat Behav.* 1993;23(4):307–319.

36. Speechley M, Stavraky KM. The adequacy of suicide statistics for use in epidemiology and public health. *Can J Public Health.* 1991;82(1):38–42.

36

The US Air Force Suicide Prevention Program: Implications for Public Health Policy

Kerry L. Knox, PhD, Steven Pflanz, MD, Gerald W. Talcott, PhD, Rick L. Campise, PhD, Jill E. Lavigne, PhD, Alina Bajorska, MS, Xin Tu, PhD, and Eric D. Caine, MD

Objectives. We evaluated the effectiveness of the US Air Force Suicide Prevention Program (AFSPP) in reducing suicide, and we measured the extent to which air force installations implemented the program.

Methods. We determined the AFSPP's impact on suicide rates in the air force by applying an intervention regression model to data from 1981 through 2008, providing 16 years of data before the program's 1997 launch and 11 years of data after launch. Also, we measured implementation of program components at 2 points in time: during a 2004 increase in suicide rates, and 2 years afterward.

Results. Suicide rates in the air force were significantly lower after the AFSPP was launched than before, except during 2004. We also determined that the program was being implemented less rigorously in 2004.

Conclusions. The AFSPP effectively prevented suicides in the US Air Force. The long-term effectiveness of this program depends upon extensive implementation and effective monitoring of implementation. Suicides can be reduced through a multi-layered, overlapping approach that encompasses key prevention domains and tracks implementation of program activities.

Although much is known about risk factors for suicide, there are few examples of multifaceted, sustainable programs for reducing morbidity and mortality attributable to suicide and suicidal behaviors. The Air Force Suicide Prevention Program (AFSPP) has been found to have achieved significant relative risk reductions of rates of suicide and other violence-related outcomes, including accidental death and domestic violence.[1] The AFSPP, now in its 13th year, is an example of a sustained community-based effort that directly addresses suicide as a public health problem.

The AFSPP, launched in 1996 and fully implemented by 1997,[1] emphasizes leadership involvement and a community approach to reducing deaths from suicide. The program is an integrated network of policy and education that focuses on reducing suicide through the early identification and treatment of those at risk. It uses leaders as role models and agents of change, establishes expectations for airman behavior regarding awareness of suicide risk (i.e., policymaking), develops population skills and knowledge (i.e., education and training), and investigates every suicide (i.e., outcomes measurement). The program represents the air force's fundamental shift from viewing suicide and mental illness solely as medical problems and instead seeing them as larger service-wide community problems (Gen T. S. Moorman Jr, US Air Force, personal communication, June 2001).

The program's approach is predicated on current knowledge that individuals at risk exhibit warning signs and that intervention at an early stage lowers risk and results in improved outcomes. Thus, the program aims to reduce stigma and encourage early help-seeking behavior by changing social norms through education and policy. This is achieved at the community level by changing the community's knowledge, values, beliefs, attitudes, and behaviors concerning distress, help-seeking, and suicide. The AFSPP affirms and encourages help-seeking behavior, normalizes the experience of distress, promotes the development of coping skills, fights the stigma associated with receiving mental health care, and educates the community about the absence of negative career consequences for seeking and receiving treatment. The program also seeks to improve outcomes in putative distal risk factors for suicide, including family violence, alcohol and substance use, diminishing work performance, and depression. The result over the years has been the creation of an atmosphere of responsibility and accountability for reducing deaths from suicide that includes new expectations for behavior at the community and individual levels.

With little theoretical guidance available in 1996 to shape the program, the air force developed an overlapping programmatic design, resulting in far-reaching enhanced capacity of organizational responsiveness in critical areas at multiple levels. These overlapping components became known formally as the

11 Initiatives of the Air Force Suicide Prevention Program, which are described briefly in the box on the next page and in detail online (AFPAM 44–160; available at http://afspp.afms.mil/idc/groups/public/documents/afms/ctb_056459.pdf).

We studied the effect of the AFSPP on air force suicide rates from 1997, when the program was fully implemented, through 2008. We examined rates in the context of a 27-year period, from 1981 through 2008, during which time there have been 3 military conflicts and a major downsizing of the air force during the early 1990s. This 27-year period provides an important historical perspective on suicide rates in an organization that underwent rapid, widespread change in force structure and that dealt with the onset and continuation of Operation Enduring Freedom in Afghanistan in 2001 and Operation Iraqi Freedom in 2003. We also conducted a naturalistic experiment from 2004 through 2006, when we measured the implementation of program components during and after a transient increase in suicide rates.

METHODS

An intervention regression model[2] was applied to evaluate the influence of the AFSPP on quarterly suicide rates over time, and to create forecasts for future quarters. This type of time-series model has independent variables marking intervention periods and autoregressive errors that model the stochastic dependency of observations over time. All analyses were conducted using SAS software[3] applied to data from air force administrative databases.

Quarterly suicide rates were calculated per 100 000 for the active duty air force population from 1981 through 2007, and forecasted rates were calculated for each quarter of 2008. Each quarterly suicide rate was modeled as a regression with separate pre- and postintervention means and with first-order autoregressive errors (where the current error term is a fraction of the previous error term plus a random disturbance), using the ARIMA procedure.[2] This model compares the preintervention quarterly mean suicide rate for all previous time periods to the postintervention mean quarterly suicide rate for all quarters following the start date of the intervention.

An autocorrelation plot and the white noise test were used to check for stationarity and autocorrelation. Both first-order autoregressive and first-order moving average models were estimated.[2] The autoregressive model provided a better fit. The model was further examined for outliers, and its residuals were tested for any remaining autocorrelation. Six outliers were detected and entered into the model as points with different means.

The intervention regression model controlled for historical trends and seasonality, as well as for statistical white noise. The size of the air force population, which decreased over the study period, was confounded with time. To determine whether population size was correlated with suicide rates independently of the intervention, we modeled the annual suicide rate as a function of annual population size and an indicator of the start of the AFSPP in 1997, using a regression model weighted by the population size and with autocorrelated errors using SAS Proc Mixed.[3] The model was repeated using the change in population size. Lastly, population risk indicators were established from historical patterns, to detect early triggers of changes in the pattern of suicide rates.

In 2002 we began discussing how the AFSPP was implemented across the many installations of the air force, and we sought to view it within a developing theoretical prevention framework.[4] In 2004 we began using an implementation appraisal survey to measure implementation of AFSPP program activities associated with each of the 11 Initiatives (see the box on this page). In 2006 we further refined the survey into checklist form. The 11 Initiatives were purposely established to provide an overlapping organizational framework, but not necessarily a theoretical framework. Therefore, we clustered items on the implementation appraisal instruments into 7 prevention domains: (1) leadership involvement, (2) continuous professional military training, (3) development of guidelines for commanders, (4) ongoing community education, (5) development of integrated delivery system and community action information boards, (6) enhancement of community mental health services, and (7) instituting policies.

The items in the domains are best described as "operational measurements," after the work of Hand[5]; this kind of measure is also called an "indicator measure" by Fayers and Hand.[6] As Fayers and Hand[6] state, in contrast to psychometric measures, the goal of using indicator measures is to construct an index that consists of the combined values of the measured variables. We then used these indexes to calculate an implementation score for each of the 7 prevention domains. (To preserve the most information for analyses of implementation levels, data were analyzed at the installation level.)

THE 11 INITIATIVES OF THE US AIR FORCE SUICIDE PREVENTION PROGRAM

1. *Leadership involvement:* Air force leaders actively support the entire spectrum of suicide prevention initiatives in the air force community. Regular messages from the chief of staff of the air force, other senior leaders, and base commanders motivate the air force community to fully engage in suicide prevention efforts.

2. *Addressing suicide prevention through professional military education:* Suicide prevention education is included in all formal military training.

3. *Guidelines for commanders on use of mental health services:* Commanders receive training on how and when to use mental health services, and their role in encouraging early help-seeking behavior.

4. *Community preventive services:* Community prevention efforts carry more impact than treating individual patients 1 at a time. The Medical Expense and Performance Reporting System was updated to effectively track and encourage prevention activities.

5. *Community education and training:* Annual suicide prevention training is provided for all military and civilian employees in the air force.

6. *Investigative interview policy:* The period following an arrest or investigative interview is a high-risk time for suicide. Following any investigative interview, the investigator is required to "hand off" the individual directly to the commander, first sergeant, or supervisor. The unit representative is then responsible for assessing the individual's emotional state and contacting a mental health provider if any question about the possibility of suicide exists.

7. *Trauma stress response (originally critical incident stress management):* Trauma stress response teams were established worldwide to respond to traumatic incidents such as terrorist attacks, serious accidents, or suicide. These teams help personnel deal with the emotions they experience in reaction to traumatic incidents.

8. *Integrated Delivery System (IDS) and Community Action Information Board (CAIB):* At the air force, major command, and base levels, the CAIB and IDS provide a forum for the cross-organizational review and resolution of individual, family, installation, and community issues that impact the readiness of

the force and the quality of life for air force members and their families. The IDS and CAIB help coordinate the activities of the various base helping agencies to achieve a synergistic impact on community problems and reduce suicide risk.

9. *Limited Privilege Suicide Prevention Program:* Patients at risk for suicide are afforded increased confidentiality when seen by mental health providers (Limited Privilege Suicide Prevention Program). Additionally, Limited Patient-Psychotherapist Privilege was established in 1999, limiting the release of patient information to legal authorities during Uniform Code of Military Justice proceedings.

10. *IDS Consultation Assessment Tool (originally the Behavioral Health Survey):* The IDS Consultation Assessment Tool allows commanders to assess unit strengths and identify areas of vulnerability. Commanders can use this tool in collaboration with IDS consultants to design interventions to support the health and welfare of their personnel.

11. *Suicide Event Surveillance System:* Information on all air force active duty suicides and suicide attempts are entered into a central database that tracks suicide events and facilitates the analysis of

This permitted us to measure operationally whether an air force installation carried out the activities described in the box on the previous page, which are the direct result of complying with the 11 Initiatives. Each question was assigned a score of 1 if a respondent answered "yes" and 0 otherwise.

The data were weighted according to the number of implementation indicators from the 11 Initiatives that were grouped within each of the 7 prevention domains. Levels of implementation were then determined across all installations, and the scores were represented as the percentage of the maximum possible score for each of the 7 domains. Air force leaders and installation commanders completed the 11 Initiatives survey in 2004 and the 11 Initiatives checklist in 2006, using administrative records of activities monitored at each installation. Data were reported anonymously to minimize the potential for reporting bias and were compiled both at the base level and at the level of the 9 major commands, which are the operational units of the service.

RESULTS

Figure 1 depicts the observed quarterly suicide rate from 1991 through 2008. The horizontal lines represent the mean pre- and postintervention quarterly suicide rates, and the deviations from this mean are depicted as outliers across the decades. The estimated mean suicide rate per quarter during the intervention period was 2.387 per 100 000, compared with 3.033 per 100 000 for the preintervention mean, for a change of 0.646 ($P < .01$). The estimated correlation coefficient between consecutive quarterly observations is 0.431 ($P < .001$), and the estimated variance of the disturbance term is 0.513. During the postintervention period, in the third quarter of 2004, there was a significant upward spike in suicide rates ($P < .001$); subsequently, suicide rates fell and have remained within the expected range of the low rates seen soon after initial implementation of the program.

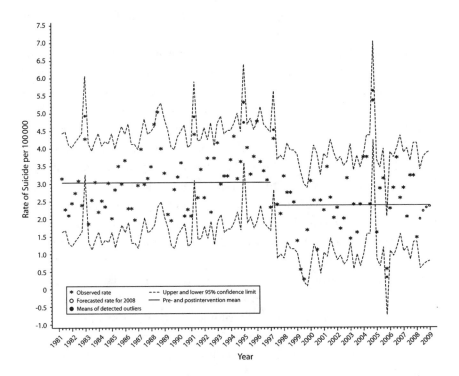

Figure 1. Quarterly suicide rates: US Air Force, 1981–2008.

Note. The US Air Force Suicide Prevention Program was implemented in 1997.

We observed an inverse relationship between population size and suicide rates in the preintervention period: a smaller population size tended to be associated with a higher suicide rate than that observed for a larger population size. All population sizes above 500 000 occurred during the period from 1981 through 1990, with the population declining during the remainder of the preintervention period. The regression model for the pre- and postintervention periods included an indicator of implementation of the AFSPP in 1997, in addition to population size. It showed a linear nonsignificant relationship between the rate and the population size, with a negative slope of -1.38 ($P > .05$). Because the population size and the intervention period are confounded, the regression intervention effect (-4.9; $P < .05$) is larger than in the bivariate analysis (-2.9; $P < .05$) unadjusted for population size. A similar trend was found when the relationship between the change in population size and suicide rate was investigated.

To give air force leadership tools for early detection of future increases in suicide rates, we developed risk indicators on the basis of the forecasted suicide rate for 2008 (9.3 per 100 000). Rates less than or equal to 1 standard deviation from the forecast rate (< 12.1 per 100 000) were identified as indicators of concern. Rates greater than 1 standard deviation from the forecast rate (12.1–14.8 per 100 000) were defined as indicators of warning, and rates greater than 2 standard deviations from the forecast rate (> 14.8 per 100 000) were identified as critical indicators of a change in the pattern of suicide rates.

Installations reported variation in the extent to which they implemented the AFSPP's suicide prevention activities as specified by the 11 Initiatives. Figures 2 and 3 show the levels of implementation across the 7 prevention domains in 2004 and 2006, respectively. These results suggest an overall higher level of AFSPP implementation in 2006 than in 2004. Median implementations for the 7 prevention domains in 2004 were all below 90%, and the lowest was 56% (Figure 2). In comparison, during 2006 the overall implementation values for 2 of the 7 prevention domains (continuous professional military training and enhancement of community mental health services) were 100% for 95% of all bases. For prevention activities in the 5 other prevention domains in 2006, at least half of the bases were found to have high levels of implementation (Figure 3).

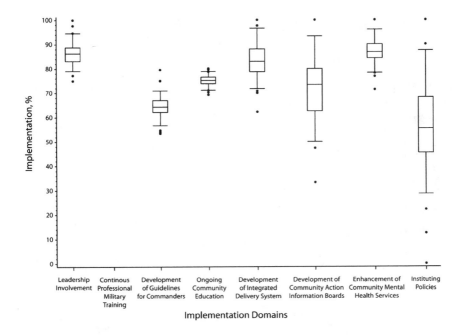

Figure 2. Levels of US Air Force Suicide Prevention Program (AFSPP) implementation, distributed across installations, in 2004.

Note. Horizontal lines represent the 5th, 25th, 50th, 75th, and 95th percentiles. Dots represent points beyond the 95th percentile.

DISCUSSION

In recent years there has been a marked increase in research on translating the findings of efficacy and effectiveness studies into actual health practices.[7,8] The AFSPP provides an opportunity to study the implementation of public health practices intended to reduce deaths from suicide. This opportunity is unique in 3 ways. First, the AFSPP was developed well before implementation science was acknowledged as a field of study. Second, the current operational structure of the AFSPP evolved over time, even though its principal initiatives were described at the outset; thus, attention to sustained implementation of its core components emerged iteratively. Third, this public health prevention program was not originally developed on a theoretical basis, which is now recommended as the best way to strengthen the credibility of measured outcomes.[7] In spite of this latter shortcoming, the subsequent identification of

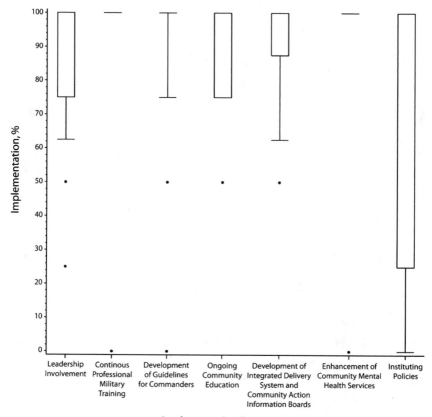

Figure 3. Levels of the US Air Force Suicide Prevention Program (AFSPP) implementation, distributed across installations, in 2006.

Note. Horizontal lines represent the 5th, 25th, 50th, 75th, and 95th percentiles. Dots represent points beyond the 95th percentile.

theoretical prevention domains for the AFSPP proved to be relatively straightforward.

The effects of the AFSPP are inevitably confounded with the activation of the air force for warfare, beginning immediately after the attacks of September 11, 2001, and accelerating into the wars in Afghanistan and Iraq. The possibility that these conflicts had an effect on suicide rates, regardless of any changes in program content or implementation, cannot be ruled out. Military morale is expected to be higher at the start of a conflict, particularly after a domestic attack, but as these 2 conflicts continued, morale may have suffered from a variety of factors, including stop-loss measures that barred service personnel from leaving the military at the end of their enlistments early in the war, the absence of any new attacks in the United States, and the cumulative effects of repeated deployments on military personnel and family members in areas such as relationships and finances. It is beyond the scope of this study to elucidate any contributions from these factors.

The upward spike in suicide rates observed during 2004 (Figure 1) raised important questions about whether the 2 ongoing wars, a decreasing force size, or diminished implementation of the AFSPP had taken its toll upon the program's presumed effectiveness. Our data did not allow us to estimate exactly when implementation efforts diminished; rather, they only gave us a snapshot at the end of 2004, a time when implementation likely had been diminishing for several years in the face of heavy demands from both the Afghanistan and Iraq wars. Regardless, air force leadership felt it was imperative to address the possibility that diminished implementation of the program played a role in the increase in suicide rates and initiated actions to ensure community-wide compliance with all of the components of the program. In 2006, levels of implementation were again measured. When suicide levels in 2004 and 2006 were compared with levels of implementation in 2004 and 2006, it appeared that diminished implementation of the AFSPP may have played a role in the reversal of the program's apparent effectiveness.

The air force now measures compliance with established AFSPP procedures on an annual basis. Organizational capacity for monitoring compliance with the program is now coupled with development of population risk indicators that are used to monitor suicide rates for identification of early shifts in patterns of suicide rates. There are limitations to this approach, but it reflects the importance of close tracking of programmatic activities for reducing deaths from suicide and the critical need to move beyond descriptive, epidemiologic studies of suicide risk.

The AFSPP has been continuously and incrementally improved since its launch, including the adoption of formalized prevention domains in 2004. The measures of implementation that were introduced in 2004 and refined for 2006 represent ongoing continuous quality improvement efforts. Given this drive to enhance effectiveness as rapidly as possible, the 2004 and 2006 measures evaluated the same key implementation prevention domains but were obtained somewhat differently. Although studies have demonstrated that this approach is appropriate when effecting changes in large organizations, it results in incrementally different measures being taken at each time point.[6] This is a limitation of the current study when viewed from the perspective of prevention science or therapeutic trials. This limitation is addressed to some degree through the development of theoretical prevention domains that remained constant over time under which the measures were grouped and compared. To date, however, there has been no external validation of these domains and measures. These data are being used as early-generation studies of implementation of a multicomponent suicide prevention program to inform the next generation of implementation studies, which should include such external validation measures.

If the relationship between suicide rates and population size in the air force were linear, as it appears to be when corrected for the intervention effect of the AFSPP, a higher suicide rate would have been expected during the postintervention years (1997–2008), when the air force population was declining. However, we are mindful of the nonsignificant inverse relationship between population size and suicide rate when left uncorrected for the intervention effect, rendering this inference somewhat tentative. We also recognize that a reduction in the number of service members with mental health problems could limit any conclusion regarding a sustainable programmatic impact over time. However, air force–specific data from the Department of Defense Survey of Health Related Behaviors found that, in 1998, 9.5% of air force personnel received mental health care; in 2002, 13.5% received mental health care; and in 2005, 13.3% received mental health care, suggesting that the air force is not decreasing its population of personnel with mental health problems.[9-11] It also is worth noting in this regard that the air force encourages early help-seeking behavior for a mental health problem, and 97% of air force personnel who seek mental health care do not experience any negative consequences to their military careers as a result.[12]

Knowledge about risk factors for suicide includes evidence that aggression, impulsivity, risk-taking, acute and chronic stresses (often including interpersonal or occupational related stress[13-18]), and alcohol or substance use[19,20] are powerfully associated with suicidal behaviors, which are moderated in their expression by gender and age. Despite these compelling data, there has been no reduction in overall suicide rates in the US civilian population since the 1940s, when national rates fell after the Great Depression and during the nation's involvement in World War II. Thus, many policymakers and clinicians remain uncertain whether systematic approaches to reducing deaths from suicide are feasible and effective. The AFSPP is the first long-term sustained effort of its kind to serve as an example of what communities can accomplish in reducing morbidity and mortality attributable to suicidal behaviors if there is ongoing commitment to do so.

Because of the wars in Afghanistan and Iraq, we can expect a large population of combat veterans to experience mental health disorders, and many of these individuals may not seek care. Stigma attached to mental health issues is a pervasive cultural phenomenon in the general US population, and it is even more pronounced in the military. The potential reluctance of military personnel to seek help because of stigma may become particularly significant in light of a recent report based on a prospective study of a US military cohort of 77 047 military active duty, reserve, and National Guard personnel by Smith et al.[21] These investigators found that deployed individuals who experienced combat exposure had a 3-fold increase in new onset of self-reported posttraumatic stress disorder. In a study by Boscarino,[22] veterans with posttraumatic stress disorder continued to be at heightened risk for suicide 30 years after separation from the service.

These findings highlight the importance of the role of specific combat exposures. It will be critical for clinicians who encounter returning military personnel to be trained to recognize the early risk factors and warning signs of suicidal behaviors, and specifically those associated with combat exposures. Although an earlier study[23] carried out among combat-exposed Vietnam veterans found a significant dose–response effect related to being wounded, it is unlikely that many physicians and clinicians are aware of the importance of assessing trauma exposure among those who have served. The larger challenge for communities worldwide is whether the pervasive stigma associated with mental health disorders and psychosocial problems will be overcome as a result of acceptance that these significant, adverse mental health outcomes are a normal human response to the exposures associated with serving in the military.

In conclusion, the US Air Force showed, through its efforts to reduce deaths from suicide, that (1) it is possible to reduce the rate of suicide across a period of years using a multifaceted, overlapping, community-based approach, and (2) reductions in suicide rates cannot be simply maintained by virtue of a program's inherent momentum. Programmatic efforts must be continuously supported and monitored to ensure sustained effects. This may mean that many communities and organizations will not easily be able to launch large-scale suicide prevention efforts on a scale comparable to the AFSPP, especially in developing countries.[24] We suspect that there may be real limitations on the feasibility of an exact replication of the AFSPP to other settings. Nevertheless, the enduring public health message from 12 years of this program is that suicide rates can be reduced, and that program success requires interventions to be consistently supported, maintained, and monitored for compliance. This is a message that all communities and organizations worldwide can embrace while considering how to appropriately structure programs and interventions at a local level.

ABOUT THE AUTHORS

Kerry L. Knox and Jill E. Lavigne are with the Canandaigua VA Medical Center, US Department of Veterans Affairs, Canandaigua, NY, and the Department of Psychiatry, University of Rochester Medical Center, Rochester, NY. Steven Pflanz is with the 579th Medical Operations Squadron, Bolling Air Force Base, Washington, DC. Gerald W. Talcott is with the 59th Mental Health Squadron, Lackland Air Force Base, San Antonio, TX. Rick L. Campise is with the 1st Medical Operations Squadron, Langley Air Force Base, Hampton, VA. Alina Bajorska is with the Department of Community and Preventive Medicine, University of Rochester Medical Center, Rochester. Xin Tu is with the Department of Biostatistics and Computational Biology, University of Rochester Medical Center, Rochester. Eric D. Caine is with the Department of Psychiatry, University of Rochester Medical Center, Rochester.

CONTRIBUTORS

K. L. Knox conceptualized and directed the study. K. L. Knox, S. Pflanz, G. W. Talcott, R. L. Campise, and E. D. Caine established the formal prevention domains that guided the development of implementation measures. K. L. Knox, J. E. Lavigne, and X. Tu supervised the data analysis. A. Bajorska carried out the data analysis. All authors participated in interpreting the results and writing and editing the article.

ACKNOWLEDGMENTS

This project was supported by National Institute of Mental Health (grants K01 MH055317, R01 MH075017-01A1, and P20 MH071897).

Note. The funding agency was not involved in the design and conduct of the study; collection, management, analysis, and interpretation of the data; and preparation, review, or approval of the article.

HUMAN PARTICIPANT PROTECTION

This study received approval from the institutional review board at the University of Rochester and the Wilford Hall institutional review board for the US Air Force.

REFERENCES

1. Knox KL, Litts DA, Talcott GW, Feig JC, Caine ED. Risk of suicide and related adverse outcomes after exposure to a suicide prevention program in the US Air Force: cohort study. *BMJ.* 2003;327(7428):1376–1380.

2. Box GEPP, Jenkins GM, Reinsel GC. *Time Series Analysis: Forecasting and Control.* Hoboken, NJ: John Wiley & Sons; 2008.

3. SAS Institute. *SAS/STAT 9.1 User's Guide.* Cary, NC: SAS Institute; 2004.

4. Knox KL, Conwell Y, Caine ED. If suicide is a public health problem, what are we doing to prevent it? *Am J Public Health.* 2004;94(1):37–45.

5. Hand DJ. Statistics and the theory of measurement. *J R Stat Soc Ser A Stat Soc.* 1996;159(3):445–492.

6. Fayers PM, Hand DJ. Causal variables, indicator variables and measurement scales: an example from quality of life. *J R Stat Soc Ser A Stat Soc.* 2002;165(2):233–261.

7. Rychetnik L, Frommer M, Hawe P, Shiell A. Criteria for evaluating evidence on public health interventions. *J Epidemiol Community Health.* 2002;56(2):119–127.

8. Wang S, Moss JR, Hiller JE. Applicability and transferability of interventions in evidence-based public health. *Health Promot Int.* 2005;21(1):76–83.

9. Bray RM, Sanchez RP, Ornstein ML, et al. *Department of Defense Survey of Health Related Behaviors Among Active Duty Military Personnel: 1998.* Washington, DC: US Dept of Defense; 1999.

10. Bray RM, Hourani LL, Rae KL, et al. *Department of Defense Survey of Health Related Behaviors Among Active Duty Military Personnel: 2002.* Washington, DC: US Dept of Defense; 2003.

11. Bray RM, Hourani LL, Olmsted KL, et al. *Department of Defense Survey of Health Related Behaviors Among Active Duty Military Personnel: 2005.* Washington, DC: US Dept of Defense; 2006.

12. Campise RL, Rowan Anderson B. A multisite study of Air Force outpatient behavioral health treatment-seeking patterns and career impact. *Mil Med.* 2006;171(11):1123–1127.

13. Conner KR, Cox C, Duberstein PR, Tian L, Nisbet PA, Conwell Y. Violence, alcohol, and completed suicide: a case-control study. *Am J Psychiatry.* 2001;158(10):1701–1705.

14. Beautrais AL, Joyce PR, Mulder RT. Precipitating factors and life events in serious suicide attempts among youths aged 13 through 24 years. *J Am Acad Child Adolesc Psychiatry.* 1997;36(11):1543–1551.

15. Duberstein PR, Conwell Y, Caine ED. Interpersonal stressors, substance abuse, and suicide. *J Nerv Ment Dis.* 1993;181(2):80–85.

16. Mahon MJ, Tobin JP, Cusack DA, et al. Suicide among regular-duty military personnel: a retrospective case-control study of occupation-specific risk factors for workplace suicide. *Am J Psychiatry.* 2005;162(9):1688–1696.

17. Helmkamp JC. Occupation and suicide among males in the US Armed Forces. *Ann Epidemiol.* 1996;6(1):83–88.

18. Marzuk PM, Nock MK, Leon AC, et al. Suicide among New York City police officers, 1977–1996. *Am J Psychiatry.* 2002;159(12):2069–2071.

19. Conner KR, Duberstein PR, Conwell Y. Age-related patterns of factors associated with completed suicide in men with alcohol dependence. *Am J Addict.* 1999;8(4):312–318.

20. Ilgen MA, Harris A, Moos RH, Tiet QQ. Predictors of a suicide attempt one year after entry into substance use disorder treatment. *Alcohol Clin Exp Res.* 2007;31(4):635–642.

21. Smith TC, Wingard DL, Ryan MA, Kritz-Silverstein D, Slymen DJ, Sallis JF; Millennium Cohort Study Team. Prior assault and posttraumatic stress disorder after combat deployment. *Epidemiology.* 2008;19(3):505–512.

22. Boscarino JA. Postraumatic stress disorder and mortality among US Army veterans 30 years after military service. *Ann Epidemiol.* 2006;16(4):248–256.

23. Bullman TA, Kang HK. The risk of suicide among wounded Vietnam veterans. *Am J Public Health.* 1996;86(5):662–667.

24. Hawton K, van Heeringen K. Suicide. *Lancet.* 2009;373(9672):1372–1381.

37

A Prospective Study of Depression Following Combat Deployment in Support of the Wars in Iraq and Afghanistan

Timothy S. Wells, DVM, PhD, MPH, Cynthia A. LeardMann, MPH, Sarah O. Fortuna, MD, Besa Smith, PhD, MPH, Tyler C. Smith, PhD, MS, Margaret A. K. Ryan, MD, MPH, Edward J. Boyko, MD, MPH, and Dan Blazer, MD, PhD

Objective. We investigated relations between deployment and new-onset depression among US service members recently deployed to the wars in Iraq and Afghanistan.

Methods. We included 40 219 Millennium Cohort Study participants who completed baseline and follow-up questionnaires and met inclusion criteria. Participants were identified with depression if they met the Primary Care Evaluation of Mental Disorders Patient Health Questionnaire criteria for depression at follow-up, but not at baseline.

Results. Deployed men and women with combat exposures had the highest onset of depression, followed by those not deployed and those deployed without combat exposures. Combat-deployed men and women were at increased risk for new-onset depression compared with nondeployed men and women (men: adjusted odds ratio [AOR] = 1.32; 95% confidence interval [CI] = 1.13, 1.54; women: AOR = 2.13; 95% CI = 1.70, 2.65). Conversely, deployment without combat exposures led to decreased risk for new-onset depression compared with those who did not deploy (men: AOR = 0.66; 95% CI = 0.53, 0.83; women: AOR = 0.65; 95% CI = 0.47, 0.89).

Conclusions. Deployment with combat exposures is a risk factor for new-onset depression among US service members. Post-deployment screening may be beneficial for US service members exposed to combat.

Depression is one of the most prevalent and costly of all public health problems.[1,2] Estimates of the 12-month and lifetime prevalence for *Diagnostic and Statistical Manual of Mental Disorders, Fourth Edition (DSM-IV)*[3] major depressive disorders is 5.3% to 6.6% and 13.2% to 16.2%, respectively.[4,5] Much of the burden associated with depression results from comorbidities and reduced ability to maintain employment. Estimates predict that by 2020 depression will be second only to ischemic heart disease as a cause of disability.[6] Even those with minor depression have higher levels of impairment based on measures of functional status and social health, and incur higher rates of medical services utilization.[7]

Female gender and heredity are reported risk factors for depression.[4,8] Women are twice as likely to be diagnosed with depression as men, which may be the result of differences in biological vulnerabilities and environmental experiences.[9] Individuals experiencing threats to personal safety, such as living in unsafe neighborhoods, and individuals living close to the World Trade Center following the events of September 11, 2001, were found to be at increased risk for depression.[10,11]

Deployments pose unique and often stressful situations to military personnel. Although the association between deployment and posttraumatic stress disorder (PTSD) has been investigated,[12–20] little is known regarding the risk for depression. One cross-sectional survey that utilized previously studied UK veterans at high risk for mental disorders found depression more common than posttraumatic stress disorder.[21] Another cross-sectional study utilizing National Comorbidity Survey data found an increased risk for major depressive disorders among male participants with combat experience.[22] These findings are supported by other population-based studies that observed an increased risk for mental disorders among 1991 Gulf War veterans,[23,24] and 1991 Gulf War or Bosnia veterans[25]; however, none were of longitudinal design.

More recently, members of the US Army and US Marine Corps were at increased risk for depression upon return from combat duties in Afghanistan and Iraq, compared with soldiers who completed questionnaires within 1 week prior to deployment.[13] However, questionnaires were administered anonymously, making it difficult to identify new-onset depression upon return from deployment. Similarly, a cross-sectional survey of Canadian Forces identified significant associations between depression and exposure to combat or atrocities.[26] Finally, depression following deployment may be comorbid with PTSD[27] and other mental disorders.[25]

Per Department of Defense policy, all members are screened for mental disorders before deployment.[28,29] Screening includes a review of medical records and an interview with a credentialed provider. Diagnosis or symptoms of depression and PTSD must be assessed for deployment suitability. Disqualifying mental health conditions include, among others, bipolar disorder and psychotic disorders, and disqualifying medications include, but are not limited to, lithium, antipsychotics, and anticonvulsants. Also, those with changes in mental disorder treatment with less than 3 months of stability, or other concerns regarding fitness for duty while deployed, are disqualified.

The Millennium Cohort is the largest-ever population-based prospective study of a military population designed to improve the scientific knowledge of the long-term health effects associated with military service.[30] Between 2001 and 2008, 3 panels of US service members were enrolled into the study. Baseline enrollment for the 3 panels ended with 31% of those invited consenting to participate in the 21-year study. The first enrollment cycle was conducted between July 2001 and June 2003, with more than 77 000 individuals completing either a postal or Internet questionnaire. Between 2004 and 2006, approximately 71% of the first panel members completed a follow-up questionnaire. Investigations of potential reporting biases showed no differential in health care utilization in the year prior to enrollment[31]; strong test–retest reliability[32]; reliable reporting of vaccinations,[33,34] occupations,[35] and deployments[36]; and minimal differences between participants choosing submission by Internet survey or paper submission.[37] Analyses of potential responder bias in ongoing follow-ups continue.

The Millennium Cohort questionnaire includes, among other questions, mental health measures based on 2 standardized scoring instruments: the Primary Care Evaluation of Mental Disorders Patient Health Questionnaire (PHQ)[38] and the Medical Outcomes Study Short Form 36-Item Health Survey for Veterans.[39] We used Millennium Cohort Study data to investigate the association of new-onset depression and deployment in support of the wars in Iraq and Afghanistan.

METHODS

The Millennium Cohort Study was launched in 2001 to collect and evaluate population-based data on behavioral and occupational risks related to military service that may be associated with poor health.[30,40] The first panel of invited Millennium Cohort Study participants was randomly selected from all US military personnel serving in October 2000. To ensure sufficient power to detect differences in smaller subgroups, those with previous deployment to Kosovo, Bosnia, or Southwest Asia; Reserve and National Guard members; and women were oversampled. Through a modified Dillman approach, 77 047 consenting participants enrolled in the first panel of the Millennium Cohort Study.[41] The methodology of the study has been described elsewhere in detail.[30] Of the 77 047 enrolled in this first panel, 55 021 (71.4%) completed the follow-up questionnaire between June 2004 and February 2006. Those completing the follow-up questionnaire were slightly more likely to be born in 1969 or earlier, married, more highly educated, officers, and non-Hispanic White compared with participants who completed the baseline survey.

The population for this study included participants in the first panel of Millennium Cohort Study who had complete demographic, behavioral, and military-specific data and who completed the baseline and follow-up questionnaires. We excluded participants from the final sample if, at baseline, they reported ever having a diagnosis for depression, met the criteria for mild or other depression, or reported taking medicine for anxiety, stress, or depression. We also excluded those completing the baseline questionnaire after deployment, completing either questionnaire while on deployment, or not answering questions on depression diagnosis or symptoms or use of medication for anxiety, stress, or depression.

The Defense Manpower Data Center provided demographic and military-specific data from electronic personnel files, including gender, birth date, highest education level, marital status, race/ethnicity, deployment experience, pay grade, service component (active duty or Reserve/National Guard), service branch (US Army, US Air Force, US Navy, US Coast Guard, or US Marine Corps), and military occupations. Race/ethnicity was classified by the Defense Manpower Data Center, and was incorporated into analyses because of differences in prevalence and incidence for depression by race/ethnicity.[42,43]

Depression Data

The PHQ, embedded in the Millennium Cohort questionnaire, provides a psychosocial assessment based on scores of several health concepts.[38,44,45] For this study, we used the PHQ to assess depression. Sensitivity and specificity have been reported as high for the PHQ-defined major depressive disorder (sensitivity = 0.93; specificity = 0.89).[46] Major depressive disorder, as measured by 9 items from the PHQ, corresponds to the depression diagnosis from the *DSM-IV*.[47] Participants used a 4-point Likert scale to rate the severity of each depressive symptom from "not at all" to "nearly every day" during the previous 2 weeks prior to questionnaire completion. For this investigation, we defined participants as having new-onset depression at follow-up if they met the following 2 criteria: (1) endorsed having a depressed mood or anhedonia and (2) responded "more than half the days" or "nearly every day" to at least 5 of the 9 items, where suicidal ideation was counted if present at all.[44]

Deployment Status

We considered participants who had completed a deployment in support of the wars in Iraq and Afghanistan between the baseline and follow-up questionnaires to be deployed. We further categorized deployment status on the basis of self-reported exposure to combat at follow-up. We classified participants as deployed with combat exposure if they reported at least one combat experience in the past 3 years, including witnessing death, trauma, prisoners of war, or refugees. We identified those who deployed and did not report any of these experiences in the past 3 years as deployed without combat exposure.

Posttraumatic Stress Disorder

The Millennium Cohort questionnaire includes the PTSD Checklist–Civilian Version, a 17-item self-report measure of PTSD symptoms.[48,49] Participants used a 5-point Likert scale (from 1 = not at all to 5 = extremely) to rate the severity of each intrusion, avoidance, and hyperarousal symptom during the past 30 days. Following standard procedures, we scored participants as having PTSD symptoms at baseline if they reported a moderate or higher level of at least 1 intrusion symptom, 3 avoidance symptoms, and 2 hyperarousal symptoms at baseline.[3] We defined participants as having a PTSD diagnosis at baseline if they reported ever having a diagnosis of PTSD from a health care professional.

Statistical Analysis

We completed a descriptive investigation to examine deployment status; demographic, behavioral, and occupational characteristics; and baseline PTSD symptoms or diagnosis with new-onset depression, stratified by gender. To calculate associations between deployment status and new-onset depression, we used multivariable logistic regression, adjusting for demographic, behavioral, and occupational variables, as well as baseline PTSD symptoms or diagnosis. We defined alcohol misuse by positive endorsement of 1 or more CAGE (cut down, annoyed, guilt, eye-opener) questions,[50] which is noted as "CAGE/alcohol" hereafter. Because of known associations between smoking and depression,[51,52] and smoking and deployment,[53] there were concerns these relations may interact. We investigated this by entering a first-order multiplicative interaction term of deployment by smoking status into the regression model. We performed regression diagnostics, including examining covariates for multicollinearity and goodness-of-fit tests. We conducted all data analyses with SAS version 9.1.3 (SAS Institute Inc, Cary, NC).

RESULTS

There were 55 021 Millennium Cohort participants who completed the 2001–2003 and 2004–2006 questionnaires. We excluded individuals with indicators of depression at baseline (n = 6537), who deployed prior to completing the 2001–2003 questionnaire (n = 1853), who completed a questionnaire while deployed (n = 2553), or who did not have complete data (n = 3859), leaving 40 219 Cohort members for inclusion in this study. We conducted separate analyses for the 30 041 men and 10 178 women who met study criteria. We categorized men and women as not deployed (22 126 men and 8543 women), deployed without combat exposures (3940 men and 891 women), or deployed with combat exposures (3975 men and 744 women). Study participants had, on average, completed the baseline survey 404.1 days prior to deployment (range = 1 to 1402 days), and had completed the follow-up survey 349.4 days, on average, after returning from deployment (range = 1 to 1366 days).

Compared with nondeployers, deployed men and women were proportionately more likely to be younger and serving on active duty (Table 1). Men and women deployed without combat exposures were proportionately more likely to have some college education, be in the US Air Force, and have occupations listed as "other" (i.e., all other occupations excluding combat, health care, service, supply, and functional specialists) compared with the other groups. Conversely, men and women deployed with combat exposures were

Table 1. Demographic Characteristics of Participants (N = 40 219), by Deployment Status: Millennium Cohort Study, 2001–2006

Baseline Characteristic	Men (n = 30 041)			Women (n = 10 178)		
	Not Deployed (n = 22 126), No. (%)	Deployed Without Combat Exposures (n = 3940), No. (%)	Deployed With Combat Exposures (n = 3975), No. (%)	Not Deployed (n = 8543), No. (%)	Deployed Without Combat Exposures (n = 891), No. (%)	Deployed With Combat Exposures (n = 744), No. (%)
Birth year						
Pre-1960	6 599 (29.8)	854 (21.7)	634 (16.0)	2073 (24.3)	100 (11.2)	95 (12.8)
1960-1969	9 371 (42.4)	1813 (46.0)	1663 (41.8)	3147 (36.8)	323 (36.3)	249 (33.5)
1970-1979	5 687 (25.7)	1156 (29.3)	1494 (37.6)	2785 (32.6)	370 (41.5)	321 (43.2)
1980-present	469 (2.1)	117 (3.0)	184 (4.6)	538 (6.3)	98 (11.0)	79 (10.6)
Education						
High school or less	9 342 (42.2)	1309 (33.2)	2025 (50.9)	3532 (41.3)	372 (41.8)	388 (52.2)
Some college	5 597 (25.3)	1517 (38.5)	801 (20.2)	2132 (24.9)	308 (34.6)	134 (18.0)
College degree	7 187 (32.5)	1114 (28.3)	1149 (28.9)	2880 (33.7)	211 (23.7)	222 (29.8)
Marital status						
Never married	4 505 (20.4)	834 (21.2)	1066 (26.8)	3024 (35.4)	386 (43.3)	355 (47.7)
Married	16 546 (74.8)	2897 (73.5)	2727 (68.6)	4460 (52.2)	405 (45.5)	294 (39.5)
Divorced	1 075 (4.9)	209 (5.3)	182 (4.6)	1059 (12.4)	100 (11.2)	95 (12.8)
Race/ethnicity						
Non-Hispanic White	16 344 (73.9)	3021 (76.7)	2754 (69.3)	5391 (63.1)	544 (61.1)	429 (57.7)
Non-Hispanic Black	2 094 (9.5)	348 (8.8)	353 (8.9)	1736 (20.3)	193 (21.7)	145 (19.5)
Other	3 688 (16.7)	571 (14.5)	868 (21.8)	1416 (16.6)	154 (17.3)	170 (22.9)
Smoking						
Never smoker	13 156 (59.5)	2427 (61.6)	2333 (58.7)	5587 (65.4)	581 (65.2)	469 (63.0)
Past smoker	5 710 (25.8)	911 (23.1)	915 (23.0)	1861 (21.8)	174 (19.5)	152 (20.4)
Current smoker	3 260 (14.7)	602 (15.3)	727 (18.3)	1095 (12.8)	136 (15.3)	123 (16.5)

(continued on next page)

Table 1. (continued)

Baseline Characteristic	Men (n = 30 041)			Women (n = 10 178)		
	Not Deployed (n = 22 126), No. (%)	Deployed Without Combat Exposures (n = 3940), No. (%)	Deployed With Combat Exposures (n = 3975), No. (%)	Not Deployed (n = 8543), No. (%)	Deployed Without Combat Exposures (n = 891), No. (%)	Deployed With Combat Exposures (n = 744), No. (%)
CAGE/alcohol[a]						
No	17 884 (80.8)	3197 (81.1)	3203 (80.6)	7595 (88.9)	787 (88.3)	651 (87.5)
Yes	4 242 (19.2)	743 (18.9)	772 (19.4)	948 (11.1)	104 (11.7)	93 (12.5)
Baseline PTSD[b]						
No	21 762 (98.4)	3903 (99.1)	3905 (98.2)	8380 (98.1)	884 (99.2)	732 (98.4)
Yes	364 (1.7)	37 (0.9)	70 (1.8)	163 (1.9)	7 (0.8)	12 (1.6)
Military rank						
Enlisted	15 674 (70.8)	2899 (73.6)	2805 (70.6)	5977 (70.0)	715 (80.3)	536 (72.0)
Officer	6 452 (29.2)	1041 (26.4)	1170 (29.4)	2566 (30.0)	176 (19.8)	208 (28.0)
Service component						
Reserve/National Guard	10 057 (45.5)	1561 (39.6)	1456 (36.6)	4401 (51.5)	366 (41.1)	351 (47.2)
Active duty	12 069 (54.6)	2379 (60.4)	2519 (63.4)	4142 (48.5)	525 (58.9)	393 (52.8)
Branch of service						
US Army	10 321 (46.7)	948 (24.1)	2539 (63.9)	4262 (49.9)	342 (38.4)	516 (69.4)
US Air Force	6 113 (27.6)	2125 (53.9)	849 (21.4)	2475 (29.0)	399 (44.8)	153 (20.6)
US Navy/Coast Guard	4 597 (20.8)	720 (18.3)	284 (7.1)	1625 (19.0)	139 (15.6)	65 (8.7)
US Marine Corps	1 095 (5.0)	147 (3.7)	303 (7.6)	181 (2.1)	11 (1.2)	10 (1.3)

(continued on next page)

Table 1. (continued)

	Men (n = 30 041)			Women (n = 10 178)		
Baseline Characteristic	Not Deployed (n = 22 126), No. (%)	Deployed Without Combat Exposures (n = 3940), No. (%)	Deployed With Combat Exposures (n = 3975), No. (%)	Not Deployed (n = 8543), No. (%)	Deployed Without Combat Exposures (n = 891), No. (%)	Deployed With Combat Exposures (n = 744), No. (%)
Occupational category						
Combat specialists	5 496 (24.8)	927 (23.5)	1301 (32.7)	491 (5.8)	83 (9.3)	65 (8.7)
Health care specialists	1 705 (7.7)	120 (3.1)	311 (7.8)	2198 (25.7)	68 (7.6)	183 (24.6)
Service supply and functional	5 524 (25.0)	828 (21.0)	838 (21.1)	3706 (43.4)	418 (46.9)	261 (35.1)
Other occupations	9 401 (42.5)	2065 (52.4)	1525 (38.4)	2148 (25.1)	322 (36.1)	235 (31.6)
Cumulative length of deployments[c]						
0 d	22 126 (100.0)	...	...	8543 (100.0)	...	...
1-180 d	...	2694 (68.4)	1670 (42.0)	...	567 (63.6)	345 (46.4)
181-270 d	...	757 (19.2)	932 (23.5)	...	165 (18.5)	157 (21.1)
≥ 271 d	...	489 (12.4)	1373 (34.5)	...	159 (17.9)	242 (32.5)

Note. PTSD = posttraumatic stress disorder. Deployed defined as at least 1 deployment in support of the wars in Iraq and Afghanistan between the baseline and follow-up questionnaire. Percentages are rounded and may not sum to 100.

[a] At baseline, participant self-reported ever feeling at least 1 of the following: (1) a need to cut back on drinking; (2) annoyed at anyone who suggested cutting back on drinking; (3) a need for an "eye-opener," or early morning drink; and (4) guilty about drinking.

[b] Self-reported a PTSD diagnosis or screened positive for PTSD symptoms at baseline.

[c] Number of total days deployed in support of the wars in Iraq and Afghanistan between the baseline and follow-up questionnaire.

proportionately more likely to have a high school education or less, be serving in the US Army, and to be combat specialists, compared with nondeployed men and women. Deployed women were more likely to have never been married compared with nondeployed women. In addition, deployed men and women who reported combat exposures were proportionately more likely to have been deployed 181 days or more compared with those deployed without combat exposures.

Men and women deployed with combat exposures had the highest occurrence of new-onset depression, (5.7% and 15.7%, respectively), followed by those not deployed (3.9% and 7.7%, respectively), whereas participants deployed without combat exposures exhibited the lowest occurrence (2.3% and 5.1%, respectively; Tables 2 and 3). This trend remained consistent when we assessed demographic, behavioral, and military-related characteristics for new-onset depression (Tables 2 and 3). Across all 3 groups, men with the highest percentages of new-onset depression were proportionately more likely to be born in 1980 or later, less educated, other than married, current smokers, enlisted, and serving in the US Marine Corps or US Army. Furthermore, they were more likely to positively endorse CAGE/alcohol questions and have PTSD symptoms or diagnosis at baseline. Similar to men, women with the highest odds of new-onset depression across all 3 deployment categories included those who were more likely to be current smokers, positively endorse CAGE/alcohol questions, have PTSD symptoms or diagnosis at baseline, be enlisted, and have a high school education or less (Table 3).

After we adjusted for deployment status, birth year, education, marital status, race/ethnicity, smoking status, positive CAGE/alcohol question responses, baseline PTSD symptoms or diagnosis, rank, service component, service branch, and occupation, both men and women deployed with combat exposure were significantly more likely to develop new-onset depression than were those not deployed (odds ratio [OR] = 1.32; 95% confidence interval [CI] = 1.13, 1.54; and OR = 2.13; 95% CI = 1.70, 2.65, respectively; Table 4). In contrast, men and women deployed without combat exposures were less likely to develop new-onset depression than were those who did not deploy (OR = 0.66; 95% CI = 0.53, 0.83; and OR = 0.65; 95% CI = 0.47, 0.89, respectively). In the adjusted model, men and women who were past or current smokers, had PTSD symptoms or diagnosis at baseline, positively endorsed CAGE/alcohol questions, or were enlisted had higher odds for new-onset

Table 2. Percentage of New-Onset Depression Among Male Participants, by Deployment Status: Millennium Cohort Study, 2001–2006

Baseline Characteristics	Not Deployed, No. (%)	Deployed Without Combat Exposures, No. (%)	Deployed With Combat Exposures, No. (%)
Total	872 (3.9)	92 (2.3)	225 (5.7)
Birth year			
Pre-1960	219 (3.3)	22 (2.6)	26 (4.1)
1960–1969	346 (3.7)	38 (2.1)	85 (5.1)
1970–1979	280 (4.9)	26 (2.3)	90 (6.0)
1980–present	27 (5.8)	6 (5.1)	24 (13.0)
Education			
High school or less	471 (5.0)	48 (3.7)	165 (8.2)
Some college	212 (3.8)	26 (1.7)	38 (4.7)
College degree	189 (2.6)	18 (1.6)	22 (1.9)
Marital status			
Never married	211 (4.7)	22 (2.6)	76 (7.1)
Married	610 (3.7)	63 (2.2)	136 (5.0)
Divorced	51 (4.7)	7 (3.4)	13 (7.1)
Race/ethnicity			
Non-Hispanic White	671 (4.1)	71 (2.4)	167 (6.1)
Non-Hispanic Black	85 (4.1)	6 (1.7)	22 (6.2)
Other	116 (3.2)	15 (2.6)	36 (4.2)
Smoking			
Never smoker	422 (3.2)	50 (2.1)	107 (4.6)
Past smoker	247 (4.3)	22 (2.4)	51 (5.6)
Current smoker	203 (6.2)	20 (3.3)	67 (9.2)
CAGE/alcohol[a]			
No	655 (3.7)	73 (2.3)	176 (5.5)
Yes	217 (5.1)	19 (2.6)	49 (6.4)
Baseline PTSD[b]			
No	809 (3.7)	87 (2.2)	209 (5.4)
Yes	63 (17.3)	5 (13.5)	16 (22.9)
Military rank			
Enlisted	730 (4.7)	73 (2.5)	199 (7.1)
Officer	142 (2.2)	19 (1.8)	26 (2.2)
Service component			
Reserve/National Guard	404 (4.0)	34 (2.2)	94 (6.5)
Active duty	468 (3.9)	58 (2.4)	131 (5.2)

(continued on next page)

Table 2. (*continued*)

Baseline Characteristics	Not Deployed, No. (%)	Deployed Without Combat Exposures, No. (%)	Deployed With Combat Exposures, No. (%)
Branch of service			
US Army	485 (4.7)	31 (3.3)	170 (6.7)
US Air Force	185 (3.0)	35 (1.7)	32 (3.8)
US Navy/Coast Guard	160 (3.5)	21 (2.9)	11 (3.9)
US Marine Corps	42 (3.8)	5 (3.4)	12 (4.0)
Occupational category			
Combat specialists	188 (3.4)	15 (1.6)	55 (4.2)
Health care specialists	81 (4.8)	4 (3.3)	18 (5.8)
Service supply and functional	233 (4.2)	24 (2.9)	50 (6.0)
Other occupations	370 (3.9)	49 (2.4)	102 (6.7)
Cumulative length of deployments[c]			
0 d	872 (3.9)	...	...
1–180 d	...	57 (2.1)	96 (5.8)
181–270 d	...	23 (3.0)	53 (5.7)
≥ 271 d	...	12 (2.5)	76 (5.5)

Note. PTSD = posttraumatic stress disorder. Deployed defined as at least 1 deployment in support of the wars in Iraq and Afghanistan between the baseline questionnaire and follow-up questionnaire.
[a]At baseline, participant self-reported ever feeling at least 1 of the following: (1) a need to cut back on drinking; (2) annoyed at anyone who suggested cutting back on drinking; (3) a need for an "eye-opener," or early morning drink; and (4) guilty about drinking.
[b]Self-reported a PTSD diagnosis or screened positive for PTSD symptoms at baseline.
[c]Number of total days deployed in support of the wars in Iraq and Afghanistan between the baseline and follow-up questionnaire.

depression. Additionally, women with new-onset depression were more likely to be born in 1970 or later, married or divorced, non-Hispanic White, active duty, and in the US Army or US Navy/Coast Guard. Men who were born in 1980 or later, served in the US Army, and worked in health care, service supply, or functional occupations had higher odds for new-onset depression.

No interaction was observed between smoking status and deployment status, nor was there interaction between baseline PTSD symptoms or diagnosis and deployment as related to depression. Additionally, length of deployment was collinear with deployment status, and excluded from the main

Table 3. Percentage of New-Onset Depression Among Female Participants, by Deployment Status: Millennium Cohort Study, 2001–2006

Baseline Characteristics	Not Deployed, No. (%)	Deployed Without Combat Exposures, No. (%)	Deployed With Combat Exposures, No. (%)
Total	654 (7.7)	45 (5.1)	117 (15.7)
Birth year			
Pre-1960	125 (6.0)	3 (3.0)	19 (20.0)
1960–1969	212 (6.7)	13 (4.0)	32 (12.9)
1970–1979	258 (9.3)	24 (6.5)	52 (16.2)
1980–present	59 (11.0)	5 (5.1)	14 (17.7)
Education			
High school or less	326 (9.2)	25 (6.7)	73 (18.8)
Some college	161 (7.6)	14 (4.6)	18 (13.4)
College degree	167 (5.8)	6 (2.8)	26 (11.7)
Marital status			
Never married	234 (7.7)	18 (4.7)	49 (13.8)
Married	327 (7.3)	22 (5.4)	54 (18.4)
Divorced	93 (8.8)	5 (5.0)	14 (14.7)
Race/ethnicity			
Non-Hispanic White	449 (8.3)	30 (5.5)	74 (17.3)
Non-Hispanic Black	108 (6.2)	9 (4.7)	26 (17.9)
Other	97 (6.9)	6 (3.9)	17 (10.0)
Smoking			
Never smoker	363 (6.5)	24 (4.1)	68 (14.5)
Past smoker	175 (9.4)	10 (5.8)	25 (16.5)
Current smoker	116 (10.6)	11 (8.1)	24 (19.5)
CAGE/alcohol[a]			
No	560 (7.4)	38 (4.8)	95 (14.6)
Yes	94 (9.9)	7 (6.7)	22 (23.7)
Baseline PTSD[b]			
No	615 (7.3)	44 (5.0)	114 (15.6)
Yes	39 (23.9)	1 (14.3)	3 (25.0)
Military rank			
Enlisted	517 (8.7)	43 (6.0)	98 (18.3)
Officer	137 (5.3)	2 (1.1)	19 (9.1)
Service component			
Reserve/National Guard	312 (7.1)	20 (5.5)	54 (15.4)
Active duty	342 (8.3)	25 (4.8)	63 (16.0)
Branch of service			
US Army	361 (8.5)	23 (6.7)	89 (17.3)
US Air Force	147 (5.9)	16 (4.0)	16 (10.5)

(continued on next page)

Table 3. (*continued*)

Baseline Characteristics	Not Deployed, No. (%)	Deployed Without Combat Exposures, No. (%)	Deployed With Combat Exposures, No. (%)
US Navy/Coast Guard	133 (8.2)	6 (4.3)	12 (18.5)
US Marine Corps	13 (7.2)	0 (0.0)	0 (0.0)
Occupational category			
Combat specialists	37 (7.5)	3 (3.6)	5 (7.7)
Health care specialists	158 (7.2)	5 (7.4)	18 (9.8)
Service supply and functional	281 (7.6)	18 (4.3)	59 (22.6)
Other occupations	178 (8.3)	19 (5.9)	35 (14.9)
Cumulative length of deployments[c]			
0 d	654 (7.7)	...	...
1–180 d	...	26 (4.6)	45 (13.0)
181–270 d	...	7 (4.2)	23 (14.7)
≥ 271 d	...	12 (7.6)	49 (20.3)

Note. PTSD = posttraumatic stress disorder. Deployed defined as at least 1 deployment in support of the wars in Iraq and Afghanistan between the baseline questionnaire and follow-up questionnaire.
[a]At baseline, participant self-reported ever feeling at least 1 of the following: (1) a need to cut back on drinking; (2) annoyed at anyone who suggested cutting back on drinking; (3) a need for an "eye-opener," or early morning drink; and (4) guilty about drinking.
[b]Self-reported a PTSD diagnosis or screened positive for PTSD symptoms at baseline.
[c]Number of total days deployed in support of the wars in Iraq and Afghanistan between the baseline and follow-up questionnaire.

analysis. However, to assess the significance of deployment length, we conducted a subanalysis incorporating deployment length with data of those deployed to examine the association between deployment length and new-onset depression. In this analysis, deployment length was not statistically significant.

DISCUSSION

We used Millennium Cohort Study data to identify more than 30 000 male and 10 000 female US service members who were free of depression at baseline. To our knowledge, this is the first population-based longitudinal study with baseline data prior to deployment to report a temporal association between combat exposure among deployed US service members and new-onset depression compared with nondeployed peers. However, finding an increased

Table 4. Multivariable Logistic Regression Adjusted Odds Ratio (AOR) of Depression, by Gender: Millennium Cohort Study, 2001–2006

Baseline Characteristics	Men, AOR (95% CI)	Women, AOR (95% CI)
2001–2006 deployment status[a]		
No deployment (Ref)	1.00	1.00
Deployed without combat exposures	0.66 (0.53, 0.83)	0.65 (0.47, 0.89)
Deployed with combat exposures	1.32 (1.13, 1.54)	2.13 (1.70, 2.65)
Birth year		
Pre-1960 (Ref)	1.00	1.00
1960–1969	1.06 (0.90, 1.24)	1.00 (0.80, 1.24)
1970–1979	1.20 (0.99, 1.45)	1.39 (1.10, 1.76)
1980–present	1.56 (1.10, 2.21)	1.61 (1.13, 2.28)
Education		
High school or less (Ref)	1.00	1.00
Some college	0.90 (0.75, 1.07)	1.03 (0.84, 1.27)
College degree	0.85 (0.68, 1.07)	1.10 (0.85, 1.43)
Marital status		
Never married (Ref)	1.00	1.00
Married	0.99 (0.84, 1.17)	1.25 (1.05, 1.49)
Divorced	1.22 (0.92, 1.62)	1.49 (1.16, 1.92)
Race/ethnicity		
Non-Hispanic White (Ref)	1.00	1.00
Non-Hispanic Black	0.88 (0.72, 1.08)	0.73 (0.59, 0.90)
Other	0.84 (0.71, 1.01)	0.75 (0.60, 0.93)
Smoking		
Never smoker (Ref)	1.00	1.00
Past smoker	1.18 (1.02, 1.36)	1.30 (1.09, 1.55)
Current smoker	1.52 (1.31, 1.77)	1.35 (1.10, 1.66)
CAGE/alcohol[b]		
No (Ref)	1.00	1.00
Yes	1.19 (1.04, 1.37)	1.27 (1.03, 1.57)
Baseline PTSD[c]		
No (Ref)	1.00	1.00
Yes	4.29 (3.34, 5.50)	2.98 (2.07, 4.28)
Military rank		
Enlisted	1.67 (1.31, 2.11)	1.65 (1.26, 2.16)
Officer (Ref)	1.00	1.00
Service component		
Reserve/National Guard (Ref)	1.00	1.00
Active duty	1.01 (0.88, 1.15)	1.21 (1.03, 1.42)

(continued on next page)

Table 4. (*continued*)

Baseline Characteristics	Men, AOR (95% CI)	Women, AOR (95% CI)
Branch of service		
US Army	1.52 (1.27, 1.82)	1.64 (1.33, 2.01)
US Air Force (Ref)	1.00	1.00
US Navy/Coast Guard	1.13 (0.91, 1.40)	1.55 (1.21, 2.00)
US Marine Corps	1.11 (0.81, 1.52)	0.88 (0.48, 1.60)
Occupational category		
Combat specialists (Ref)	1.00	1.00
Health care specialists	1.52 (1.20, 1.93)	1.09 (0.77, 1.55)
Service supply and functional	1.20 (1.01, 1.43)	1.09 (0.78, 1.54)
Other occupations	1.09 (0.93, 1.28)	1.04 (0.74, 1.47)

Notes. CI = confidence interval; PTSD = posttraumatic stress disorder. Odds ratios for men and women are adjusted for all variables listed.
[a]Deployment defined as at least 1 deployment in support of the wars in Iraq and Afghanistan between the baseline questionnaire and follow-up questionnaire. Combat exposure defined as reporting at least 1 combat-like exposure on the follow-up questionnaire.
[b]At baseline, participant self-reported ever feeling at least 1 of the following: (1) a need to cut back on drinking; (2) annoyed at anyone who suggested cutting back on drinking; (3) a need for an "eye-opener," or early morning drink; and (4) guilty about drinking.
[c]Self-reported a PTSD diagnosis or screened positive for PTSD symptoms at baseline.

risk for a mental disorder associated with combat exposure is not unique, as Smith et al. observed similar findings for PTSD with Millennium Cohort data.[14]

Other research, though cross-sectional in design, has found similar depression risk with exposure to combat or witnessing atrocities among members of the Canadian military.[26] Although PTSD was associated with increased length of deployment among Vietnam veterans[54] and UK veterans serving in Afghanistan or Iraq,[55] this trend was not found for depression in this study. Additionally, a large historical prospective study found an inverse association between mental health hospitalizations and US servicewomen who were members of the US Navy or US Marine Corps serving in combat support occupations.[56] These contrasting observations may be caused by underlying differences in PTSD and depression risk factors, or because the Vietnam study was conducted on a relatively small sample many years after the war's end, making it difficult to rule out misclassification of exposure or outcome.

In this study, deployed men and women without combat exposures were significantly less likely to develop depression than were nondeployed men and women. This finding may suggest that individuals who are healthier and at less risk for depression are more likely to deploy and, thus, mitigate stress-related effects of deployment[57-60] among men and women who do not face combat exposures. In other words, deployment with low probability of exposure to combat (or the effects of combat, such as being in the line of fire or handling casualties, prisoners, or treating the wounded) may not be significantly stressful to the majority of US service members.

Military hardiness, the context-specific adaptation of psychological hardiness,[61] has been observed to moderate the impact of deployment stressors on depression.[62] Military hardiness may also partially explain the observation that male combat specialists were at lower risk for depression than either health care specialists or men whose duties include service supply and functional support, after adjustment for a number of variables, including combat exposure. It is possible that combat specialists are more mentally prepared for deployment-related stresses either through training or selection factors for their positions. Medical personnel have significant exposure to the after effects of the trauma of combat but may not be as well-prepared to cope with the effects of this exposure because of different training or constitutional make-up. Another possibility is that the range and type of combat stressors medical personnel experience are fundamentally different in unmeasured ways than those experienced by combat specialists. Men working in service supply and functional-support occupations conduct convoy and other duties that randomly and frequently put them in dangerous situations, and similarly may not have the advantages of combat specialist training or constitution.

The reporting of baseline PTSD symptoms or diagnosis was associated with new-onset depression in adjusted models for both female and male US service members. Finding comorbid PTSD and depression following exposure to traumatic events has received significant attention in the scientific literature.[63-68] However, the causes of this comorbidity remain poorly understood.

One study found that trauma variables known to be related to PTSD development, such as type and horror of the trauma, were also related to the occurrence of comorbid mental disorders, including depression, generalized anxiety disorder, and agoraphobia.[69] Similarly, depression was observed to develop with or without comorbid PTSD following exposure to a traumatic event.[66,70] Some believe that PTSD and depression comorbidity can be largely explained by common genetic influences.[71,72] Further research to unravel this comorbidity is paramount as comorbid PTSD and depression have been reported to increase dysfunction,[63,64] health care utilization,[65] and the risk for suicide.[65,68] Data from the Millennium Cohort Study have contributed to the understanding of PTSD among US military populations.[14,15,73] Following the publication of this article and as additional cohort data become available, subsequent analyses will investigate PTSD and depression comorbidity.

Other risk factors for depression observed in this study were consistent with previous reports that used data from military and civilian populations.[4,5,73–75] In adjusted models, male and female US service members were at increased risk for depression if they were younger, past or current smokers, positively endorsed CAGE/alcohol questions, and had served in the US Army. Additionally, women who were married or divorced, non-Hispanic White, active duty, and served in the US Navy/Coast Guard were at increased risk of depression. The increased risk of depression among married women compared with never-married women may be related to postpartum depression,[76] separation anxiety associated with leaving family members while deployed, or a lack of social support in the deployed setting. Although few studies have examined increased separation anxiety or increased lack of social support among deployed married women, animal studies provide evidence that separation may induce depression,[77,78] and studies have found an association between sense of belonging and depression.[79,80] It is also plausible that differences exist in role expectations and family or social support for married male and female deployed service members. For example, married women may be expected to resume routine family care while attempting to cope with the events of the deployment, more so than their male counterparts.

Limitations to these analyses should be noted. A population accounting for 31% of invited cohort members as well as self-report of exposures and symptoms has the potential to introduce bias. However, multiple investigations of possible reporting and selection biases in baseline Millennium Cohort data suggest reliable reporting, minimal response bias, and a representative sample of military personnel, including deployers.[14,15,30–35,37,73,81] Use of the PHQ along with the *DSM-IV* criteria has shown to correlate well with a physician's assessment of depression symptoms,[32] and the PHQ is internally valid in Millennium Cohort members.[32] However, the use of a standardized instrument for self-reported data as a surrogate for depression diagnosis is imperfect. Finally, the definition of combat exposure in this study was quite broad, encompassing a number of stressful events that often accompany combat, but do not necessarily indicate actual engagement in combat operations (i.e., exchanging fire with an enemy).

Despite limitations, these analyses offer the first large, prospective epidemiological investigation of new-onset depression symptoms in combat-deployed military men and women. The large sample of both men and women along with adjustment for multiple potential confounding variables allowed for a robust investigation of the association between deployment and new-onset depression. Depression is often underreported in electronic health care databases among populations that do not readily access care for mental disorders, making it often advantageous to use self-reported measures.

In summary, male and female US service members who deployed and reported combat exposures were at increased risk for depression compared with nondeployed service members, after adjustment for baseline PTSD symptoms or diagnosis and other potentially confounding variables. Conversely, men and women who deployed and did not report combat exposures were at lower risk for depression than nondeployed men and women. These findings support hypotheses that stress associated with combat may lead to depression, and that stress related to deployment, in the absence of combat exposure, may be mitigated by selective deployment of service members who are at decreased risk for the development of depression in comparison with nondeployed men and women.

ABOUT THE AUTHORS

Timothy S. Wells and Sarah O. Fortuna are with the US Air Force Research Laboratory, Wright-Patterson AFB, OH. Cynthia A. LeardMann, Besa Smith, Tyler C. Smith, and Margaret A. K. Ryan are with the Department of Defense Center for Deployment Health Research, Naval Health Research Center, San Diego, CA. Edward J. Boyko is with the Seattle Epidemiologic Research and Information Center, Veterans Affairs Puget Sound Health Care System, Seattle, WA. Dan Blazer is with Duke University Medical Center, Durham, NC.

CONTRIBUTORS

T. S. Wells led the design, analyses, and article development. C. A. LeardMann contributed to the design, conducted most of the analyses, and assisted with article writing. S. O. Fortuna assisted with design, made recommendations during the analyses, and wrote the introduction of the article. B. Smith, T. C. Smith, M. A. K. Ryan, E. J. Boyko, and D. Blazer made significant contributions to the design, helped to guide analyses, and provided critical review of the article.

ACKNOWLEDGMENTS

This work represents report 08-06, supported by the Department of Defense, under work unit no. 60002. The views expressed in this article are those of the authors and do not reflect the official policy or position of the Department of the Navy, Department of the Army, Department of the Air Force, Department of Defense, Department of Veterans Affairs, or the US Government.

In addition to the authors, the Millennium Cohort Study Team includes Lacy Farnell, Gia Gumbs, Isabel Jacobson, Molly Kelton, Travis Leleu, Jamie McGrew, Katherine Snell, Steven Spiegel, Kari Welch, Martin White, James Whitmer, and Charlene Wong from the Department of Defense Center for Deployment Health Research, Naval Health Research Center, San Diego, CA; Paul J. Amoroso, from the Madigan Army Medical Center, Tacoma, WA; Gary D. Gackstetter, from the Department of Preventive Medicine and Biometrics, Uniformed Services University of the Health Sciences, Bethesda, MD, and Analytic Services Inc, Arlington, VA; Gregory C. Gray, from the College of Public Health, University of Iowa, Iowa City; Tomoko I. Hooper, from the Department of Preventive Medicine and Biometrics, Uniformed Services University of the Health Sciences; and James R. Riddle, from the US Air Force Research Laboratory, Wright-Patterson Air Force Base, OH. We are indebted to the Millennium Cohort Study participants, without whom these analyses would not be possible. We thank Scott L. Seggerman and Greg D. Boyd from the Management Information Division, Defense Manpower Data Center, Seaside, CA. Additionally, we thank Michelle Stoia from the Naval Health Research Center. We also thank the professionals from the US Army Medical Research and Materiel Command, especially those from the Military Operational Medicine Research Program, Fort Detrick, MD. We appreciate the support of the staff of the Henry M. Jackson Foundation for the Advancement of Military Medicine, Rockville, MD.

HUMAN PARTICIPANT PROTECTION

This research has been conducted in compliance with all applicable federal regulations governing the protection of human subjects in research, and was approved by the institutional review board, Naval Health Research Center, San Diego, CA (Protocol NHRC.2000.007).

REFERENCES

1. Stoudemire A, Frank R, Hedemark N, Kamlet M, Blazer D. The economic burden of depression. *Gen Hosp Psychiatry*. 1986;8(6):387–394.

2. Greenberg PE, Kessler RC, Birnbaum HG, et al. The economic burden of depression in the United States: how did it change between 1990 and 2000? *J Clin Psychiatry*. 2003;64(12):1465–1475.

3. *Diagnostic and Statistical Manual of Mental Disorders, Fourth Edition*. Washington, DC: American Psychiatric Association; 1994.

4. Hasin DS, Goodwin RD, Stinson FS, Grant BF. Epidemiology of major depressive disorder: results from the National Epidemiologic Survey on Alcoholism and Related Conditions. *Arch Gen Psychiatry*. 2005;62(10):1097–1106.

5. Kessler RC, Berglund P, Demler O, et al. The epidemiology of major depressive disorder: results from the National Comorbidity Survey Replication (NCS-R). *JAMA*. 2003;289(23):3095–3105.

6. Murray CJ, Lopez AD. Alternative projections of mortality and disability by cause 1990–2020: Global Burden of Disease Study. *Lancet*. 1997;349(9064):1498–1504.

7. Wagner HR, Burns BJ, Broadhead WE, Yarnall KS, Sigmon A, Gaynes BN. Minor depression in family practice: functional morbidity, co-morbidity, service utilization and outcomes. *Psychol Med*. 2000;30(6):1377–1390.

8. Ebmeier KP, Donaghey C, Steele JD. Recent developments and current controversies in depression. *Lancet*. 2006;367(9505):153–167.

9. Kessler RC. Epidemiology of women and depression. *J Affect Disord*. 2003;74(1):5–13.

10. Cutrona CE, Wallace G, Wesner KA. Neighborhood characteristics and depression: an examination of stress processes. *Curr Dir Psychol Sci*. 2006;15(4):188–192.

11. Galea S, Ahern J, Resnick H, et al. Psychological sequelae of the September 11 terrorist attacks in New York City. *N Engl J Med.* 2002;346(13):982–987.

12. Hoge CW, Auchterlonie JL, Milliken CS. Mental health problems, use of mental health services, and attrition from military service after returning from deployment to Iraq or Afghanistan. *JAMA.* 2006;295(9):1023–1032.

13. Hoge CW, Castro CA, Messer SC, McGurk D, Cotting DI, Koffman RL. Combat duty in Iraq and Afghanistan, mental health problems, and barriers to care. *N Engl J Med.* 2004;351(1):13–22.

14. Smith TC, Ryan MA, Wingard DL, Slymen DJ, Sallis JF, Kritz-Silverstein D. New onset and persistent symptoms of post-traumatic stress disorder self reported after deployment and combat exposures: prospective population based US military cohort study. *BMJ.* 2008;336(7640):366–371.

15. Smith TC, Wingard DL, Ryan MA, Kritz-Silverstein D, Slymen DJ, Sallis JF. Prior assault and posttraumatic stress disorder after combat deployment. *Epidemiology.* 2008;19(3):505–512.

16. Milliken CS, Auchterlonie JL, Hoge CW. Longitudinal assessment of mental health problems among active and reserve component soldiers returning from the Iraq war. *JAMA.* 2007;298(18):2141–2148.

17. Ismail K, Kent K, Brugha T, et al. The mental health of UK Gulf war veterans: phase 2 of a two phase cohort study. *BMJ.* 2002;325(7364):576.

18. Unwin C, Blatchley N, Coker W, et al. Health of UK servicemen who served in Persian Gulf War. *Lancet.* 1999;353(9148):169–178.

19. Orcutt HK, Erickson DJ, Wolfe J. A prospective analysis of trauma exposure: the mediating role of PTSD symptomatology. *J Trauma Stress.* 2002;15(3):259–266.

20. Orcutt HK, Erickson DJ, Wolfe J. The course of PTSD symptoms among Gulf War veterans: a growth mixture modeling approach. *J Trauma Stress.* 2004;17(3):195–202.

21. Iversen A, Dyson C, Smith N, et al. 'Goodbye and good luck': the mental health needs and treatment experiences of British ex-service personnel. *Br J Psychiatry.* 2005;186:480–486.

22. Prigerson HG, Maciejewski PK, Rosenheck RA. Population attributable fractions of psychiatric disorders and behavioral outcomes associated with combat exposure among US men. *Am J Public Health.* 2002;92(1):59–63.

23. The Iowa Persian Gulf Study Group. Self-reported illness and health status among Gulf War veterans. *JAMA.* 1997;277(3):238–245.

24. Dlugosz LJ, Hocter WJ, Kaiser KS, et al. Risk factors for mental disorder hospitalization after the Persian Gulf War: U.S. Armed Forces, June 1, 1991–September 30, 1993. *J Clin Epidemiol.* 1999;52(12):1267–1278.

25. David AS, Farrin L, Hull L, Unwin C, Wessely S, Wykes T. Cognitive functioning and disturbances of mood in UK veterans of the Persian Gulf War: a comparative study. *Psychol Med.* 2002;32(8):1357–1370.

26. Sareen J, Cox BJ, Afifi TO, et al. Combat and peacekeeping operations in relation to prevalence of mental disorders and perceived need for mental health care: findings from a large representative sample of military personnel. *Arch Gen Psychiatry.* 2007;64(7):843–852.

27. Erickson DJ, Wolfe J, King DW, King LA, Sharkansky EJ. Posttraumatic stress disorder and depression symptomatology in a sample of Gulf War veterans: a prospective analysis. *J Consult Clin Psychol.* 2001;69(1):41–49.

28. Individual protection and individual unit deployment policy, Oct 2001 (with updates through Jan 2009) [policy letter]. MacDill AFB, FL: US Department of Defense, Commander, Central Command; 2009.

29. Policy guidance for deployment-limiting psychiatric conditions and medications, Nov 2006 [policy letter]. Washington, DC: US Department of Defense, Assistant Secretary of Defense for Health Affairs; 2006.

30. Ryan MA, Smith TC, Smith B, et al. Millennium Cohort: enrollment begins a 21-year contribution to understanding the impact of military service. *J Clin Epidemiol.* 2007;60(2):181–191.

31. Wells TS, Jacobson IG, Smith TC, et al. Prior health care utilization as a potential determinant of enrollment in a 21-year prospective study, the Millennium Cohort Study. *Eur J Epidemiol.* 2008;23(2):79–87.

32. Smith TC, Smith B, Jacobson IG, Corbeil TE, Ryan MA. Reliability of standard health assessment instruments in a large, population-based cohort study. *Ann Epidemiol.* 2007;17(7):525–532.

33. Smith B, Leard CA, Smith TC, Reed RJ, Ryan MA. Anthrax vaccination in the Millennium Cohort: validation and measures of health. *Am J Prev Med.* 2007;32(4):347–353.

34. LeardMann CA, Smith B, Smith TC, Wells TS, Ryan MA. Smallpox vaccination: comparison of self-reported and electronic vaccine records in the Millennium Cohort Study. *Hum Vaccin.* 2007;3(6):245–251.

35. Smith TC, Jacobson IG, Smith B, Hooper TI, Ryan MA, For The Millennium Cohort Study Team. The occupational role of women in military service: validation of occupation and prevalence of exposures in the Millennium Cohort Study. *Int J Environ Health Res.* 2007;17(4):271–284.

36. Smith B, Wingard DL, Ryan MA, Macera CA, Patterson TL, Slymen DJ. US Military deployment during 2001-2006: comparison of subjective and objective data sources in a large prospective health study. *Ann Epidemiol.* 2007;17(12):976–982.

37. Smith B, Smith TC, Gray GC, Ryan MA. When epidemiology meets the Internet: Web-based surveys in the Millennium Cohort Study. *Am J Epidemiol.* 2007;166(11):1345–1354.

38. Spitzer RL, Williams JB, Kroenke K, et al. Utility of a new procedure for diagnosing mental disorders in primary care. The PRIME-MD 1000 study. *JAMA.* 1994;272(22):1749–1756.

39. Ware JE, Sherbourne CD. The MOS 36-item short-form health survey (SF-36). I. Conceptual framework and item selection. *Med Care.* 1992;30(6):473–483.

40. Gray GC, Chesbrough KB, Ryan M, et al. The Millennium Cohort Study: a 21-year prospective cohort study of 140,000 military personnel. *Mil Med.* 2002;167(6): 483–488.

41. Dillman DA. *Mail and Telephone. Surveys: The Total Design Method.* Vol xvi. New York, NY: Wiley; 1978.

42. Sclar DA, Robison LM, Skaer TL. Ethnicity/race and the diagnosis of depression and use of antidepressants by adults in the United States. *Int Clin Psychopharmacol.* 2008;23(2):106–109.

43. Riolo SA, Nguyen TA, Greden JF, King CA. Prevalence of depression by race/ethnicity: findings from the National Health and Nutrition Examination Survey III. *Am J Public Health*. 2005;95(6):998–1000.

44. Spitzer RL, Kroenke K, Williams JB. Validation and utility of a self-report version of PRIME-MD: the PHQ primary care study. Primary Care Evaluation of Mental Disorders. Patient Health Questionnaire. *JAMA*. 1999;282(18):1737–1744.

45. Spitzer RL, Williams JB, Kroenke K, Hornyak R, McMurray J. Validity and utility of the PRIME-MD patient health questionnaire in assessment of 3000 obstetric-gynecologic patients: the PRIME-MD Patient Health Questionnaire Obstetrics-Gynecology Study. *Am J Obstet Gynecol*. 2000;183(3):759–769.

46. Fann JR, Bombardier CH, Dikmen S, et al. Validity of the Patient Health Questionnaire-9 in assessing depression following traumatic brain injury. *J Head Trauma Rehabil*. 2005;20(6):501–511.

47. Kroenke K, Spitzer RL, Williams JB. The PHQ-9: validity of a brief depression severity measure. *J Gen Intern Med*. 2001;16(9):606–613.

48. Blanchard EB, Jones-Alexander J, Buckley TC, Forneris CA. Psychometric properties of the PTSD Checklist (PCL). *Behav Res Ther*. 1996;34(8):669–673.

49. Weathers FW, Litz BT, Herman DS, Huska JA, Keane TM. The PTSD Checklist (PCL): reliability, validity, and diagnostic utility. Paper presented at: Annual Meeting of International Society for Traumatic Stress Studies; October 1993; San Antonio, TX. Available at: http://www.pdhealth.mil/library/downloads/PCL_sychometrics.doc. Accessed October 9, 2009.

50. Bush B, Shaw S, Cleary P, Delbanco TL, Aronson MD. Screening for alcohol abuse using the CAGE questionnaire. *Am J Med*. 1987;82(2):231–235.

51. Wiesbeck GA, Kuhl HC, Yaldizli O, Wurst FM. Tobacco smoking and depression-results from the WHO/ISBRA study. *Neuropsychobiology*. 2008;57(1–2):26–31.

52. Martini S, Wagner FA, Anthony JC. The association of tobacco smoking and depression in adolescence: evidence from the United States. *Subst Use Misuse*. 2002;37(14):1853–1867.

53. Smith B, Ryan MA, Wingard DL, Patterson TL, Slymen DJ, Macera CA. Cigarette smoking and military deployment: a prospective evaluation. *Am J Prev Med*. 2008;35(6):539–546.

54. Dohrenwend BP, Turner JB, Turse NA, Adams BG, Koenen KC, Marshall R. The psychological risks of Vietnam for U.S. veterans: a revisit with new data and methods. *Science.* 2006;313(5789):979–982.

55. Rona RJ, Fear NT, Hull L, et al. Mental health consequences of overstretch in the UK armed forces: first phase of a cohort study. *BMJ.* 2007;335(7620):603.

56. Lindstrom KE, Smith TC, Wells TS, et al. The mental health of U.S. military women in combat support occupations. *J Womens Health (Larchmt).* 2006;15(2):162–172.

57. Gaylord KM. The psychosocial effects of combat: the frequently unseen injury. *Crit Care Nurs Clin North Am.* 2006;18(3):349–357.

58. Adler AB, Huffman AH, Bliese PD, Castro CA. The impact of deployment length and experience on the well-being of male and female soldiers. *J Occup Health Psychol.* 2005;10(2):121–137.

59. Bartone PT, Adler AB, Vaitkus MA. Dimensions of psychological stress in peacekeeping operations. *Mil Med.* 1998;163(9):587–593.

60. Vogt DS, Pless AP, King LA, King DW. Deployment stressors, gender, and mental health outcomes among Gulf War I veterans. *J Trauma Stress.* 2005;18(2):115–127.

61. Lambert CE, Lambert VA. Psychological hardiness: state of the science. *Holist Nurs Pract.* 1999;13(3):11–19.

62. Dolan CA, Adler AB. Military hardiness as a buffer of psychological health on return from deployment. *Mil Med.* 2006;171(2):93–98.

63. Shalev AY, Freedman S, Peri T, et al. Prospective study of posttraumatic stress disorder and depression following trauma. *Am J Psychiatry.* 1998;155(5):630–637.

64. Zatzick D, Jurkovich GJ, Rivara FP, et al. A national US study of posttraumatic stress disorder, depression, and work and functional outcomes after hospitalization for traumatic injury. *Ann Surg.* 2008;248(3):429–437.

65. Campbell DG, Felker BL, Liu CF, et al. Prevalence of depression-PTSD comorbidity: implications for clinical practice guidelines and primary care-based interventions. *J Gen Intern Med.* 2007;22(6):711–718.

66. Gerrity MS, Corson K, Dobscha SK. Screening for posttraumatic stress disorder in VA primary care patients with depression symptoms. *J Gen Intern Med.* 2007;22(9):1321–1324.

67. Grieger TA, Cozza SJ, Ursano RJ, et al. Posttraumatic stress disorder and depression in battle-injured soldiers. *Am J Psychiatry.* 2006;163(10):1777–1783, quiz 1860.

68. Oquendo M, Brent DA, Birmaher B, et al. Posttraumatic stress disorder comorbid with major depression: factors mediating the association with suicidal behavior. *Am J Psychiatry.* 2005;162(3):560–566.

69. Maes M, Mylle J, Delmeire L, Altamura C. Psychiatric morbidity and comorbidity following accidental man-made traumatic events: incidence and risk factors. *Eur Arch Psychiatry Clin Neurosci.* 2000;250(3):156–162.

70. North CS, Nixon SJ, Shariat S, et al. Psychiatric disorders among survivors of the Oklahoma City bombing. *JAMA.* 1999;282(8):755–762.

71. Koenen KC, Fu QJ, Ertel K, et al. Common genetic liability to major depression and posttraumatic stress disorder in men. *J Affect Disord.* 2008;105(1–3):109–115.

72. Scherrer JF, Xian H, Lyons MJ, et al. Posttraumatic stress disorder; combat exposure; and nicotine dependence, alcohol dependence, and major depression in male twins. *Compr Psychiatry.* 2008;49(3):297–304.

73. Riddle JR, Smith TC, Smith B, et al. Millennium Cohort: the 2001-2003 baseline prevalence of mental disorders in the U.S. military. *J Clin Epidemiol.* 2007;60(2):192–201.

74. Grieger TA, Fullerton CS, Ursano RJ, Reeves JJ. Acute stress disorder, alcohol use, and perception of safety among hospital staff after the sniper attacks. *Psychiatr Serv.* 2003;54(10):1383–1387.

75. Johnson EO, Breslau N. Is the association of smoking and depression a recent phenomenon? *Nicotine Tob Res.* 2006;8(2):257–262.

76. Rychnovsky JD. Postpartum fatigue in the active-duty military woman. *J Obstet Gynecol Neonatal Nurs.* 2007;36(1):38–46.

77. West M, Rose SM, Spreng S, Verhoef M, Bergman J. Anxious attachment and severity of depressive symptomatology in women. *Women Health.* 1999;29(1):47–56.

78. Levine S, Lyons DM, Schatzberg AF. Psychobiological consequences of social relationships. *Ann N Y Acad Sci.* 1997;807:210–218.

79. Hagerty BM, Williams RA. The effects of sense of belonging, social support, conflict, and loneliness on depression. *Nurs Res.* 1999;48(4):215–219.

80. Choenarom C, Williams RA, Hagerty BM. The role of sense of belonging and social support on stress and depression in individuals with depression. *Arch Psychiatr Nurs.* 2005;19(1):18–29.

81. Wells TS, LeardMann CA, Smith TC, et al. Self-reported adverse health events following smallpox vaccination in a large prospective study of US military service members. *Hum Vaccin.* 2008;4(2):127–133.

PART VIII

Warning Signs for Suicide

38

What Are the Warning Signs for Suicide?

George A. Gellert, MD

Three-quarters of all suicide victims gave some warning signs or cues of their intent to a family member or friend. Between 20% and 50% of suicide victims had attempted suicide previously. Not all suicide attempts are intended to result in death, but they are always expressions of great distress that should be addressed rapidly and aggressively. Talking about suicide, discussing or searching for methods of committing suicide, and wanting to end one's life are all examples of "suicidal ideation" and are important warning signs. People who exhibit this behavior often will subsequently try to end their lives. It is a myth that people who talk about suicide do not actually do it; in fact, they do. They may act as if they are saying goodbye forever or going away. Extraordinary focus on or discussion about death and dying could be suicidal ideation. Dramatic personality changes, such as a quiet and shy person becoming very outgoing and sensationalistic, could indicate a potential for suicide.

Increased alcohol or drug use is often a suicide warning sign. Expressing a sense of lack of purpose in life; feeling trapped, guilty, anxious, and agitated; being unable to sleep or sleeping all the time; feeling hopelessness and withdrawing from friends, family, and society; experiencing uncontrolled anger or rage; engaging in recklessness and risk-taking behavior; and experiencing dramatic mood changes could singly or in combination indicate an elevated risk for suicide.

If someone you know is going through a very stressful period, having difficult relationships, or failing to meet important personal goals, keep an eye out for signs of crisis. Listen for statements that describe feelings of depression and helplessness. These individuals often will express great loneliness and hopelessness. They will be very pessimistic and will have feelings of guilt and self-reproach. Persons who are suffering with painful or terminal diseases should be closely monitored for suicide warning signs. Bereaving spouses are also at increased risk for suicide. Watch persons who are putting their affairs in order, giving away cherished possessions, paying off debts, or changing a will. This may indicate planning for suicide. A decreased interest in work or hobbies is an important sign, particularly in people who are generally career-oriented or otherwise active. A sudden and intense lift in spirits may not mean that the depression has lifted but that the person is feeling relief at knowing that their problems will soon end (through suicide).

Although the majority of people with depression will never attempt suicide, most suicide victims experience depression before attempting suicide. Depression should be a concern if a number of the following behaviors persist for more than two weeks: sadness, crying, apathy, depressed mood, and feelings of worthlessness. There may be a change in appetite; loss of weight and disturbed sleep; slowed speech, thinking process, and movement; loss of interest in and pleasure derived from usual activities; decreased sex drive; and diminished concern about personal appearance. Fatigue and loss of energy are common, and the person may have difficulty remembering, making decisions, or concentrating. Depression that is characterized by agitation or anxiety or by alcohol and drug abuse should be especially concerning.

CAN SUICIDE BE PREVENTED?

Yes. Suicide can be prevented. Many suicides are preventable, and most suicidal people want desperately to live. However, they are unable to see alternatives to their problems. Although some suicides occur without any recognizable warning signs, most do not. Most suicidal people give definite warning signs of their suicidal intentions, but those who have close contact with them are often not aware of the significance of such warnings or do not know what to do.

The depression, substance abuse, changes in affect and behavior, and emotional crises that often precede suicide can be recognized and treated. Identifying individuals at increased risk of suicide and treating them clinically are perhaps the most important and promising prevention strategies for suicide. Both psychotherapy and drug therapy (e.g., antidepressants) are available and may work effectively for a person who wants to end his or her life.

The treatment of depression is effective 60%–80% of the time. (However, antidepressant therapy in depressed children and adolescents can actually increase the risk of suicidal thinking and behavior, and thus, their clinical use must be balanced against heightened suicidality in these age groups.) Programs to train health care workers and teachers in schools to recognize individuals at risk for suicide have been found to be helpful in making sure people receive appropriate care and treatment. However, not all individuals commit suicide because of an underlying mental illness, major life stress, or unlivable situation.

A number of strategies are widely used to prevent suicide, though few of these have been evaluated for their actual impact. One of the best ways to prevent suicide is to reduce the availability of methods to commit suicide. Because it is sometimes carried out on impulse, reducing the availability of the means for suicide can decrease its frequency. In particular, reducing the easy availability of guns and pharmaceuticals may be of value. Eliminating access to guns in the home, even if these are locked away and unloaded, can make suicide harder to complete, particularly among adolescents. People often feel ambivalent about committing suicide, and if the means for it are not readily available, the impulse may pass.

The US Department of Health and Human Services has articulated 11 goals within a national strategy for suicide prevention. These are summarized as follows:

- Goal 1: Promote awareness that suicide is a public health problem that is preventable
- Goal 2: Develop broad-based support for suicide prevention
- Goal 3: Develop and implement strategies to reduce the stigma associated with being a consumer of mental health, substance abuse, and suicide prevention services
- Goal 4: Develop and implement suicide prevention programs
- Goal 5: Promote efforts to reduce access to lethal means and methods of self-harm

- Goal 6: Implement training for recognition of at-risk behavior and delivery of effective treatment
- Goal 7: Develop and promote effective clinical and professional practices
- Goal 8: Improve access to and community linkages with mental health and substance abuse services
- Goal 9: Improve reporting and portrayals of suicidal behavior, mental illness, and substance abuse in the entertainment and news media
- Goal 10: Promote and support research on suicide and suicide prevention
- Goal 11: Improve and expand surveillance systems

Most communities have suicide prevention hotlines; however, the effectiveness of these has not been clearly shown. Because some individuals who are about to attempt suicide are ambivalent about dying, if given an opportunity to reach out for help and support, people may do so. Help is readily available by just picking up the phone and calling a local suicide emergency hotline. The number to call in your locality can be found in the telephone directory or on the internet, by asking the information operator servicing your phone, or by contacting the agencies listed at the end of this book.

In addition to suicide hotlines, many communities have suicide prevention or crisis intervention centers. These organizations combine a number of services that can be used by people who are suicidal, including telephone hotlines and counseling. Suicide prevention centers help to reduce the loneliness that an individual is experiencing and can provide a means of entry into the mental health care system. A suicide hotline or crisis center, however, should not be a substitute for obtaining mental health care from a professional with specific expertise in this problem.

Various kinds of health care providers offer suicide prevention and treatment services. Universities, high schools, and religious organizations also may provide assistance. Early identification and treatment of depression in elderly persons are important to preventing suicide among this at-risk group. Early recognition of and response to major stresses and conflicts among adolescents and the young may help to decrease their rates of suicide.

WHAT DO I DO IF I THINK SOMEONE I KNOW MAY BE SUICIDAL?

If you know someone who you think may be suicidal, you should respond to the signs that he or she is at risk. Do not be afraid to get involved. The social taboo against suicide often leads people to avoid doing things to help another that they would readily do if the person were physically sick or near death. All suicide threats and attempts should be taken very seriously. Listen attentively to the person. Try not to act shocked. It is imperative that you remain actively engaged with that individual and help them to obtain appropriate services and support. Be sure to get professional help; do not try to solve the problem by yourself, and do not act as the person's only counsel and support. Available data suggest that the best way to prevent an individual from taking his or her own life is to obtain psychiatric care. Some people may require hospitalization with continual observation and monitoring for a time. Appropriate treatment of alcohol or drug abuse is essential.

You may have to accompany the suicidal person to a psychiatric facility, hospital emergency department, or doctor's office. The person may be unwilling to seek help, which is often a reflection of being hopeless, having given up on life, and believing that he or she cannot be helped. But he or she can, and if he or she is not willing or able to seek help on his or her own and with your assistance, you should get help independently. This is not disloyalty, but a sign of true friendship and love. Remember that his or her judgment is impaired in the current state of mind, and that he or she can be restored to a normal and healthy life. Before you leave the person, make sure that he or she has received professional help from qualified mental health professionals or that the risk of suicide has dissipated.

If you are aware of someone in your environment who may be suicidal and is expressing suicidal thoughts, you can help this person contact any of the resources in your community or listed at the end of this chapter. Do not be afraid to ask a person if he or she is thinking about suicide. Ask whether a method has been selected. This will not encourage suicide but will convey that someone genuinely cares and is willing to listen and help. Contrary to popular belief, talking to someone about suicide does not "put ideas into their head." If an elderly person is depressed or a younger person is in a stressful situation that may precipitate a suicide, you can engage local resources and services in your community to help that person.

Do not be judgmental. Never dare suicidal persons to complete the act as a way to test their seriousness. It is not wise to argue in an effort to convince them not to commit suicide, or that their situation in life is actually satisfactory or fortunate, or that they will hurt their family if they kill themselves. People considering suicide need to feel more worthy and less guilty. Do not lecture about the value of living, and avoid being glib. Instead communicate that you care about the person and are very concerned. Ensure the person that he or she is not alone, and that the desire to commit suicide will pass. Explain that depression can be treated effectively and that other life problems can be solved. The message that you want to convey is that a suicide crisis is temporary, the pain can be survived and will pass, and help is available. Above all, be sure that your suicidal family member or friend gets attention from a mental health professional.

Stay with a suicidal person until help is available. Never leave a person at risk alone, even briefly. Remove drugs, sharp objects, and other items that can be used to inflict injury on oneself. If the person already has a weapon or other means of suicide at hand, call 911 emergency services for assistance. If the person talks about using a firearm that he or she owns for suicide, call the police so they may remove the firearm. Even after treatment has begun, it is important for you to stay involved with your family member or friend. He or she will need support during treatment. After the person has received help and is no longer imminently suicidal, help the person make appointments with a medical doctor and a therapist. If you live with the individual and medication is involved in his or her treatment plan, help ensure that he or she takes it regularly, and watch for side effects that need to be communicated to the doctor. If you do not live with the person, follow up with him or her on a regular basis to make sure that he or she is doing okay.

There are instances of individuals who, for the purposes of drama or getting attention, will talk about committing suicide with little actual intent or risk of attempting the act. However, the fact remains that many individuals who actually commit violence against themselves give clear indication beforehand, either in their behavior or by verbally expressing their desire to end their lives. It is better to be misled and falsely alarmed by someone not likely to actually commit suicide than to dismiss an individual as a craver of attention who attempts it or succeeds.

WHAT DO I DO IF I FEEL SUICIDAL?

Many people consider suicide at some time in their lives. This is not that unusual, unless the feelings and thoughts about ending life persist. You should not feel guilty or ashamed for considering suicide. If you feel suicidal, or are considering ending your life for some reason, you should seek help first by confiding in someone you trust. There are many people and service agencies that can help you through this difficult time. You can be helped back to a healthier perspective and state of mind. If you call the National Suicide Prevention Lifeline at (800) 273-TALK (8255), you will be routed to someone to speak with on a suicide telephone hotline in your community. Also you can call the National Hopeline Network at (800) SUICIDE (784-2433). The Deaf Suicide Hotline number is (800) 799-4TTY (4889).

You may be depressed, and this treatable problem can impel you to suicide. Your family represents a first line of support, as do your friends and colleagues. However, if you are unable to ask these people for help or for some reason you are uncomfortable in asking them for help, then it is very easy for you to reach out by yourself and obtain confidential professional services. In your community there is likely to be a suicide telephone hotline or crisis intervention center. If not, a hospital, a religious organization such as a church, or another community agency can assist in connecting you with appropriate service providers. You can find out how to reach any of these from your local telephone directory or by calling the information operator. The local police department or 911 also can be called for information about the suicide prevention center and services in your community.

There is help available to you, and that assistance can make a difference to your outlook and life. If you are reading this book, then obviously you are ambivalent enough about taking your life to at least consider getting help. Don't stop there. Call your local suicide hotline and talk with someone in your community who can help. Some friendly help and professional support in this difficult period will help you to overcome this challenge, improve your outlook over the long term, and live.

HOW DO I COPE WITH THE LOSS OF A LOVED ONE TO SUICIDE?

The 32,000 Americans who complete suicide each year leave behind many spouses, children, friends, and other loved ones who must grieve and work through their bereavement. These so-called suicide survivors may suffer from complex and serious emotional states and reactions. Depression is quite common, with fatigue, withdrawal, inability to concentrate, disturbed sleeping and eating patterns, and a general disinterest in life. Anger may occur and can be directed at family members or oneself, or possibly the loved one who died. Guilt about not preventing the suicide can be significant, along with an agonizing and persistent desire to understand why the loved one killed himself or herself. It seems that some feelings of guilt are unavoidable for most suicide survivors, but try not to allow guilt to dominate your experience. No one is to blame for most suicides. Shame also is experienced by some, and the stigma of suicide may be hard to avoid in social situations.

Over time these emotions decrease in intensity and become less intrusive. It is important to recognize these reactions in yourself and others. Just knowing that you are not alone in experiencing these feelings helps. Some of these feelings and states of mind are adaptive and can help you to overcome the sense of loss and the pain associated with losing a loved one through suicide. Emotional numbness helps to screen out pain and allows it to be managed in a gradual manner.

The American Suicide Foundation recommends a number of strategies for coping with the loss of a loved one through suicide. Keep close to other people during this period. Don't let yourself become isolated. Talk to loved ones about the suicide and seek their help. Help them to overcome the awkwardness and helplessness that they may feel. Share your feelings of loss and pain. Recognize the different ways in which others grieve, some of which may be very different from your own. Do not fail to realize that children will experience many of the same emotions and confusion as adults regarding the loss, and with similar intensity. Do not obsess about trying to understand the reasons for the suicide, and do not let this activity consume you. Slowly allow yourself to enjoy life again, and don't think that enjoying life is somehow disloyal or a betrayal of the lost person.

Support groups exist for suicide survivors. They can provide relief and an environment for communicating feelings and learning ways to strengthen oneself while moving forward and beyond the suicide. Groups also help overcome some of the isolation that survivors experience. Individual counseling with a mental health professional or a member of the clergy is another resource available to suicide survivors.

WHERE CAN I GET MORE INFORMATION AND HELP?

In searching for information and local resources on suicide prevention and treatment of mental health problems such as depression, you may contact a number of community service organizations, including your personal or family physician, local health department, local medical centers and hospitals, and other social service providers. For information on suicide prevention services in your community, look in the Yellow Pages under "Human Services Organizations" or "Social Service Organizations."

Talk to your spouse, another family member, a close friend, or a clergyman aswell. If you are feeling suicidal, call your local police department or 911 and ask that they put you through immediately to a suicide crisis center or hotline.

To find a suicide crisis center near you, visit http://suicidehotlines.com/ on the internet or contact the National Suicide Hotline at (800) SUICIDE (784-2433) or (800) 273-TALK (8255).

Appendix 2 at the back of the book is a bibliography for further reading on each of the violence topics discussed in this volume, organized chapter by chapter.

The following are national organizations and useful internet websites that can refer you to specific services in your local community.

NATIONAL ORGANIZATIONS

American Association of Suicidology (202) 237-2280
American Foundation for Suicide Prevention (888) 333-2377
American Psychiatric Association (888) 35-PSYCH (77924)
American Psychological Association (800) 374-2721; TYY (202) 336-6123
Anxiety Disorders Association of America (240) 485-1001
Centers for Disease Control and Prevention National Center for Injury Prevention and Control (800) CDC-INFO (232-4636)
Depression and Bipolar Support Alliance (800) 826-3632
LGBT Youth Suicide Hotline (866) 4-U-TREVOR (88-7386)
National Alliance on Mental Illness (703) 524-7600
National Center for Victims of Crime (800) FYI-CALL
National Clearinghouse for Alcohol and Drug Information (877) SAMHSA-7; Spanish (877) 767-8432; TDD (800) 487-4889
National Crime Prevention Council (202) 466-6272

National Hopeline Network (800) SUICIDE (784-2433)

National Institute of Justice National Criminal Justice Reference Service (800) 851-3420

National Mental Health Association 703-684-7722

National Organization for Victim Assistance (800) 879-6682

National Suicide Prevention Lifeline (800) 273-TALK (8255)

USEFUL INTERNET WEBSITES

American Association of Suicidology: www.suicidology.org

American Foundation for Suicide Prevention: www.afsp.org

American Psychiatric Association: www.psych.org

American Psychological Association: www.apa.org

Befrienders: www.befrienders.org

Boys Town: www.boystown.org

Centers for Disease Control and Prevention: www.cdc.gov/safeusa/suicide.htm

Crystal Palace: http://www.crystal.palace.net/~llama/selfinjury

Depression and Bipolar Support Alliance: www.dbsalliance.org

Mental Health America: www.nmha.org

National Alliance on Mental Illness: www.nami.org

National Center for Health Statistics: www.cdc.gov/nchs/fastats/suicide.htm

National Institute of Health National Library of Medicine: www.nlm.nih.gov/ medlineplus/suicide.html

National Institute of Justice, National Criminal Justice Reference Service: www.ncjrs.gov

National Institute of Mental Health: www.nimh.nih.gov

National Organization for Victim Assistance: www.trynova.org

Save: www.save.org

Screening for Mental Health, Inc.: www.mentalhealthscreening.org

Suicide.org: www.suicide.org

Suicide and Suicide Prevention: http://www.psycom.net/depression.central.suicide.html

Suicide Hotlines by State: http://www.suicide.org/suicide-hotlines.html

Suicide Hotlines by State: http://suicidehotlines.com

Yahoo Suicide Resource: http://dir.yahoo.com/Society_and_Culture/death_and_dying/suicide

Adapted from *Confronting Violence: Answering Questions About the Epidemic Destroying America's Homes and Communities*, 3rd Edition